Fixing Your Feet: Injury Prevention and Treatments for Athletes

1st Edition 1997
2nd Edition 2000
3rd Edition 2004
4th Edition 2006
5th Edition 2011
6th Edition 2016

Manufactured in the United States of America
Distributed by Publishers Group West

Library of Congress Cataloging-in-Publication Data

Names: Vonhof, John, author.
Title: Fixing your feet : prevention and treatments for athletes / John Vonhof.
Description: Sixth edition. | Birmingham, AL : Wilderness Press, 2016. | Includes bibliographical
    references and index.
Identifiers: LCCN 2016007498 | ISBN 9780899978307 (paperback)
Subjects: LCSH: Foot—Care and hygiene. | Running injuries—Prevention. | Hiking injuries—
    Prevention. | BISAC: SPORTS & RECREATION / Reference. | HEALTH & FITNESS /
    Reference.
Classification: LCC RD563 .V63 2016 | DDC 617.5/85—dc23
LC record available at http://lccn.loc.gov/2016007498
ISBN: 978-0-89997-830-7; eISBN: 978-0-89997-831-4

Published by: 🐾 **WILDERNESS PRESS**
              An imprint of AdventureKEEN
              2204 First Ave. S, Ste. 102
              Birmingham, AL 35233
              800-443-7227; FAX 205-326-1012
              info@wildernesspress.com

Visit wildernesspress.com for a complete listing of our books and for ordering information. Contact us at our website, at facebook.com/wildernesspress1967, or at twitter.com/wilderness1967 with questions or comments. To find out more about who we are and what we're doing, visit blog.wildernesspress.com.

Many of the designations used by manufacturers and sellers to distinguish their products are claimed as trademarks. Where those designations appear in this book and the author is aware of a trademark claim, they are identified by initial capital letters. These products are listed in alphabetical order for the sake of simplicity. The order does not imply one product is more helpful or less helpful than another.

SAFETY NOTICE: Although Wilderness Press and the author have made every attempt to ensure that the information in this book is accurate at press time, they are not responsible for any loss, damage, injury, or inconvenience that may occur as a result of using this book. The information contained here is no substitute for professional advice or training. Readers are encouraged to seek medical help whenever possible.

FIXING YOUR FEET

Injury Prevention and Treatments for Athletes

John Vonhof

6th Edition

 WILDERNESS PRESS . . . *on the trail since 1967*

Dedication

This sixth edition of *Fixing Your Feet* is dedicated to two people I hold in high regard:

J. Martin Carlson, MS, CPO, FAAOP, and founder and president of Tamarack Habilitation Technologies, Inc., for his academic research and writings on the role of shear in blister formation. He has made me rethink how blisters form, and has paved the way for a better understanding of blister formation, and prevention and treatment.

Rebecca Rushton, a podiatrist from Western Australia, whom I trust and whose friendship I value. She has also championed blister prevention and the relationship of shear to blister formation and treatment. Rebecca wrote the foreword to this edition.

Acknowledgments

Thank you to the people who have learned foot-care skills to help others. It takes a special kind of person to work on someone else's dirty feet. Thanks for the hours spent honing your skills and the long hours spent in aid stations, often under less-than-desirable conditions—and in many cases, sharing what you have learned and your questions.

Thank you to the thousands of athletes who, over the life of this book, have shared their experiences, asked for foot-care help, and given me encouragement to keep writing about *Fixing Your Feet.*

Again, I give special thanks to my wife, Kathie, for her continued patience through yet another rewrite and research process, and my son, Scott, who, after one of my 12-hour track runs in 1996, gave me the original idea for this book. Thank you to my daughter Wendy for helping with the research for this edition.

Thank you, Lisa Butler, whose poem "Foot Fetish" has graced these pages for many editions.

Thanks to the staff of AdventureKEEN and Wilderness Press for believing in the ongoing potential for this sixth edition of *Fixing Your Feet.* They make it look great, correct my errors, and continue to take it to a high level of professionalism.

My Motivation

Run with perseverance the race marked out for you. —*Hebrews 12:1*

Contents

Foreword

With a quarter of the body's bones, the feet are sophisticated pieces of architecture. Each foot is an intricate network of bones, muscles, tendons, ligaments, nerves, and skin. Quite simply, they are a mechanical marvel. But the demands of an active lifestyle can exceed their ability to remain uninjured. At some stage, they will let you know enough is enough.

Athletes recognize the importance of happy and healthy feet to their enjoyment and success in their chosen activity. There is a healthy respect there. Treat your feet well and the sky is the limit. Ignore or mistreat them and they'll provide an unending mental and physical strain that will threaten not only your result, but also your very ability to finish.

In spite of a healthy respect, many athletes don't know how to do foot care. In my experience, foot care falls down in one of three areas. Either preventive foot care is ignored or inadequate; troubleshooting is confused, limited to whatever is on hand and often counterproductive; or treatment is rushed and disorderly, again, limited to the inadequate array of supplies on hand.

For 19 years, John has worked tirelessly in educating athletes on all matters feet. As a retired paramedic, an emergency room technician, an orthopedic technician, and a former ultrarunner himself, he has both the background and the experience to offer expert insight and advice on foot care. John volunteers at some of the most epic races around the world and treats athletes from beginner to elite. We talk regularly about our shared interest, foot blisters. He's seen his fair share. Make no mistake; many athletes would not have seen the finish line had it not been for his efforts.

John is only one man. Yet the reach of his teachings is wide, thanks in no small part to his book, *Fixing Your Feet: Injury Prevention and Treatments for Athletes.* Now in its sixth edition, *Fixing Your Feet* cements its position as "the bible" for active people of all persuasions. With information on almost every foot-care product that exists, and many I've never heard of, his book is a worldwide favorite on the subject for a reason. John uses his vast experience in managing feet in race situations and talking to runners about their experience to provide valuable practical advice in an easy-to-understand format. In this new edition, there is a new chapter, "Blister Prevention: The New Paradigm," with sections on blister formation, shear and its role in blisters, and a short history of blister studies. There's new important information on maceration and techniques on blister treatments, a lot of new foot-care tips, new products, and more—none of which is to be missed.

Having a healthy respect for your feet is one thing. Knowing how to treat them right is another. Quite simply, if you're interested in looking after your feet better, so you can enjoy your sport and achieve to your potential, this book is required reading and an essential piece of your kit.

Rebecca Rushton BSc (Pod)
Podiatrist, Esperance Podiatry, Western Australia
Australian Multiday Ultramarathon Foot-Care Specialist
Founder of Blister Prevention, blisterprevention.com.au

Fixing Your Feet

Introduction

*"One thing is for sure: when one's feet hurt . . .
it definitely gets one's attention."*
—Denise Jones, the Badwater Blister Queen

Helping people has been my motivation for more than 20 years of learning as much as possible about foot care. I love to see athletes able to finish their races without foot problems. That hasn't changed.

Over the past 20 years I have stressed many things over and over. Things haven't changed. Here's my short list.

- First and foremost, you are responsible for your feet.

- You need to find what works for your feet.

- What works for you may not work for the next person.

- We are each an experiment of one when it comes to foot care.

- Anyone can learn how to do high-quality foot care.

- Blisters are still the number one foot-care problem athletes face.

- Toenail and skin care are two of the most important parts of foot care.

- Foot care is often the most overlooked part of preparing for a race.

I want to emphasize that *Fixing Your Feet* is not a book to be read from front to back. I encourage you to start with the chapter on "Getting the Most out of *Fixing Your Feet*" to learn how to gain the most benefit from the book and learn how one athlete applied what he learned. It's right after this Introduction. Then look over the table of contents to find and read the chapters that address any areas you currently struggle with. Then go back and spend time in each of the four parts: Foot Basics, Footwear Basics, Prevention, and Treatments. Study them to gain a complete education on good foot-care techniques and skills. We live in a popular do-it-yourself culture, and this should extend to learning how to manage your own feet. Subscribe to my free blog at fixingyourfeet.com/blog to get up-to-date information on foot-care products and services, as well as techniques.

This sixth edition of *Fixing Your Feet* is not a magic bullet. Reading the book will help you learn what you can do. But you still must learn how to do it—and that requires hands on your feet, and maybe even the feet of others. It's the old give-a-man-a-fish-versus-teach-a-man-to-fish concept. You'll learn by doing.

In each edition, the foreword has presented a perspective that emphasized a unique and valuable point:

■ Our feet are our primary mode of transportation and require our attention and preparation.

—**Billy Trolan, MD, first edition**

■ Most of our foot problems could have been avoided with proper care.

—**David Hannaford, DPM, second edition**

■ Our feet will take us to new challenges and adventures if we make the conscious choice to care for them.

—**Dan Barger, the Primal Quest Expedition Race founder, third edition**

■ If your feet are happy, you're happy. If your feet are miserable and want to quit, you are miserable and want to quit.

—**Demetri "Coup" Coupounas, fourth edition**

■ Our feet connect us to the surrounding terrain, propelling us toward our next destination. Take care of your feet and the world is yours to enjoy. Ignore your feet and life can be a miserable experience.

—**Brian J. Krabak, MD, fifth edition**

■ Treat your feet well and the sky is the limit. Ignore or mistreat them and they'll provide an unending mental and physical strain that will threaten not only your result, but also your very ability to finish.

—**Rebecca Rushton, BSc (podiatrist), sixth edition**

This sixth edition has an important new chapter, "Blister Prevention: The New Paradigm." It contains new findings on blister formation and introduces the concept of shear, which in turn changes the way we look at blister prevention. In addition, there are updates and changes throughout every chapter, including coverage of new products and new techniques.

In the publishing world, not many books make it to a sixth edition. *Fixing Your Feet* has done so because it continues to offer solutions.

Fixing Your Feet is for you—solutions for your feet. I would love to hear from you. Send me an e-mail at john@fixingyourfeet.com and let me know your story about your feet.

Foot Fetish

My feet are runner's feet;
a little rough around the edges,
with black nails on the toes where I have nails at all
Lovingly decorated with bright colors.

My toes are warriors, of a sort.
They carry the entire continent of my body on adventures
and rise to challenges that could crush them.
Some days they are worn and calloused,
but they are strong and fierce adversaries for the
rocks they overtake.

My arches are the springboard of my soul.
They give me lift with every step I take
and cushion all my landings.
They are always ready
when I want to jump for joy.

My heels respond when the shepherd
of my spirit nips at them to run.
They strike again and again,
to thwart frustration,
to redeem the day.

My feet are runner's feet;
a little rough around the edges,
but they are strong
and they are willing
and oh, I love them.

—Lisa Butler, ultrarunner

Getting the Most Out of
Fixing Your Feet

In the 19 years since *Fixing Your Feet* first came out, I have answered many questions about foot care. I have patched thousands of feet at ultramarathons, multiday stage races, adventure races, marathons, and walking events. If there is one thing I have learned, it is this: the majority of athletes wait until they have problems to learn how to care for their feet.

When problems develop, everything becomes reactive—working to solve an existing problem. Preventing foot problems is being proactive—working to solve problems before they develop. Being proactive takes time up front. Being reactive takes time and resources often when they are not available or when using them may jeopardize the outcome of the event. I prefer proactive.

So here you are, holding this book in your hands. Maybe it's the first time you've seen it or maybe you had one of the earlier editions. The question is how can you get the most value out of it?

I would start by skimming the contents, the foreword, and the introduction. That will give you a feel for the depth of information inside. Then, read the chapters that catch your attention—maybe because you are dealing with those particular issues.

After that, read "Part One: Foot Basics" and "The Magic of Fit" chapter in "Part Two: Footwear Basics."

If you are new to learning about foot care, set aside some time to read through "Part One: Foot Basics" and "Part Two: Footwear Basics." They are the starting point for everything else in the book. Especially read all of "Part Two: Footwear Basics" if you are shopping for shoes.

After that, if you are currently experiencing foot problems, read the appropriate sections in "Part Four: Treatments"—then go back and read "Part Three: Prevention." Otherwise, read the "Prevention" and "Treatments" sections to get a well-rounded understanding of foot care. You'll get more out of the book that way. If you want to learn how to do foot care for others or as part of a medical team, focus on the "Prevention" and "Treatments" sections.

Anytime you see products that sound interesting, check them out on the listed websites. Not all of the products are right for you, but I guarantee that many are.

Nathan's story below is a perfect example of how to get the most out of *Fixing Your Feet*.

Nathan's Story

As I was finishing the material for the fifth edition, I received an e-mail from Nathan Wilson, who lives in the Kimberley region of northwest Australia. The week before, he had finished the seven-day, 250K stage race known as Racing the Planet: Australia. Previously Nathan had finished some marathons and ultramarathons, the longest one being 100K. Of the 185 starting competitors in Racing the Planet: Australia, only 118 completed the race, and most competitors had problems with blisters from the first day.

Three months before the race, Nathan bought *Fixing Your Feet*. He read it and learned a great deal about what he needed to do in preparation for this grueling event. Importantly, he learned how to deal with the problems he had experienced in earlier races. He learned how to pretape his feet and had the right tapes. He taped his feet three times during the race. He carried seven pairs of Injinji toe socks and Teko merino wool blend socks to wear over the toe socks. He used a lubricant at the start of each day. He used Sorbothane insoles for added shock absorption. For river crossings, he took off his shoes and socks and, once on the other side, cleaned his feet and reapplied lubricant. Each evening he cleaned his shoes and insoles. When he got into camp each day, he dried his feet and coated them with iodine and, in one instance, benzoin, to dry them further. He watched his electrolytes to avoid swelling of his feet and hands. For him, the race was an enjoyable experience.

Nathan was proactive from the beginning. Contrast that to others, who did not have adequate protection for the wet conditions, did not know how to use the contents of their "required" foot-care kit, did not pretape, used the wrong tape, had not conditioned their feet and bodies for the weight of their packs, and were reactive to problems.

Nathan wrote, "I realized that the part of the book that focused on working on your feet prior to a large event really had an impact on me. After reading people's stories of soaking their feet, removing calluses, and filing their toenails, I was motivated to do the same on a near-daily basis. It also motivated me to work on my ankle strength and my calves to help my feet. I suppose if I had not done this prep work, all of the taping, lubricants, toe socks, and so on would have helped some, but it might not have made such a difference. A lot of people have asked about the race and the blisters 'I must have had.' I just laugh and tell them that I didn't get a single one."

Nathan thanked me for getting him through Racing the Planet: Australia, a very tough event. I commend Nathan for doing things right. I hold Nathan up as an example of how to use the material in this book. I could not have found a better illustration of being proactive. I challenge you to do likewise.

The Best of 20 Years of Foot Care

In 1996 I spent a year writing the first edition of *Fixing Your Feet*. In the 20 years since then, I have learned a lot that is worth repeating. This chapter comes from my experiences, learned in the field and shared in my blog. You may find some of this repeated elsewhere in the book, and there is a reason for that. This is important stuff. It includes answers to questions and comments I also hear over and over. Allow me to share a bit of what I have learned. I also encourage you to check out and subscribe to my *Fixing Your Feet* blog by going to fixingyourfeet.com.

Five Tidbits of Wisdom

1. Taking care of your feet is your job. Do not count on someone else to take care of your feet.

2. Fit is key. Shoes that are too short or that are wrong for the event will make your feet hurt and lead to problems.

3. Your feet must be conditioned to endure the rigors and stresses of your chosen sport or sports. Train in race conditions in the shoes and socks you will wear on race day. Work up to distances that you will tackle in your event.

4. A little toenail care goes a long way in preventing blisters and black toenails. Properly trimmed and filed nails will not catch on socks and will be less likely to lead to toe blisters.

5. Calluses can and usually do lead to problems with blisters or with the thickened and hardened skin folding up on itself when it becomes macerated from being wet. They will become painful.

The Golden Rule for Your Feet

The signature line on Mike's e-mail caught my eye: "Treat your feet as you would have yourself be treated." As a runner, he had e-mailed me about one of my blog posts, and his mention of "running's golden rule" caught my attention.

Mike says, "I think it means the same as the Golden Rule: Take care of your feet and they will take care of you; treat your feet with respect and kindness and they'll support you in tough times; be a best friend to your feet and they'll be your best friend when you need one most."

I like that. Too often we relegate our feet to the end of the line. Sure, we buy good footwear and socks, but that's it—we forget about the feet themselves. We forget quality toenail care and then wonder why we get black toenails. We forget about callus control and then wonder why we have to deal with blisters underneath them. We fail to deal with corns, athlete's foot, and other problems common to feet. We get blisters but don't take time to figure out why we get them or learn measures to prevent and treat them.

We forget the golden rule: "Treat your feet as you would have yourself be treated." Actually, it is pretty easy. A few minutes a day is all it takes.

Basic Foot Care: It's Your Job

In January 2006 I had the opportunity to serve on the medical team at the Coastal Challenge, a seven-day, 150-mile stage race in Costa Rica. Some 51 athletes from around the world were there to experience the trails, roads, beaches, and rain forests of a beautiful country. The people were warm and very friendly. The food was great. The scenery was fantastic; the wildlife, colorful and exotic; and the weather, hot and humid. We had great fun.

I made some observations over the course of seven days. What I want to share here is pretty basic—but what many forget.

You are responsible for your feet. Not me. Not the medical crew, if there is one. It's your job. Let me explain.

You should have a foot-care kit appropriate for the length (both in miles and days) and type of event. Having a foot-care kit means that you also know how to pretape to prevent hot spots and blisters, repair any blisters you get, apply any patches you have, care for your toenails, and manage calluses or any other unique features of your feet.

The medical staff doing foot care at the Costa Rica race had lineups every evening. Three of us were patching feet. We had a lot of materials but quickly went through much of it. It is difficult to patch feet in the evening and then be expected to patch feet at the aid stations the next day, and then again that evening. We would have run out of materials in a few days. Fortunately, some of the runners had their own materials and patched their own feet. I commend them. They really helped us.

You also need to come into an event with feet that are properly prepared. That means reducing your calluses so they aren't as thick. The little calluses on the bottom of your toes can quickly become bothersome. Those on your heels can ruin your whole event. Work on your toenails so they won't create toe blisters and black toenails. See the "Toe Problems" chapter for more on toenails. Put miles on your feet to condition them for the rigors of the event you will be doing. Running 20 miles a week will not prepare you effectively for doing a 150-mile, seven-day event. Also, prepare your feet by having quality shoes and socks—not ones that are worn down.

So what's the bottom line? It's your job to be prepared. It is not the job of the medical staff to patch you up every night and every morning, and at every aid station during the event—especially when your feet are not prepared coming into the event. Many times we can work small miracles, but please work with us. Then watch us as we work and take the time to learn so the next time you can help us out.

Lisa Bliss, MD, the former Badwater Ultramarathon medical director, supports my comments. "If runners think we are there for blister care, then they will not take the time or effort to learn about it themselves and train appropriately in advance of the race," she says. "I don't mind helping; I just don't want runners to be helpless about prevention and treatment."

Self-Education

Podiatrist Rob Conenello, who managed feet at the seven-day Sahara Race in Egypt, said, "I would go daily to the athletes' tents to help them prevent injury. The key is to educate the participants on how to tape themselves and care for small problems."

Self-education takes many forms. It's getting your feet in the best shape and condition possible for the events you do. It's getting inside your footwear. Literally. Check the insoles. It may be a basic, nonsupporting piece of heavy cardboard. Consider replacing them with supportive insoles. Check for bad seams and stitching in the shoe. Know your foot type and research reviews to find the best shoes. Know what makes for a well-fitting shoe.

Find what works best for your feet. Learn how your skin reacts to powders and lubricants to reduce friction. Learn how to tape your feet and patch a blister—in different ways with different products. Learn how to trim your toenails. Learn how to strengthen your feet and ankles. Learn what words such as *proprioception* and *onychocryptosis* mean and how they affect your feet.

Are Your Feet Prepared?

When I talk to runners preparing for a race, some seem to be well prepared. They know about blisters and what kind of socks to wear. They either have experience with foot issues or want to learn more. Others seem unconcerned or unprepared.

The main question I ask is, "Are your feet prepared?" The tips below can easily apply to anyone running or walking a marathon, or doing any similar event. Are they magic? No. But many people, even athletes, seem to forget the commonsense tips that can make their event a better experience.

Preparing Your Feet for a Race

BEFORE THE RACE

- Toenails too long catch on socks. Trim them short.

- File toenails smooth so no rough edges are felt.

- Use a callus file to smooth calluses.

- Clean out lint and junk from inside shoes.

- Check your shoelaces and replace if frayed.

MORNING OF THE RACE

- Apply a layer of your favorite lubricant or powder.

- Smooth your socks around your feet.

- Avoid tying laces too tightly.

DURING THE RACE

- If you feel a hot spot, apply a pad, a bit of tape, a dab of lubricant, or even an energy gel wrapper between your sock and shoe.

- Loosen shoelaces if you have pain on the top of your foot.

AFTER THE RACE

- If you have blisters, soak your feet in Epsom salts and warm water three times a day.

- Drain blisters only if they are in a pressure area.

- Trim edges of loose skin around torn and drying blisters.

- If feet are swollen, elevate and ice.

With Footwear, Try Then Adjust

A triathlete recently said after running a marathon, "My left instep is still quite bruised. It took a pounding from the stretchy triathlon shoelaces that I used and—whoops!—never adjusted quite properly. Lesson learned: too loose is better than too snug."

In other words, she put the laces in her shoes and ran in them without adjusting them to fit her feet. This is an easily made and common mistake. When you make changes to your footwear, learn to try . . . and then adjust as necessary. You can apply this same failure to other parts of your footwear.

A few don'ts when it comes to footwear:

- Don't wear new shoes for a walk, race, or hike without trying them first—it's easy to miss a bad fit, a rough inside seam, or a wrong fitting arch. Walk around the house in them for a few hours.

- Don't wear new socks in an event without first trying them inside your shoes—the socks may be thicker or thinner than your previous socks, making the fit different.

- Don't replace insoles without checking if they are thinner or thicker than the old ones, which can change the space for your feet inside your shoes.

Don't Give Up on Footwear

Maggie was having tremendous problems getting a good fit with her footwear. She wrote, "This is by far the most frustrating thing I have experienced in my quest to find my personal 'very best way.' Occasionally I have come up with a combination that has had very acceptable results, only to have the same strategy fail miserably on the next outing."

Many more people have the same problem. Some have had only a few minor problems while others have had lots. I like to hear from those who never have foot problems. They may be doing everything right, be genetically blessed with good feet, and likely have put lots of miles on their feet in order to have the right conditioning. Others, such as Maggie, have tried every idea under the sun—without success. These are the ones I love to talk to. They are dedicated to finding what works and will give up at nothing.

Maggie and others are on a quest to find the best fit, as well as the best shoe and sock combination possible. They love being outdoors, running, hiking, or walking. It is a part of who they are. But they want to do it with happy feet.

You may be frustrated as Maggie was. My advice? Don't give up. There is a solution. There are shoes out there that will fit. With the search you'll learn about fit, socks, insoles, orthotics, lacing techniques, heel counters, forefoot width, pronation, supination, shoe lasts, narrow feet, wide feet, Morton's toe, bunions, and much more. Read shoe reviews in magazines. Do web searches on different shoes with the word *reviews* in the search box. Quiz your shoe store salesperson. Ask questions. Try different pairs by different manufacturers. Don't leave the store with a shoe that doesn't feel right. Don't settle for second best. Your feet deserve the very best.

Preventing Blisters

If there is one thing I have come to know, it's this: The very best way to prevent blisters today may not work tomorrow.

I wrote the above in response to a hiker who said he knew the secret to preventing blisters. He wrote, "The very best way to prevent blisters is to wear sock liners under your socks. Nothing works better to prevent blisters."

I wrote back to him, "There is not *one* 'very best way' for everyone to prevent blisters. I've patched thousands of feet and have seen it all and heard it all. I feel there is a very best way for each of us. It may mean using powder, lubricant, liner socks, double layer socks, toe socks, pretaping, toughening your skin, keeping your skin as soft as a baby's bottom, and a host of other ideas. It may also be a combination of ways. Just understand that the very best way today may fail tomorrow. It's important to know your options."

Many others have learned this the hard way. They love their calluses, only to get deep blisters underneath. They wear the wrong socks. They fail to get the best fit possible. They don't trim toenails and then blister on the tips of their toes. They find that yesterday's solution is now today's blister. It can happen to anyone—and it usually does.

I appreciate the solutions that people find. I've found them too. I've heard the comments, "Wow! My blisters are gone. I found the best socks." That's great. I'm happy. But be careful. Take a bit of time and know your options. Socks are good but learn how to tape. Learn about insoles, fit, lacing options, and more. You know your own feet better than anyone else so you have to experiment to find what works best for you.

Let Your Feet Breathe

Are your feet comfortable? I mean, do they get to relax like the rest of you? If you are like most people, you get home from work and change into something comfortable. You know, loose-fitting clothes that are soft.

So what do you put on your feet? Socks and comfortable shoes? Flip-flops or sandals? Or maybe you even choose to go barefoot? What's the right choice?

In the same way that your body needs something comfortable, your feet do too. After a day cooped up in socks and shoes, or nylons and heels, give your feet a break. Let them out for some air. They need to breathe too. Wiggle your toes. Rub your feet. According to the American Podiatric Medical Association, our feet have approximately 250,000 sweat glands and produce as much as a pint of moisture per day. Your feet need their space and they need to be let out for air at least once a day. Be nice to your feet and let them breathe.

Miles on Your Feet

One runner whom I admire and consider a close friend is Catra Corbet. She has proven herself as the "owner" of the Ohlone Wilderness Trail. Many years she will run an Ohlone 100 or more just because she loves the trail so much. Occasionally Catra will run 200 miles on the trail! In talking to Catra after she completed one of those 200-mile runs, she mentioned that she had no blisters. I remember years ago taking a picture of her taping her toes. She used to tape every toe. I have a photo of her with a heel blister too. Now though, Catra runs blister free. What's the difference?

I believe Catra's success with blister-free feet came through the miles of running she puts on her feet. She doesn't run short runs, she doesn't run a couple of times a week—she runs a lot. Many of you know Catra, or have heard of her—and know how much she runs. She also has found the right shoes for her feet—Hokas. She also wears Drymax socks—a favorite of mine.

But it's not just Catra. I have worked medical and provided foot care at hundreds of ultramarathons, adventure races, walks, and multiday races and have seen the same thing.

At the Western States 100 Michigan Bluff 55.7-mile aid station, for example, the top 20–30 runners come through without needing any type of foot care. There may be one or two who get some type of foot care from their crew down the road, but if so, it is generally pretty minor. Most often, if anything, they just change socks or shoes.

As the race progresses and more runners come through, we begin to see runners needing help with foot care. The farther back the runners are, the more foot care they need. Not every runner, but many of them. And many of them have multiple issues. Not just one blister, but quite a few. The more problems they have, the more complex the repair, and the longer it takes to complete the fix. This becomes a huge issue if they are trying to stay ahead of the cutoffs at each aid station. I remember a runner several years ago whose feet we patched up. At the next aid station, she needed more care and wanted to get out of the aid station quickly to avoid the cutoff. That meant not doing a quality patch job—and she came back to the aid station after going a bit down the road. She knew her race was over.

So the point here is that you need to put lots of miles on your feet in order to train them for long conditions. You can run 10 miles a day, day after day, and then try and do a 50-miler, and odds are—you'll have problems. You have 10- to 15-mile feet—not 50-mile feet.

This applies to walking, running, adventure racing, hiking, any activity where you use your feet. It all boils down to how many miles you are putting on your feet.

We all can't be the top runners. Many runners don't have unlimited time to train. So what can the rest do? Make sure you get some long runs, especially closer to your race. Make sure you have the best possible fit in your shoes. Make sure you wear quality socks. Reduce your calluses. Learn proper toenail care. Change your socks and shoes as necessary for the conditions of your run or race.

What Changed?

Let's begin with a story from an unnamed runner: "I'll start by saying that I've never had problems with blisters in the past, except for one little problem four years ago. So this last weekend I start the AT100, and by mile 16 I have hot spots going on the sides of both heels. Got out the duct tape and did my thing, but by mile 32 both heels have blisters going, and I have hot spots on the balls of both feet as well. I retape, moleskin, and so on, but to no avail. By mile 48 the blister on the heel of my right foot has broken; the hot spots on the balls of my feet have turned into half-dollar-size blisters. Retape and go. At mile 57, I retape again; the side of the heel of my right foot is bleeding. Coming back into an aid station the blister on the ball of my right foot has popped and I rather painfully 'squish' with every step. By this point I've had it, and at mile 67 I drop. I did nothing different than I've ever done—same shoes, same socks, and the same lubricant. Everything was identical to my other 30 races where I've had no problems whatsoever. So what happened here?"

Blisters can be puzzling because they seem to develop on different parts of the foot at different times and for different reasons. If this happens to you, a question is in order, "What changed?"

The answer is sometimes simple and easy. Other times, it's complex. People tell me they never blistered before today, or they blistered in a new area, or had problems with their toes, or something else. Or they tell me they worked hard to rid their feet of calluses and now something happened and their feet are trashed. Some tell of bad blisters deep underneath calluses. Or bad toe blisters.

Never mind the problem. The question is always the same, "What changed?" Another angle on the question is, "What felt different?" Even if you used the same shoes, socks, and lubricant as before, other factors could be different. Perhaps there was a change in hydration, temperature, and humidity. Maybe your training changed, and you didn't put in the necessary miles before the event. Trail factors include slope, dust and grit, rocks, mud, and water. Perhaps water went down your legs while you were sponging off, or you didn't wear gaiters, or the mesh upper of the shoes allowed dust and grit inside that caused the hot spot. The insoles could be old and should be replaced if any of their fabric is folding down, or if a rough edge is exposed. The shoe's heel counter could be too rigid, or the heel counter fabric frayed, or the juncture of the insole and heel counter bothersome—all factors that could cause blisters. It could even be how tight you tied your shoes to secure your heel in place and the amount of heel movement. Socks often bunch up and cause problems. Maybe you changed to a new sock or never changed socks. How quickly after a hot spot developed and how well you taped the hot spots and blisters could also be a factor. Many times we blister more easily in certain places when walking as opposed to running, and that could also have been a factor. The lubricant you put on your feet could have worn off and was not replaced, or the lubricant softened the skin and led to blisters. Maybe your toenails were not trimmed and caught on your socks, causing toe blisters. The toe box could have also been too short or too low. Your feet could have been wet too long and the skin macerated into blisters. You could have slightly turned an ankle and thus changed your gait, causing pressure and blisters in never-before problem areas. And the list goes on.

Chances are that *something* changed. You need to figure out what it was. It could be something simple or complex or even a combination of changes.

Many athletes find that they have been fine and blister free for years and then an event comes along and their feet are trashed. Sometimes it is just one of those days. No two events are the same; few of us can do events time after time and not experience problems with legs, stomach, mind, or feet. So if your feet had been good and healthy and they blistered or had other problems, ask yourself, "What changed?"

Trimming Toenails

How hard can it be to trim your toenails? For a lot of folks, it's a huge deal and something they never do. In all the years I have been patching feet, I have observed that untrimmed toenails are the number one cause of problems leading to toe blisters and black toenails. Socks will catch on nails that are too long or that have rough edges. This puts pressure on the nail bed, leading to blisters under the toenails, blisters at the tips of the toes, or painful toenails as they are pushed back into the cuticle. Nails that are too long are also prone to pressure from a toe box that is too short or too low.

So what are some tips to keeping your toenails under control? Toenails should be trimmed straight across the nail—never rounded at the corners. Leave an extra bit of nail on the outside corner of the big toe to avoid an ingrown toenail. After trimming toenails, use a nail file to smooth the top of the nail down toward the front of the toe and remove any rough edges. If you draw your finger from the skin in front of the toe up across the nail and can feel a rough edge, the nail can be filed smoother or trimmed a bit shorter.

You can use an emery board from your drugstore, a cheap "use it a few times and toss it" file. Better yet, invest a few bucks in a nice metal file that will last a long time and serve you well. To trim your nails, there are regular nail clippers, nippers, and scissors made exclusively for thicker toenails. If your local drugstore or pharmacy doesn't stock them, check out footsmart.com for a great selection.

A little bit of care in toenail trimming goes a long way in preventing toe blisters and black toenails, as well as making your socks last longer.

The Little Toe Triangle

We each have two. Little toes, that is. The number of problems with these little appendages has impressed me. It's all about that little triangle of skin where most problems occur.

If you look at your little toes, your toes may be well rounded and soft. Or they may have the often-typical triangle look where the skin on the bottom of the triangle is hard and callused. The skin on the bottom of the toe forms the point of the triangle. The problem is that on many of our little toes, this bottom point is hard and callused skin. The hard skin is prone to blisters forming underneath as pressure from the toe box creates shear. Often this hardened skin is partially under the skin of the next toe, another pressure area. The outside of the foot, the little toe area, is often more wet and damp than the inside of the shoes, leading to macerated skin. Once softened, this skin can easily blister underneath, or worse yet, the skin can separate, leading to major skin problems.

One runner whose feet I patched at Primal Quest had struggled for the whole event with macerated skin on his feet. When he came into a transition area, the skin had stripped off the bottom point of this triangle—of both feet. I know it was painful and uncomfortable. Once patched, he continued on as best he could.

The little toe is so small that it is hard to patch well. The use of Hypafix, Micropore, or a kinesiology tape is a good choice. Even better, in my opinion, is reducing the hard callused skin. Injinji toe socks can also be helpful. Good shoes are vital too. Shoes with a good toe box that allows the toes room to wiggle are best. Once the skin has blistered, 2nd Skin is good to use as a patch. Cut it to fit the blister. Too much and it becomes bulky and rubs on the neighboring toe.

During a race or hike, be watchful of your little toes. This small but potentially troublesome triangle of skin deserves special care.

Informed Athletes

I am always happy to see informed runners and racers. They know, for the most part, what their feet need. The athletes with the fewest foot problems share the following characteristics:

- Many pretape their feet to protect against hot spots and blisters.

- Most use moisture-wicking socks.

- Most change socks and shoes when necessary and before problems set in.

■ Most know about their foot problems, knowing when they have Morton's foot, bunions, calluses, bad toenails, or anything else out of the ordinary.

■ Many have tried to rid their feet of calluses, knowing that a blister under a callus is the worst kind to get.

■ Many use a good, state-of-the-art lubricant to avoid friction.

■ Most know the importance of shoes that fit well.

■ Many file down their toenails.

Still Learning

What disturbs me is that there are still large numbers of athletes who seem to give little thought to their feet. The athletes with the most foot problems share the following characteristics:

■ They shove feet into shoes without straightening their socks.

■ They wear the wrong socks and do not look inside their socks for seams that cause toe blisters.

■ They have sacrificed fit and buy a shoe because a friend recommended it and not because it was the best shoe for their feet.

■ They try to fix blisters with Band-Aids.

■ They fail to change their socks often enough when their feet are wet.

■ They fail to trim their toenails and wonder why they get black toenails and toe blisters.

■ They fail to put in the miles that their feet need to be toughened for the rigors of racing.

■ They speed through checkpoints, feeding their faces but not tending to their feet.

As Billy Trolan, MD, said in the foreword for the first edition of *Fixing Your Feet*, "The one factor that continues to amaze me is that individuals and teams will spend vast amounts of money, time, and thought on training, equipment, and travel, but little or no preparation on their feet. Too often the result has been that within a few hours to a few days, all that work has been ruined. Ruined because the primary mode of transportation has broken down with blisters." That was written in 1997 and is still true today.

What Were You Thinking?

Tonya Olson and I were working side by side as runners came over for our help at the Michigan Bluff aid station at Western States. She was a quick learner and asked a lot of questions—which was good. Twice, she seemed perplexed, as I was also.

The first time was with a runner who had stubbed her toe, which lifted the big toenail off the nail bed. There was blood under the nail. We noticed more than blood. There was also a large buildup of residue from toenail fungus. I drained the blood blister but could do little to reduce the angle of the nail. It stuck up quite a bit. Putting pressure on the nail to try and get it to lay flatter didn't work. It hurt her too much. There was too much nail fungus buildup under the nail. That is common with nail fungus. I ended up running a strip of Kinesio-Tex tape from the top of the toe over the tip and underneath. Then I wrapped a length of tape around the toe to help hold the nail down. I talked to the runner about her toenail fungus while I worked. She was aware of the fungus, but hadn't done anything about it.

The second case was a runner who came in with macerated feet. We cleaned his feet and looked them up and down for anything to patch. Tonya pointed out a bunch of opened skin between his toes. Not a couple of tiny tears, but a lot of open skin around several toes. The skin was soft and wet, and had torn open. It looked pretty painful. It was athlete's foot. As I worked on his feet we talked to the runner. He worked in a running store. The advice I gave him was to get out of shoes during the day and let his feet air. And to start taking a proactive approach to medications to rid his feet of athlete's foot.

Both cases were interesting in that they knew that they had a preexisting problem condition with their feet. And both had chosen to do nothing, ignore the problem. Maybe it will go away on its own.

The problem was that these two runners had entered this 100-mile run; paid a large amount of money for gear, travel, crew and pacers; and spent a lot of time training—without thinking about their preexisting foot conditions: toenail fungus in the first case and athlete's foot in the second.

Each condition was not enough to end a run on a normal day. However, this was a 100-mile run. The trail was wet and full of rocks, roots, sand, and dirt, and this was a race where things "happened."

A stubbed toe led to a raised big toenail that now pressed even more on a toe box. It must have hurt—especially on the downhills. The athlete's foot led to easily opened and torn skin between the runner's toes. The wet conditions had made it worse. That open and raw skin must have hurt too.

As I worked on their feet, I talked to both and told them they needed to take care of their conditions. I really wanted to say, "What were you thinking?" Truth be told, I wanted to yell it at them, **"What were you thinking?"**

Both runners had made choices that jeopardized their finishing. When you invest all that money and energy into a race, why not make sure the two feet that are responsible for getting you there are in the best shape possible?

Part One

Foot Basics

Seeking Medical Treatment

The information and advice given in this book is provided to athletes to use in their efforts to resolve foot problems. Not all foot problems or injuries will be resolved successfully by following the tips or using the products mentioned in this book. There are times when it is important to seek professional medical help.

Never ignore an injury. Pushing through an injury or returning to your sport too soon after being injured can lead to additional injuries. You do not want to turn a temporary injury into a permanent disability. Too often athletes rely on self-diagnosis rather than consulting with a medical specialist. If during or after running or hiking you have persistent foot problems or recurring pain that you cannot resolve, seek medical treatment from a medical specialist who can provide his or her medical expertise for your problem.

Primary Medical Specialists for Feet

ORTHOPEDISTS are orthopedic surgeons, experts of the joints, muscles, and bones. This includes upper and lower extremities and the spine. Look for an orthopedist who specializes in the foot and ankle. The American Academy of Orthopaedic Surgeons and the American Orthopaedic Foot and Ankle Society can provide referrals. There are also orthopedic clinical specialists (OCS).

PODIATRISTS are doctors of podiatric medicine (DPM) who work on the feet up to and including the ankles. They specialize in human movement, and medical and surgical problems including foot diseases, deformities, and injuries, such as nail, skin, bone, tendon, and diabetic disorders. Podiatrists treat such disorders with surgery, custom-made orthotics (shoe inserts), physical therapy, injections, casting and braces, prescription medication, and medicated creams and ointments. The American Podiatric Medical Association and the American Academy of Podiatric Sports Medicine can provide referrals.

If you have chronic foot problems, or you are uncertain what your feet are trying to tell you through their pain, consider consulting a podiatrist or orthopedic surgeon. Listen to your whole body and especially your feet. Be attentive to when the pain begins and what makes you hurt more or less. Then be prepared to tell the specialist about the problem, its history, what you have done to correct it, and whether it worked or got worse.

There is a wide range of skill overlap between orthopedists and podiatrists. Both can treat most of the same foot problems. When searching for a medical specialist for your feet, talk to doctors about their training, experience, and whether they have a specialty field. Both of the two specialist fields have doctors who specialize in sports medicine, and these would be my first choice. Weigh this information when making a decision about whom to turn to for help. Additionally, a variety of other specialists can provide assistance in strengthening, alignment, rehabilitation, and footwear design and fit.

Foot Specialists

PEDORTHISTS work with the design, manufacture, fit, and modification of shoes, boots, and other footwear. Pedorthists are board certified (C.Ped.) to provide prescription footwear and related devices. They will evaluate, fit, and modify all types of footwear. A C.Ped. can help find a shoe built on a last (the form over which a shoe is constructed) that best matches a person's feet, and then construct a custom orthotic that meets his or her particular biomechanical needs and interfaces with the shoe in a way that improves its fit and performance. The American Orthotics and Prosthetics Association and the Pedorthic Footwear Association can provide information and referrals.

SPORTS MEDICINE DOCTORS specialize in sports-related injuries. They are typically doctors of internal medicine with additional training in sports medicine. When treating athletes with lower-extremity injuries that do not improve with their initial treatment, they may refer the athlete to a podiatrist or orthopedist. Most are members of the American College of Sports Medicine (which does not provide referral services).

PHYSICAL THERAPISTS (PT) are licensed to help with restoring function after illness and injury. Most work closely with medical specialists. Physical therapists use a variety of rehabilitation methods to restore function and relieve pain: massage, cold and heat therapy, ultrasound and electrical stimulation, and stretching and strengthening exercises. There are also masters of physical therapy (MPT) and doctors of physical therapy (DPT). The American Physical Therapy Association can provide referrals.

ATHLETIC TRAINERS are licensed to work specifically on sports-related injuries. Rehabilitation methods may be similar to physical therapy but can additionally focus on maintaining cardiovascular fitness while injuries heal. The National Athletic Trainers' Association can provide referrals.

MASSAGE THERAPISTS work with athletes in reducing pain and tightness in muscles, tendons, and ligaments—the body's soft tissues. The American Massage Therapy Association can provide referrals. Look for either licensed massage therapists (LMT) or board-certified in therapeutic massage and bodywork (BCTMB).

CHIROPRACTORS are doctors of chiropractic (DC) medicine who specialize in the alignment of the body's musculoskeletal system. Pelvis, back, and neck pain and muscle imbalances are often treated by a chiropractor. Some may specialize in sports injuries. There are also certified chiropractic sports physicians (CCSP). Two organizations, the American Chiropractors Association and the International Chiropractic Association, can provide referrals.

When the time comes to seek medical attention, ask others in your sport for referrals, ask at your local running or outdoors store, look in the Yellow Pages, or search online. If you have a choice, choose a sports medicine specialist over a general doctor. For contact information for the professional organizations previously mentioned, check "Medical and Footwear Specialists" on page 351.

You Can Have Healthy and Happy Feet

This chapter was suggested by a reader who commented, "Many people don't have a clue about their own feet, about how things work and why, or about regular and preventive maintenance." As athletes, feet should be one of our most important concerns. They get us where we are going and back again. We toss on a fanny pack or backpack and trot off without a thought to what that means to our feet. We shove them into shoes and boots without taking time to look at them. We add miles too fast, stress them with uneven terrain, let them become too dry or too wet, and then wonder why our feet hurt.

Think "Feet"

Many foot problems happen because we forget to think about our feet. The only way to have feet that are healthy and happy is to be proactive in foot care, to stay on top of minor problems before they become major problems. That means you buy high-quality shoes and socks, take care of your skin and toenails through self-care, condition your feet with the miles you need for the sports you will participate in, don't stress them beyond what they can do, and rest them when they need rest.

A Weekly Ritual

Once a week before putting on socks, take a few seconds to run your hands over your feet to check for anything out of the ordinary. If you find something, refer to the index to find the corresponding section in the book. Ask yourself some questions:

- Do I see any redness?

- Are there any cracks or cuts in the skin?

- Do my nails need trimming?

- Do my nails look discolored or thick?

- Is there redness or tender areas at the nail beds?

- Do I see any scaly skin?

- Does anything itch?

- Do I have any old blisters that need attention?

- Is there pain anywhere?

- Do I have any callus buildup that needs attention?

- Do I see any corns or plantar warts?

- Does anything feel funny?

Talk to Your Doctor

Your doctor can do a foot check whenever you have a physical. He or she can help catch problems before they become medical emergencies. Ask what you should watch for. Typically watch for sores that don't heal, ingrown toenails, swelling, cold feet, numbness, a burning or tingling feeling, or unresolved or abnormal pain—even melanomas. Problems with our feet can develop into long-term health issues, which can rob us of our mobility and independence. The American Orthopaedic Foot and Ankle Society says that many of the more than 4.8 million visits to doctors made each year for foot and ankle problems are problems that could have been prevented with better footwear and foot care.

Summer Foot-Care Basics

Summers are fun. We get outdoors and explore. We walk, hike, run, and participate in sports. Many of these activities, however, put added stressors on our feet. This section discusses what we should do to prepare our feet for summer.

Many of us go barefoot in the summer. If you are outside, be watchful for cuts and abrasions to your skin. Use an antibiotic ointment if necessary. Going barefoot will cause the skin on the bottom of your feet to harden and turn into calluses. The problem occurs when a blister develops under a callus. If you like calluses, try to keep them under control and not too thick. Use a pumice stone or callus file to keep them manageable. Also watch for cracks in the heels. These cracks are called fissures and can be several layers of skin deep. Once cracked, the skin has to heal from the inside out. The use of a skin moisturizer in the morning and evening can do wonders to keep your feet in shape. When applying a moisturizer or callus remover cream in the evening, occasionally wrap your feet in a plastic bag or plastic wrap to hold the cream on the foot.

When you wear flip-flops and sandals, be aware that the same rules apply here as going barefoot. You can also develop a very thick and hard "corner" of skin at the edges of the heel. Be attentive to the condition of the skin on the bottom of your feet and care for it as described previously.

Keeping skin soft can help the toes. Many of us develop a hardened layer of skin at the bottom of our toes, especially the baby toes. This can easily develop into calluses and then blister. A file and skin moisturizer can help.

Toenails need to be kept trimmed and filed smooth. Trim them straight across to avoid an ingrown nail. File the nail smooth so when you draw your finger across the tip of the nail, you can't feel rough edges. Nails that are too long or have rough edges can catch on socks and push the nail back into the nail bed. They also hit the front of the inside of the toe box, putting pressure on the nail, which can cause black nails. If the nail comes loose, be sure to keep it covered with a Band-Aid so it won't come off when pulling socks on or off.

This is a good time to drag all your shoes out of the closet and give them a once-over. Check for worn-out uppers, worn-down soles that could change your gait and cause problems, and compressed midsoles that offer no cushioning and support. Put these shoes aside and save them for gardening and chores. If the shoes are OK, check for worn-out, paper-thin insoles. Replace them to give the shoes more life.

Strong ankles make walking, hiking, and running easier. Use a wobble board or ankle exercises to strengthen these important joints. A good exercise is to stand on one foot, or even on a soft pillow, with arms outstretched; when you master this, close your eyes. Ankle exercises help to promote better balance, ankle strength, and the ability to respond in midstride to changes in the terrain.

Winter Foot-Care Basics

In the winter you still need to work on your skin and toenails, and keep calluses in check. Because you're not barefoot or in sandals as much, you may forget to check your feet as often as you do in the summer. In addition, be watchful for dry skin. The cold, snow, and ice make it important to wear good socks and keep your feet warm. The thick socks can make your feet sweat more, so be watchful for athlete's foot. The use of antifungal foot powder can help prevent problems. Winter is a good time to go through your sock drawer and toss old and worn socks. Do the same with shoes, replacing old insoles, laces, and, if necessary, tossing the shoes too.

Aging Feet

Being aware of how your feet change as you age can help you prepare and make good choices. At a meeting of the American Academy of Orthopaedic Surgeons in Orlando, experts with the Foot and Ankle Society described the variety of foot problems that emerge with age and how to tell which ones can probably not be blamed on normal aging.

Cherise M. Dyal, MD, the chief of the Foot and Ankle Division of Orthopaedic Surgery at the Montessori Medical Centre in New York, explained, "There are five things that occur naturally with aging. The size increases as your feet get longer and wider; you lose some of the padding on the bottom of your foot, so you thin out your fat pad and tend to lose some of the spring in your step; your foot tends to become a little stiffer, so you lose some of the range of motion in your foot and ankle; you tend to have some problems with balance; and there is a very mild settling of the arch that's seen as a flattening of the foot. Those are the natural changes."

It has been well documented that foot problems increase with age. A good resource as we get older is the book *Great Feet for Life: Footcare and Footwear for Healthy Aging* by Paul Langer, DPM. According to Paul, the most common foot complaints by older adults are toenail and skin problems, calluses or corns, swelling, bunions, and arthritis.

Here are some tips to deal with aging feet.

- Make sure to have your feet sized each time you buy shoes.

- Choose shoes with additional cushioning and support.

- Switch to insoles with more cushioning in the heel and support in the arch. Sorbothane and Spenco insoles with gel are good choices.

- Pay close attention to your toenails. They often thicken as you age, so be sure to keep them trimmed and filed properly.

10 Easy Steps to Happy Feet

Here are my top 10 foot-care tips to keep your feet healthy and happy. Each of these tips is explained in depth in this book.

1. Make sure your footwear fits.

2. Buy high-quality footwear.

3. Wear moisture-wicking socks.

4. Practice self-care of your feet.

5. Manage your toenails.

6. Strengthen your feet and ankles.

7. Rest your feet.

8. Condition your feet for your sport.

9. Learn how to prevent blisters.

10. Carry a small foot-care kit.

Sports and Your Feet

Running, hiking, and adventure racing place extreme demands on our feet. Soccer, football, and court sports stress the feet and ankles with their quick changes in direction and sudden stops. Skiing and snowshoeing encase our feet in unforgiving hard boots that also stress our ankles. The surfaces we play and compete on vary from dirt, rock, grass, asphalt, and concrete to wooden courts, tracks, snow, and ice. Every sport offers wide ranges of difficulty. We challenge ourselves with ultramarathons on trails or roads. We test our limits in adventure races under extreme conditions. We tackle the multisport fun of duathlons and triathlons. Whatever our sport, our feet take a beating.

A run may be a relatively short road 10K or a grueling ultrarunning event of 100 miles with thousands of feet of mountainous ascents and descents. It may be in a short- or medium-length duathlon or triathlon, or a longer Ironman or Ultraman triathlon. There are also further extremes: 24-, 48-, and 72-hour runs, six-day runs, and 1,000-mile races. The terrain may be paved roads, tracks, fire roads, trails, cross-country, or any combination. You may run without any gear, with a single water bottle, or with a fanny pack or lightweight backpack loaded with extra socks, food, and water bottles.

A hike may be a day trip with a day pack, an overnighter with a midweight 40-pound backpack, or a 10-day High-Sierra trip with a pack that tips the scales at 65 pounds. You may be a traditional backpacker with a full-size pack that carries all the comforts of home, a fast-packer with a 30-pound pack, or an ultralight backpacker with a 16-pound pack. Typical backpackers may cover 6–10 miles in a day, ultralight backpackers can easily cover 30 miles, while fast-packers may cover 40 or more miles. The hike duration may be a night in your local hills, a week in the desert, three weeks in the Sierra, or several months on the Appalachian Trail or the Pacific Crest Trail.

Many athletes are choosing multiday running and walking events. The event that started the rage is Racing the Planet's seven-day stage races, where participants carry all their own gear, including food, as they navigate 150 miles in places such as

China, the Sahara, Chile, and more. Racing the Planet's events, the newer six-day Gore-Tex TransRockies Run, and other similar events are geared for people looking for adventure and challenges, in a doable event. Of course, this multiday format also brings with it lots of foot problems.

Adventure racing has included events with names such as Primal Quest, Eco Challenge, the Raid Gauloises, and the Beast of the East. Although the list of current races has declined, they still pull in many teams. These are typically competitive team races with four participants who must all finish together. Combining sports disciplines such as trail or cross-country running, mountain biking, rappelling, climbing, kayaking, canoeing, horseback riding, swimming, glacier climbing, and others, these races pose challenges along an often unknown course with constantly changing terrain. Many are multiday events over distances up to 450 miles. In these team events, the whole team is only as fast as the feet of its slowest member. Robert Nagel, one of the world's best adventure racers, recalls his experiences in the 1996 Extreme Games: "Our team had a strong and growing lead when my feet caused us to grind to a crawl. We continued, barely, losing more than 12 hours in the process, but still managed to take third place." He remembers that ESPN continued to show tapes of his feet 16 months after the event! After that experience, he worked hard to perfect a foot-care regimen that would prevent such a disaster from happening again.

Most sports require considerable use of the feet, and participation in these sports requires an athlete to keep his or her feet happy and healthy. Many of these athletes have learned the finer points of keeping their feet in shape. They rely on the many sources of conventional wisdom about foot care. But while much of this wisdom is good, the best advice often comes from athletes who, through trial and error, have found unique solutions for the prevention and treatment of their foot problems. Ronald Moak, an Appalachian Trail thru-hiker (1977) and Pacific Crest Trail thru-hiker (2000), sums it up best: "I would like to think that after 30 years of backpacking, I'd have solved the little dilemma of my feet. But, alas, I'm not that naive." Ronald has the right idea—it's good to listen to all forms of advice and then try different things. Don't be afraid to go against conventional wisdom. Just because it didn't work for others, that doesn't mean it won't work for you.

Sport Similarities

What do the aforementioned sports have in common? Foot-stressing sports have many similarities. They pound the feet, stress the joints, and strain the muscles, often to unnatural extremes. They may take place over a day, yet often are done over several days, or even a week or more. While athletes participate in these sports, their feet become highly susceptible to hot spots, blisters, and problems with toenails, stubbed toes, bruises, sprains, strains, heel spurs, plantar fasciitis, and Achilles tendinitis. All of these sports can be more enjoyable by solving these common foot problems.

Runners put considerable weight on their feet with each step. Though hikers move more slowly than runners, they often find their feet stressed by the weight of a fully loaded hydration pack or backpack. Adventure racers may stress the feet faster in shorter events or longer over multiday events in which they compete in multiple sports and carry the special equipment they require. The longer multi-day adventure races often tax the feet more than we can imagine with the regular exposure to water, constantly changing adverse conditions, and lack of time to do proper foot care.

In *Long-Distance Hiking: Lessons from the Appalachian Trail* (Ragged Mountain Press, 1998), Roland Mueser describes what he found when he surveyed hikers:

> Problems with feet were endemic. Half of the hikers experienced blisters at the start; many of these were attributed to thrusting tender feet into stiff, heavy boots. During his first few days in Georgia, one hiker was forced into a hospital for an entire week with so many serious blisters that his trip was terminated. And even later when hikers' feet became tough-ened, the combination of rain, heavy boots, and wet socks meant trouble for one out of five on the trail. One foot-troubled backpacker reported having seven blisters at one time. And more than one hiker, squirming out of boots, was horrified to see socks soaked with blood.[1]

Studies have shown that "carrying heavy external loads (i.e., a heavy backpack) during locomotion appears to increase the likelihood of foot blisters."[2] In addition, the type of physical activity performed is a factor in the probability of blister devel-opment. As we intensify our activity and as the duration of the activity increases, frictional shear forces are increased. Heavy loads, high-intensity activities, and long-duration activities are what we do as runners, hikers, and adventure racers. In our events, most of us experience at least two of these three stressors. Ultrarunner Suzie Lister typically experiences few problems with her feet while running ultras. However, when she participated in the 1995 Eco Challenge, the added weight of a pack on her back and the multiday stresses of adventure racing caused many problems with her feet: blisters on top of blisters and swollen feet.

The similar stresses among sports make the preventive maintenance and treat-ments for blisters and other foot problems necessary for all sports. This book approaches the different disciplines—running, triathlons, hiking and backpacking, and adventure racing—as one and the same when dealing with one's feet. Proper foot care is the most important variable for a successful outing.

Differences in Terrain

The terrain is an important part of your running, hiking, and playing environ-ment. While a flat, smooth, and resilient surface may seem ideal, it is not. Most runners spend the majority of their running miles on roads and trails, while most hikers spend their time on trails. The ideal surface is one that keeps changing the stresses on our body. This will help prevent injury and make you stronger. Changing surfaces develop muscles and reflexes. Don't always choose the same surface. Mix it up.

Variations from our normal running or hiking surface can produce problems as we compensate for uphills, downhills, concave surfaces, or irregularities of the sur-face. Be aware of compensations in your stride or gait due to changes in the surface.

Dirt and Trails

Dirt and trails provide a soft running and hiking surface. Trails or fire roads can open new vistas to the adventuresome athlete. Some trails are well groomed, while others are barely maintained. Soft dirt trails provide excellent shock absorption and can be a good surface to use if recovering from an injury.

Whether running or hiking, pay close attention to rocks, roots, wet leaves, mud, and other potential trail hazards, any of which can cause a turned ankle or a fall. On rainy days, slippery mud and grasses can present problems with footing. Watch for uneven terrain, roots, and holes on grassy sections of trail. Trail dust, dirt, pebbles, and rocks can be kicked up into the sock or between the sock and the shoe. These irritants can cause hot spots, blisters, or cuts. Gaiters worn over the shoe or boot tops can help prevent this problem (see "Gaiters," page 162).

Hiking on trails while wearing a backpack presents the added problem of maintaining one's balance with a top-heavy load while negotiating rocks, roots, and uneven trail. Attention to your footing can help prevent a turned ankle. Striding uphill stretches the Achilles tendons and the calf muscles and makes the pelvis tilt forward. Going downhill increases the shock impact to the heels when landing and tilts the body backward. Constantly going up- and downhill may also cause problems with toes, toenails, heel pain, plantar fasciitis, and more.

Grass

Grass is a forgiving surface and a great choice if you are prone to road-impact injuries. Be careful of uneven grassy areas, holes from burrowing animals, the slipperiness of wet grass, and the occasional rock or glass.

Roads

Road running is the mainstay of most runners. The asphalt surface of most roads provides a softer surface than concrete sidewalks. However, roads have slanted surfaces curving down toward the sides. The convex surface puts more stress on the downward side of your shoes and your body. The foot of the higher leg rotates inward, while the foot of the lower leg rotates outward. Avoid prolonged running on slanted surfaces, or at least spend equal time on both road shoulders. Keep your eyes open for potholes and manhole covers. Of course, the biggest hazard to road runners is vehicles. Where possible, run opposite the flow of traffic and safely to one side of the road, and choose roads with wide shoulders.

Concrete and Sidewalks

Concrete is approximately 10 times harder than asphalt. While the surface is usually smooth, your bones, muscles, and connective tissue get hammered. This surface can cause foot, leg, or back pain through the jarring of the joints. Shin splints, stress fractures, and compartment syndrome are common injuries from running on concrete. Care must be taken to watch your footing on sidewalks to avoid the tapered edges of driveways and drop-offs at curbs. The use of good, cushioned shoes and gel insoles can make concrete bearable—but try at all costs to avoid running on concrete.

Courts

Court play is usually on either asphalt or wood. Tennis courts may be indoors or outdoors. Basketball, racquetball, and other indoor sports are usually on wood. While an asphalt or wood court surface is hard and unforgiving, the main foot stresses for athletes playing on them are caused by sudden, quick movements and sudden starts and stops. Cushioned or motion-control shoes, depending on your feet, will protect your ankles. A good shoe fit, coupled with moisture-wicking socks and insoles, will prevent hot spots and blisters.

Sand

Walking or running on sand is hard work. Though sand is soft, its surface is not typically flat. Your heels may sink in more than the forefoot, and the uneven sand may cause a turned ankle. If you have access to a beach, try to stay near the water on the wet and packed sand.

Snow and Ice

Walking or running in the snow or on ice can be challenging. There may be snow on top of a layer of ice. Your shoes cannot make good traction unless they have been modified with small screws or special traction gear. Falling is a hazard and muscle pulls can be common as you slip or slide.

Tracks

Most of us at some time run on tracks. True, they can be boring. Running in circles, actually in ovals, lap after lap after lap after lap may not be your idea of a good run, but there may be a time for it in your running schedule. A track allows us to calculate with accuracy how fast we are running. I have used a track for occasional speed workouts. Prior to my first 24-hour track run, I spent 3 hours running at a local high school track to get a feel for the repetitiveness of track running.

The continuous running in one direction stresses the outer leg, so if possible, change direction every now and then. Dirt tracks should always be checked for ruts and uneven surfaces that could cause you to trip. Running in the outer lanes is less stressful when rounding the curves.

Conditioning

Conditioning means more than getting your body in condition. It also means getting your feet into the best shape possible for your sport. Your feet will respond to training in the same way your legs respond. Increasing your running or hiking time by increments will allow your feet time to adapt to the added stresses of the additional mileage. Doubling your mileage too quickly can lead to potential problems. If you are working up to a marathon, an ultra, or a multiday hike, do back-to-back training days to work your feet into their best possible condition. Toned and strengthened feet can reduce the occurrence of injuries, as well as sore and tired feet.

personal experience

"In 1991, I walked through immigration in the old Stapleton International Airport in Denver, wide-eyed and fresh from Australia and sporting some nice, neat, size 9 wing tips, comfortably encasing my soft corporate toes. Years later I am outgrowing my somewhat less than nimble size 11 trail shoes, with nary a hope of ever squeezing back into my old wing tips. This rather dramatic change in foot size is due entirely to conditioning. In 1984, when I started adventure racing in Australia, I had a size 8 shoe, but the intervening 22 years spent running and hiking around for prolonged periods with a pack on my back has resulted in a physiologic adaptation.

"This is really just conditioning. The same effect can be seen in farmer's hands, which grow to quite unusual sizes over decades of manipulating heavy machinery and tools. It is not uncommon to walk into a bar in the Midwest and see the little old farmer, neatly shrunk inside his once tight-fitting Wrangler jeans, with absolutely enormous gnarled hands nursing a beer.

"So, to get these nice, big, abuse-proof peds, spend some time on them. Lots of time. So much time that they hurt really bad. I don't usually say this, but in the case of feet, no pain, no gain. Don't go out and get bloody blisters, but do go out for those really long hikes, with a pack stuffed with baguettes, Camembert, bottles of red wine, and the kitchen sink and really abuse your lower leg structures. Work the crossword every day and you will get good at it; wield a hammer all day and you will get calluses on your hands; hike with a heavy pack for hours and you'll get bigger, tougher feet!"

—Ian Adamson, adventure racer

Brick Robbins was an adequately trained runner when he started his thruhike of the Pacific Crest Trail, but he quickly found that running had not conditioned his feet. The extra weight of a backpack caused additional stress to his feet. After 100 miles his feet were sore and bruised. By the time he reached Idyllwild—another 70 miles down the trail—he had killer blisters that took another 270 miles to heal. Although his feet were in good shape from running, they needed additional conditioning for the weight of a pack. There are no shortcuts to conditioning your feet. Your feet will become conditioned to longer distances by gradually increasing your mileage.

When Karen Borski thru-hiked the Appalachian Trail in 1998, she had very few foot problems. A year before the thru-hike, however, her feet were so out of shape that after an 8-mile day hike they would be riddled with huge blisters on the sides of the heels. Wearing a pack, she found that after only a few miles, blisters would begin to develop on the soles of her feet, usually the balls of the feet where the main pressure is felt. Karen recalls that she was "so frightened and worried about these blisters that I was afraid I would not be able to thru-hike." To fix the problem, she first bought new boots that were slightly too large so that during the course of a hike, as her feet naturally swelled, they wouldn't become too tight and rub. Then she started hiking with a pack every weekend. After hobbling around for most of the following week nursing these awful blisters, she would go out and do it again. When calluses finally began to develop, she took up running on the weeknights, both to get her body in shape and to help toughen her feet.

So, what is the best way to condition your feet? Your feet must be conditioned to endure the rigors and stresses of your chosen sport or sports. Train in race conditions in the shoes and socks you will wear on race day. Do short hikes with a pack on your back before taking off to tackle a multiday hike. Use a wobble board to strengthen your ankles. Toughen your feet with barefoot walking. Work up to distances that you will tackle in your event. Work out the kinks; find the best shoes and socks for what you will be doing. Learn how to trim your toenails and reduce calluses. Discover the proper insoles that provide support to relieve your plantar fasciitis or heel pain. Strengthen your toes and ankles. In short, do your homework before you head out to tackle the big one. Your feet will thank you.

If you are training for a long hike or an adventure race, at least 60% of your training should be done while wearing your pack with about the same amount of weight as you plan to carry during your race. This works your upper and lower body and trains the muscles, tendons, and ligaments of your ankles and feet to handle the extra weight. You must also train on somewhat the same terrain you'll face during a race—rocks, sand, up- and downhills, even with wet feet. Knowing in advance how your feet respond to these conditions will help you anticipate problems. Finally, you must train for the same distances as the race itself. One or two long runs a week is much better than five or six short runs. To the undertrained, the multiple days of pounding on your feet can take a cumulative toll and make every step painful.

Biomechanics

Many athletes who have participated in extreme sports have learned firsthand how one minor problem can be magnified over time and eventually have major consequences. Typically this happens when a blister affects the gait, a backpack's weight throws off balance and stance, or stressed or weakened muscles cause an imbalance in the body's mechanics. Every athlete has different strengths and weaknesses, different degrees of flexibility, and different muscle skills and body types. These factors affect the way we walk, run, and move. Add on a fanny pack or backpack, or put a flashlight in one hand and a water bottle in the other hand, and your biomechanics change. Each time your foot lands, it absorbs about two-and-a-half times your body weight. For every mile you travel, your feet hit the ground around 800 times each.

The Importance of Alignment

You all know the foot bone is connected to the ankle bone, and the ankle bone is connected to the leg bone. True, correct alignment of all those bones at the joints keeps you moving relatively pain-free now, and prevents many degenerative changes down the road. Total body alignment is essential to the success of any athletic activity.

Even more important to the healthy functioning of the feet and their ability to carry you through life is the spine—the very specific focus of chiropractors. The spinal cord carries sensory and motor information from your feet (and everywhere else for that matter) to your brain and back again. If one of the vertebral bones is even slightly misaligned or fixated, it can affect the communication lines and your feet and brain can be broadcasting misinformation. The joints of your feet and particularly your ankles contain nerves called proprioceptors that send messages about the changes in terrain that you are walking, standing, or running on. The brain then interprets and makes the miniscule changes in every joint in your body, from the tilt of your skull to the tuck of your tailbone, to keep you upright.

Chiropractors come in many styles. I recommend one who specializes in sports chiropractic and who adjusts extremities as well as the spine. Those chiropractors are certified in orthopedics and can design a rehab program of strengthening and stretching. Always get referrals from other runners and make sure the chiropractor is a good fit for you.

—Pam Adams, chiropractor

Maryna, a holistic practitioner who was part of the medical team at the Canadian Eco Challenge, emphasizes how your whole leg and, indeed, your whole body needs to function in a unified, integrated way. She saw a lot of blisters caused by legs being out of alignment in various places from hips to knees to ankles. Misalignment causes radical changes in all phases of your footfall from strike to break over to push off. Problems can work from the legs down or from the feet up. An understanding of biomechanics will help us visualize the cause and effect.

Understanding Biomechanics

Biomechanics is the study of the mechanics of a living body, especially the forces exerted by muscles and gravity on the skeletal structure. The foot, which includes everything below the ankle, is a complicated but amazing engineering marvel. With an intricate biomechanical composition of 26 bones each, together the foot bones account for almost one-quarter the total number of bones in the entire body. Thirty-three joints make each foot flexible. About 20 muscles manage control of the foot's movements. Tendons stretch like rubber bands between the bones and muscles so that when a muscle contracts, the tendon pulls the bone. Each foot

Top view of the bones
of the foot

Side view of the bones of the foot

contains 109 ligaments that connect bone to bone and cartilage to bone and hold the whole structure together. Nerve endings make the feet sensitive. With each step you walk or run, your feet are subjected to a force of two to three times your body weight, which makes the feet prone to injury.

The big toe, commonly called the great toe, helps to maintain balance while the little toes function like a springboard. The three inner metatarsal bones provide rigid support while the two outer metatarsal bones, one on each side of the foot, move to adapt to uneven surfaces.

Your feet are each supported by three arches. The transverse arch runs from side-to-side just back from the ball of the foot. This is the major weight-bearing arch of the foot. The medial longitudinal arch runs the length of the instep, flattening while standing or running, giving spring to the gait, and shortening when you sit or lie down. The lateral longitudinal arch runs on the outside of the foot. Both longitudinal arches function in absorbing shock loads and balancing the body. These three arches of the foot are referred to singularly as the foot's arch.

Our feet have four ranges of motion. Upward motion is called dorsiflexion and downward is plantar flexion. Inward motion is known as inversion while outward motion is eversion.

With a basic understanding of the foot's construction, it becomes increasingly important to be aware of how we affect our body's biomechanics. At some point in training for an event, we need to try to mimic the event itself. Wear the same shoes and socks that you plan on wearing during the event. Wear the same clothes. Carry the same weight in a fanny pack or backpack. Even get out in the same weather. Although we may not realize it, these factors can change our stride, work different muscles, and put pressure on different body parts—including the feet.

Avoiding Biomechanical Problems

The body lines up over the foot. When the foot goes out of alignment, the ankle, knee, pelvis, and back may all follow. Analyzing the way we stand, walk, and run helps a podiatrist or orthopedist determine whether we have a mechanical misalignment and how it can be corrected. He or she will also want to see your running shoes to analyze the wear patterns on the soles.

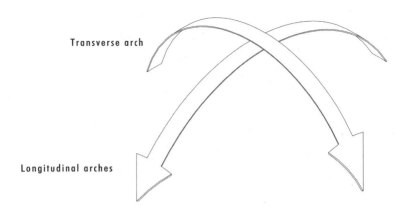

Transverse arch

Longitudinal arches

An example of biomechanics is the functioning of the foot's arch. A low arch, or flat foot, typically occurs when the foot is excessively pronated, turning it inward. A high arch supinates the foot, rolling it outward. Both of these structural variations can cause knee, hip, and back pain. When one arch flattens more than the other arch, that inner ankle moves closer to the ground. That hip then rotates downward and backward causing a shortening of that leg during walking and running. The pelvis and back both tilt lower on the shortened leg side and the back bends sideways. The opposite leg, which is now longer, is moved outward toward the side that puts added stress on its ankle, knee, and hip. The shoulder on that side then drops toward the dropped hip. All of these are compensations as the body adapts. Muscles, tendons, ligaments, and joints are stretched to their limit. The body is out of alignment. Pam Adams, a chiropractor, gives her perspective on how this all works on page 34.

The stresses on our bodies can result in inflammation, often the cause of foot pain. Running on unbalanced and uneven feet may result in fatigue. Fatigue gives way to spasms that may cause a shift in the shape of our feet. Corns, calluses, bunions, spurs, and neuromas may develop when joints are out of alignment.

Do not fall into the trap of drawing erroneous conclusions about your injuries or the type of shoes or equipment that you need for your running style. A podiatrist or orthopedist should check pain associated with running. Heel pain that we try to resolve with a heel pad may not be caused by a heel problem but by arch problems. This in turn may throw off the biomechanics of the body's alignment. If you begin a run and right away experience knee pain, you most likely have a problem with the knee. If the pain comes after running for a while, it is most likely not a knee problem but a biomechanical problem. Likewise, you may think that because you are a heavy runner, you need a shoe with lots of cushioning. Based on that decision, you buy a cushioned shoe, the most cushioning insoles, and wear thickly cushioned socks. But, in reality, what you may need is a stability control shoe. This is where the help and expertise of medical specialists comes in. They are trained to determine biomechanical problems.

In 1991 Craig Smith and his brother set out to hike 300 miles of the Continental Divide Trail. With training and planning done, they started with heavy packs that tipped the scale at almost 58 pounds each. Two days and 22 miles later, Craig had developed severe pain in both knees. Forced to abort the trip, they cached as much gear as possible before starting back. With Craig's knees wrapped with torn T-shirt strips, it took them four days to backtrack the 22 miles. It took several weeks of conditioning therapy before he could finally walk without a limp. Craig learned to pack lighter, do exercises that focus on strengthening his knees, and use a walking stick on downhills. He could have easily been a victim of biomechanical problems that centered in his knees.

Remember that most athletes have foot problems or become injured by doing too much, too soon, and too fast. To avoid biomechanical problems, use proper footwear, pace yourself, do strength training, and train in the gear you will use in your event.

CONDITIONING PRODUCTS

The **DYNA-DISC** is made of the same material as a gym ball and is inflatable with just a standard ball needle and pump. The Dyna-Disc has both smooth and knobbed sides. Perfect for balance training, lower back, pelvic stabilization, and weight-shift exercises. The company also offers balance and wobble boards. exertools.com

OPTP (ORTHOPEDIC PHYSICAL THERAPY PRODUCTS) has a wide range of devices for balance/proprioception, massage, stretching, strength training, and more. optp.com

POLES can be used to hike farther and more comfortably, absorb shock, keep your knees healthy, and help maintain balance. Walkers, hikers, backpackers, and adventure racers have discovered the benefits of poles. Made of either aluminum or carbon fiber, many models offer antishock support and carbon tips. Poles are made by **BLACK DIAMOND, KOMPERDELL, LEKI, MSR,** and **REI.** Typically called hiking or trekking poles, they can be found in sporting goods and camping stores. Some people use two, but others are comfortable using one. Check your local outdoors store for lightweight models.

WOBBLE and **ROCKER BOARDS** can be used to improve balance and strength, retrain injured muscles, improve muscle memory, and build core strength. You can get a wobble board for both feet or two smaller wobble boards, one for each foot. **SIMPLY FIT BOARDS** (simplyfitboard.com), **FITTERFIRST** (fitter1.com), and **INDO BOARD** (indoboard.com) are three companies that offer wobble boards.

Form and Health

As long as you have good form, whether walking, running, hiking, paddling, or biking—any activity where you are using your feet for movement—you stand a better-than-average chance of not injuring yourself due to a biomechanical problem. But if a pack rides wrong on your back, making you lean to the side, or if weak abs make you lean forward, or tired arms cause your shoulders to drop, or spent quads cramp up, your body is tossed out of alignment. This will ultimately work

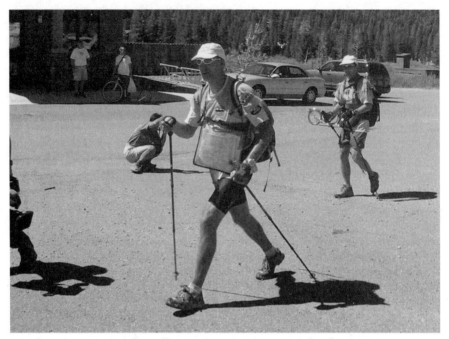

Use hiking poles for support and to help the knees.

its way down to your feet. As they compensate for your biomechanical problems, your gait and stride change, and your feet develop their own problems.

So what is gait? We'll take our definitions from Wikipedia, the free encyclopedia. Its definition is "the way locomotion is achieved using human limbs."

Wikipedia also says, "Walking is the most common human gait. It is characterized by alternating steps of left and right lower limbs. It generally provides useful speeds of progression for daily activities with near-optimal energy efficiency. . . . Running is nearly identical to walking except that the person is actually airborne once each beat. This is the chief high-speed gait of humans. The beats happen faster and the distance traveled per beat is also much higher. Running requires much more energy than walking. . . . Jogging is a sub-gait of run where the pace is much less and the legs nearly never go out of the body's center line."

Thus gait can be best described as your own particular style of walking or running, which determines the distribution of stress to various parts of your legs and feet. While there is no single proper gait that suits everyone, if you experience pain or discomfort (particularly back, hip, or knee pain) while walking or running, a gait analysis from a podiatrist or physical therapist may be in order.

Dr. Stephen M. Pribut, in an article "Gait Biomechanics" on his website, drpribut.com, explains a gait analysis: "In the gait examination, we will observe for symmetry. We will look for clues regarding leg length inequality. Arm swing asymmetry, uneven head bounce, unilateral pelvic drop, and uneven stride length are all indicators that there is a leg length inequality. Other factors to note are the heel contact point, an apparent bouncy gait, excessive pronation of the foot, early heel off, and the angle of gait."

Your best bet is to maintain good form by thinking smart and training wisely, whatever the discipline. Make sure your shoes are not worn down—replace them before they lose their support and cushion. Wear good insoles to balance the foot and provide good heel and arch support and alignment. Strengthen the ankles and knees with specific exercises. Do upper body exercises to strengthen your abs, back, and shoulders for carrying your pack. Work your arms so they can help maintain balance and proper form. Learn how to tape a sprained ankle or turned knee. Condition yourself in incremental stages without huge jumps in mileage or extremes. Train with the gear you will use in an actual race—building up to appropriate weights rather than carrying everything all at once. Use hiking poles for support and to help the knees. Learn your body's weak links and find exercises to strengthen those muscles and joints.

Every one of us, at one time or another, can fall victim to biomechanical problems as we race to extremes. Train smart and race smart, and you can stay healthy, starting with your feet.

Part Two

Footwear Basics

The Magic of Fit

The website foot.com gives the following statistic: "The average person takes about 8,000 to 10,000 steps a day, which adds up to about 115,000 miles over a lifetime. That's enough to go around the circumference of the earth four times. Ill-fitting shoes bring on problems." I agree.

Fit is key. Again, repeat after me: "*Fit is key.*" Without properly fitting shoes or boots, your feet will encounter many problems that can initiate many others. If your footwear is too loose, your feet will slide around, creating shear. If your footwear is too tight in certain areas, your feet will experience excessive pressure. Wearing too loose or too tight footwear will change the biomechanics of your foot strike, which in turn will affect your gait and throw off your whole stride and balance. This will stress your tendons and ligaments. When your feet and toes are pinched in too-tight shoes with socks that make the fit even tighter, the blood circulation is reduced. To top it all off, you will endure aches and/or pain, and will be more tired from dealing with all of the above. Sounds like fun, right? Unfortunately many athletes have resigned themselves to this type of process. They go out strong for as long as their feet last—which in many cases is not as long as they had hoped and often is well before the finish line or the end of their journey. Does it have to happen this way? You decide.

Dr. Benno, the lead author of a study on footwear in the *British Journal of Sports Medicine,* found that runners who select shoes they feel are the most comfortable are more efficient and get hurt less. Another study, by Running USA, found that fit/comfort was the top determining factor in shoe purchases. Cushioning was second.

Fit starts with properly fitting shoes with a quality insole. No matter how good your socks are or how well you apply tape or how good any other component is, if the shoes fit incorrectly, you will have problems.

In *Advanced Backpacking*, Karen Berger makes a good comment on the fit of boots—and the same advice applies to any sport shoe. "Like most marriages, the mesh between boot and foot is not always a good match. If you look at the feet of several people, you'll undoubtedly see a range of bumps and bunions, arches, and anklebones—all of which are encased in the same hard leather cage. It takes a bit of time, accommodation, and softening for boots and feet to settle into a comfortable routine."[3] Because our feet are so different, many factors go into achieving a good fit.

Rich Schick, a physician's assistant and ultrarunner, believes the key to getting the proper size shoe is the insert: "If the foot does not fit the insert, then the shoe will have to stretch to accommodate the difference or there may be excessive room in the shoe, which can lead to blisters and other foot problems." He thinks there is too much confusion about straight lasts, curved lasts, semicurved lasts, and so on:

> You don't need to know any of this if you use the insert to fit your shoes. The same holds true for the proper width of shoe. Simply remove the insert from the shoe and place your heel in the depression made for the heel [in the insert]. There should be an inch to an inch and a half from the tip of your longest toe to the tip of the insert. None of your toes or any part of the foot should lap over the sides of the insert. If they do, is it because the insert is too narrow or is it because of a curved foot and straight insert or vice versa? The foot should not be more than about a quarter inch from the edges of the insert either. This includes the area around the heel, or the shoe may be too loose. Check to see if the arch of the insert fits in the arch of your foot. Finally, if all the above criteria are met, then try on the shoe. The only remaining pitfalls are tight toe boxes and seams or uppers that rub.

Even after buying shoes that fit well, be alert to changes inside your shoes as you walk, run, and hike. Jason Pawelsky, with Tamarack, the maker of the popular ENGO patches, reminds, "We all know that changing conditions (terrain, temperature, distance, and so on) can make even the best-fitting pair of shoes feel and perform differently so there is no perfect fit 100% of the time. The challenge is to get runners, hikers, and team sports players to not only recognize that, but to react proactively."

Learning from Shoe Reviews

We can learn a lot from shoe reviews. Whether the reviews are in magazines or websites, or posted in online forums and blogs, they can be helpful to hear what others have to say about shoes you are considering. RunRepeat.com is a website that features running shoe comparisons. In late 2015 they ran the numbers from 134,867 customer reviews of 391 running shoes from 24 brands. Shoes were ranked from one to five stars based on satisfaction. Interestingly, their conclusion was that expensive shoes are not any better than more moderately priced shoes. This means inexpensive running shoes are often better rated then expensive ones. They pointed out that perceived shoe quality is very subjective and the study was not scientifically based. One possible finding from the comparison is that runners who buy more expensive shoes likely have higher expectations and are more critical in their reviews.

Be Careful Out There

The newspaper and mail often bring us ads from discount sports and department stores. They typically advertise shoes with names that are unknown to the well-read athlete. Who has heard of these shoes? Many major shoe companies make shoes aimed at these stores. They may be good shoes, but I wouldn't buy them for serious walking or running.

While most athletes are careful and know enough to buy running shoes at a running store, many more people are not. Pity the beginning walker or runner who buys shoes without the quality help from a qualified salesperson. They'll get no help with fit—important things such as foot type, toe box space, arch support, and heel counter grip, to say nothing of shoe type, such as motion control, cushioning, and so on. They'll get no help finding the right shoes for whatever they plan to run and no information about the shoe's life expectancy.

They take their shoes home, lace them up, and start running. A small percentage of them will still be going a year later. But many more will have quit because their feet hurt, or after wearing the shoes down—and not knowing when to get new ones—they got injured and quit.

If you know someone who is starting to run or even walk seriously, take a moment and share a bit of your experience on buying good footwear. Many shoe companies make midrange or even cheap shoes, and I don't want these substandard shoes to have a negative influence on people wanting to get out and exercise. We all have to be careful out there.

Many shoe and boot companies suggest specific models that are best for certain types of activities and sports, and for certain types of feet. They do this because many shoes are made for a specific type of foot—and many people have feet that will work better with one type of shoe than another. Look for the buyer's guides in the magazines of your sport. Runners can find shoe reviews in *Runner's World*, *Trail Runner*, and *UltraRunning*. Backpackers and hikers can check out *Backpacker* magazine's reviews, and *Outside* magazine's Buyer's Guide for helpful information.[4] Wear Tested Gear Reviews (weartested.org) is another good site with reviews. Many online shoe retailers also offer phone advice support or online guides. For information on shoe reviews and gear review sources, see page 350 in the appendix. Other sport-specific magazines may offer similar reviews. Many websites are now posting reviews, and some offer reader comments or reviews.

The September 2015 *Runner's World* Shoe Finder asked up front if readers knew the type of shoe that worked best for them. If so, they were guided to a four-section grid based on more shoe, less shoe, and more cushioning, less cushioning. Each box of the grid contained shoes recommended for that more/less choice. Other readers were asked questions about body mass index, running mileage, and injury experience, after which they too were directed to one of the four boxes to find their recommended shoes. Each shoe reviewed was also rated for heel cushioning, forefoot cushioning, and flexibility; and the shoe's weight and heel and forefoot heights were given. Unfortunately, these guides of suggested shoes usually only include 12–18 shoe models.

It's a good starting point, but I would use the guides as a reference point to shop at my local running store and get their personal insights.

Can there be more than one shoe that is right for your feet? Are there perfect shoes? Christopher Willett went through four pairs of shoes on his 2003 Pacific Crest Trail thru-hike (2,600-plus miles) and bought them as he went. Wearing size 15 running shoes, he didn't really have the option of buying from an outfitter along the trail. He would call or use the Internet from various towns along the way and have new shoes and socks sent up trail. He started in Brooks Adrenaline GTS and liked them in the hot 563-mile Southern California section. He wished the next shoe, the Asics Eagle Trail, had a more protective sole but liked the tread. While the New Balance 806s were structurally good, he felt they had a poor tread design; it is the only shoe that he would not wear again. He finished the last 670 miles in the Asics Gel Trabuco V and liked their durability and tread. Would one of the shoes have worked for his whole thru-hike? If they had been the NB 806s, the answer would be no. Probably any of the other three would have worked the whole way, but Chris might have had problems sticking with one shoe given the varying weather and terrain of the trail. Even the most perfect shoe can have small issues: breathability, tread design, cushioning, sole protection, and so on. Each of these issues can make them perfect for one set of conditions and wrong for another.

Know Your Feet

With knowledge of biomechanics and your specific foot type, you can make a better choice than shopping blindly. When shopping for shoes or boots, try on several different pairs from several different companies. This will help you identify those that initially feel good versus those that just don't feel quite right. Knowing how different shoes and boots fit your feet will help in the final selection.

A biomechanically efficient athlete lands on the back outside of the heel and rolls inward (pronation) to absorb shock. The foot flattens as the motion moves forward, rolls through the ball of the foot, and rotates outward (supination) to the push off. Overpronation is the inward roll of the foot as you roll off the heel. Many runners nowadays land on their forefeet rather than heels.

| Under-pronation | Neutral | Over-pronation | Severe overpronation |

There are two main schools of advice for preparing to purchase shoes. One school suggests asking a friend to watch or even to videotape your feet as you walk or run to determine how they land and your general form. This information and the wear patterns on your old shoes can help you decide whether you should look for shoes that compensate for underpronation, overpronation, or severe overpronation, or whether you can get by with shoes for neutral pronators. Use this information to select shoes from one of four categories: neutral-cushioned shoes for underpronators, stability or motion-control shoes for overpronators, motion-control shoes for severe overpronators, and neutral shoes for neutral pronators.[5]

Another school of advice suggests that you first consider your running and biomechanical needs, including your most common running surface, and then select one of five categories that best matches your needs: motion control, stability, cushioned, lightweight training, or trails. Secondly, determine whether your foot type is flat-, normal-, or high-arched (discussed below). Use this information to select shoes from within that category.[6]

Take your old shoes with you when you shop for new shoes. The wear patterns on the soles can help you or the salesperson determine how you run and the best shoes for your running style. Normal wear is on the outer heel and across the ball of the foot. Pronators show wear both on the outer heel and the inner forward side of the shoe. Supinators typically show wear on the heel to the forefoot along the outer edge of the shoe.

The key to a good fit in running shoes is to know your foot type. To determine this, walk on a hard surface with wet, bare feet to see your imprint.

The Three Arch Types

FLAT-ARCHED FEET leave an imprint that is almost completely without an inward curve at the arch. Looking down their leg, these athletes will typically see their feet turned outward like a duck's feet. They will typically do best in a semicurved or straight last shoe that offers good stability and/or motion control. They are often overpronators. The use of an arch support is usually helpful.

NORMAL-ARCHED FEET leave an imprint that shows the forefoot and heel connected, but with an inward curve at the arch. Standing and looking down their leg, these athletes will see their ankles and feet follow the vertical line down their lower leg. These athletes will typically do best in a semicurved last shoe because they are generally efficient in their gait. They might benefit from a cushioned or stability shoe with moderate control features. They are normal pronators.

HIGH-ARCHED FEET leave an imprint that shows the forefoot and heel connected by a very narrow curve at the arch. If your feet are turned inward, you will typically do best in a curved last shoe with good cushioning. Athletes with high arches are typically underpronators and should avoid motion-control shoes.

A common problem when buying shoes and boots is that people will tell the salesperson, "I wear a size 9.5." Well that may or may not be true. Over time, our feet change, typically getting larger. The fat pads on the bottom of our feet become

Flat arch   Normal arch   High arch

thinner as we get older. We may get bunions or our calluses may thicken and affect fit. You may have been a 9.5, but now you may be a 10 or 10.5.

It's very important to get your feet sized each time you purchase a new pair of shoes. The Brannock Device is the tool that stores use to measure your feet to determine shoe size. Be sure to measure each foot. Measure sitting and standing—although standing is the most important measurement. Many of us have one foot a bit larger than the other foot and you should always buy shoes to fit the larger foot. It also measures the width of your foot. Correct fitting properly positions the ball of the foot joint at the widest part of the shoe so the toes have the room they need.

This easy measurement is important to get the best fit possible. Remember, though, after measuring your feet and trying on a pair of shoes, they still may not feel right. Shoes can vary in construction, and one company's shoes may run smaller or larger than those of another company. Once on your feet, the shoes need to feel comfortable. If not, move up or down a half size and see if that helps.

Shop around until you find running shoes that feel right on your feet. A correct fit will help in blister prevention. Valerie Doyle remembers her fight to beat blisters. When she learned how to buy shoes that fit properly, she found they solved her blister problem. The same applies to fitting boots. Studies have found that tight footwear can increase the forces exerted by the shoe or boot on the foot, increasing blister probability, while loose-fitting footwear increases the movement of the foot inside the shoe or boot, causing increased shear forces on the foot, which in turn increases blister probability.[7]

Walk in the shoes or boots for a while to be sure they are comfortable. Some shoes and boots will be higher at the ankle and may put pressure on your ankle bones. Others will not bend at the same forefoot and toe point, making an uncomfortable heel to toe transition or pinching the toes. There may also be a seam inside the shoe or boot that rubs your foot and creates pressure and a potential blister. Pay close attention to the overall fit.

Fitting shoes means more than simply handing you a size 9 shoe and pushing down on the toe and saying, "Yup, it has enough room." When trying on shoes, the toe box (the front part of the shoe that covers the toes) is one of the most important parts of your shoe, and a good salesperson will make sure to emphasize this factor. Those little (or large) toes at the end of your feet need room, both height and width. The right toe box can save your toes. The wrong toe box can cost you your toenails.

In shoes with the right toe box, your toes will feel comfortable and have room to wiggle and breathe. Shoes with the wrong toe box will squeeze your toes—giving them no room to wiggle and breath. This squeezing may happen from the sides and/or the top. The side squeeze will push your toes together and maybe even underneath each other. A squeeze from the top will put pressure on your toenails. When going downhill, this pressure often results in subungual hematomas or black toenails. If your nails are not trimmed properly and are too long, jamming the toes into the front of the shoe will put additional pressure on the nails and cause nail bed problems.

One rule of thumb is that when standing in your shoes, you need a thumb's width of space between the end of your longest toe and the front inside of the shoe. Generally this works. You may want more space when you are going to be involved in a multiday race, hike, or event. In that case, consider buying shoes a size or two larger than normal. You'll note I said "space between the end of your longest toe." For the majority of us, that means your big toe. But for about 15% of the population, it means the toe next to the big toe. This is a condition called Morton's foot or Morton's toe. This condition, usually hereditary, requires shoes to be fit to that toe.

If you have narrow or wide feet, consider shopping for shoes or boots that offer variable lacing capabilities. These shoes and boots will have lace eyelets that are not lined up in an up-and-down row but spaced horizontally farther apart. See "Lacing Options" (page 167) for information on how to lace for different types of feet.

The American Academy of Orthopaedic Surgeons gives suggestions for buying shoes. Foremost, they remind us that shoes should always conform to the shape of your feet; your feet should never be forced to conform to the shape of a pair of shoes. Their suggestions apply equally well to buying boots.

Components of a Good Fit

Fit can be achieved with simply a little common sense and a bit of luck. Out of all the shoes and boots to choose from, there is more than one brand and style that will fit your feet well.

Buying Footwear

Buying shoes has evolved to a level of complexity never before seen. Buyers have to study the latest issue of their favorite running, ultrarunning, adventure racing, triathlete, or outdoors magazine or website, or try to read through the materials posted on manufacturers' websites to comprehend the language they're speaking. Does Impact Quotient Technology really matter to you or me? Does IQS really guide my foot "from heel to toe in a much more natural, comfortable stride"? I know what a truss is, so is a Trusstic System something similar?

We're not buying a car, just a pair of shoes. But the complexity of the selection process has been turned up several notches. If you want to find the best

Commonsense Tips for Trying on Shoes

- Try on and fully lace both shoes.

- The shoes should feel comfortable. You should feel no discomfort in any part of the shoe's fit.

- The shoes should feel natural and move with your foot and not force your feet to conform to the shoes.

- Feel around the inside of the shoe for rough spots where the parts of the uppers are stitched together.

- Your toes should have plenty of room to move and wiggle, and the toe box should not be too short in height or length. Aim for at least 0.5–1 inch of space between your longest toe and the front interior of the shoe.

- The tops of feet shouldn't be pinched when the shoes are laced properly.

- Your little toe should not be pinched by the shape of the front of the shoe. Likewise, your big toe joint should fit at the widest point of the shoe.

- Be sure the shoe's counter (the part that wraps around your ankle and heel) does not rub your foot wrong. Your heels should be snug in the heel counter of the shoe and should have little up and down movement. There should be a firm grip of the shoe to your heel, but not too firm.

- The arch of each foot should be supported, but the shoe arch should not be too high, or too far backward or forward, for your foot type.

- The shoe's shape (last) should be comfortable and not overly curved or straight for your foot type.

- The shoes should fit well with the same type of socks you will be wearing in your training and/or race event.

- The shoes should flex well for the type of terrain you will encounter and at the right point of your foot. This will help provide support to your ankles and prevent uncomfortable heel-to-toe transition or pinching of the toes.

- The shoes should provide adequate protection for the bottom of your feet from rocks and uneven terrain.

- The fit of the shoe should come from the shoes themselves, not from tying the laces.

- The laces should stay tied the way you like them without coming undone.

- The shoes should have outsoles for the type of event or race you will be doing. They should help keep your feet in place inside the shoes.

- If the insoles that come in the shoe are weak and flimsy, replace them when you are buying the shoes—get a pair that provides support and cushioning.

- If you will be using orthotics or special insoles, make sure that they fit in the shoes without pushing your feet too high in the shoes' uppers or too far forward.

shoes, you now have to read the fine print—and understand what the fine print means. Many of the aforementioned acronyms and terms are puzzling unless you read further. Some of the shoe companies' websites are very helpful, offering images and understandable explanations of what these things mean. But some are downright useless.

The bottom line: We need to find a shoe that fits well, lasts more than a few miles, and doesn't rub us the wrong way. And after we buy the shoes and find that we love them, we hope they don't discontinue them in six months when the new models are released. There is something to be said for brand loyalty. I have it and I suspect many of you also do—especially when you've found a pair that fits well.

In today's marketplace, we are in a shoe buyer's heaven. Everywhere we turn, there's a shoe store, and in almost every magazine and on every website, there are ads galore for new shoes and boots. But are all things equal? Here is where I chime in with a big resounding NO.

First, we are faced with the typical mall store, usually a chain shoe store that employs people without any degree of knowledge of how to fit shoes. Many times, they also sell shoes that one would never find elsewhere. Some shoe companies sell shoes to these stores that are not found in running stores and running magazines. They are different, not as well made, yet are perfect for the typical mall shopper.

Specialty outdoor stores, such as running, backpacking, and camping stores, carry shoes that are well made and well known. This is important because we can find reviews of these shoes online and in sport-specific magazines. This allows us to shop with a high degree of knowledge that the shoes we buy are made for our sport and will perform well. These stores also have salespeople who can fit shoes and help you choose between several pairs.

There are running shoes (and this means road shoes and trail shoes), walking shoes, cross trainers, and other sport-specific shoes. I can walk in running shoes but would not run in walking shoes. I can run and walk in most cross trainers, but you would be wise to not use walking and running shoes for a serious game of basketball or other court sport. I can run on trails in most road shoes, although I may sacrifice traction and support. While I can also run on roads in trail shoes, they are often clunky, heavier, and not as flexible.

My preference is to use shoes for what they are intended. I have road and trail shoes and I use them for their intended purpose. Your choice in footwear is important. When shopping for shoes, look for those made for your sport. When participating in sports, use shoes designed for that specific sport.

Personally, I would never buy shoes from any source without trying them on, and walking in them, running a short bit, or using them on an incline board. I prefer to frequent my local running stores, walking stores, and hiking or outdoor stores. I often check out Internet sites where shoes are also sold. If I recognize a particular shoe and know that it fits my foot, I might buy from one of these sites, but with rare exceptions, I buy from my local stores. I value the service, the help with fit, and their look at my gait as I try out the new shoe. They will measure my feet, look at my old shoes (so yes, take your old shoes along), ask what I will be using the shoes for, ask about my foot type, ask about any injury history, and maybe which shoes I have worn in the past. When they bring out the shoes, they will often point out the shoe's features. They'll have me try on the shoes, and they will check for correct spacing in the toe box (both length and height). They will ask me to walk in the shoes and maybe even to go outside and run to get a feel for the shoes. My bottom line: I want a shoe that works on my foot, a shoe that fits as well as possible, and a shoe that's right for whatever sport I throw at it—and that requires the help of a good salesperson.

Buy your shoes wherever you want, but remember, fit is one of the most important elements of using your shoes and boots without problems. Your local shoe store is dedicated to providing you with high-quality choices in shoes and service you can't get through mail order. There is more than one pair of shoes for your feet. There may be a half dozen models that will fit well. The experts at your local store will help you select several brands and models to come up with a good final choice.

Tips for Buying Footwear

Whether buying shoes for running, hiking, court sports, or soccer, it is important to get a good fit. When you purchase footwear, consider the whole picture, not just the shoe or boot you hold in your hand. Your footwear must work with your choice of socks, insoles, and orthotics (if your wear them), and also with the activity you will be using them for. Hiking boots that feel OK when you walk around the store may feel different when you get home and try them when carrying a 30- to 40-pound pack on your back.

Here are some suggestions for buying shoes and boots.

- Use shoe buying guides as just that—do not eliminate a shoe from your consideration until you have tried it on.

- Try shoes in a range of prices—don't save a buck at the expense of your feet. The differences between several pairs of shoes can be amazing.

- Judge a shoe by how it fits on your foot, not by the marked size.

- When going to try on or buy shoes, take a pair of your socks along rather than rely on the store's basket of socks that have been on who knows how many feet.

- Do not buy a pair assuming that they will fit better later, unless they are leather boots. In most cases, today's shoes and boots require no breaking-in period.

- Have your feet sized each time you buy new footwear. Measure both sitting and standing to determine your elongation factor.

- Fit new shoes to your larger foot and your longest toe.

- Try on shoes at the end of the day, preferably after running or walking, because your feet normally swell and become larger after you have been standing and sitting all day.

Footwear purchasers frequently forget to allow enough toe space when buying shoes and boots. When your foot is in the shoe, the arch naturally flattens. Since your heel is held in place by the shoe's counter, your foot can only move forward. If the shoe does not have this bit of extra space in the toe box, the toes become cramped. Toenail problems, blisters, and calluses may develop.

Our Aging Feet

As we age, our feet change. Make no mistake, that fat pad on the bottom of your foot is getting thinner as you get older. Our feet spread out, getting longer and wider, so we may move up a size or more in footwear. Additionally, we usually become a bit stiffer in the joints. Your arch may also flatten more than normal. Just because we are aging doesn't mean that our feet have to hurt or that we have to stop walking, running, or whatever our activity is. As long as we remember how our feet change as we age and buy footwear that fits, we can stay physically active. So the natural question is, "What should we do?" Here are three steps to keep your aging feet happy.

- Have your feet measured each time you buy shoes.

- Buy shoes that fit the shape of your foot and have a wide and long enough toe box.

- Invest in a good pair of insoles that provide cushioning and support.

Tips for Hard-to-Fit Feet

When you shop for shoes or boots, you may find it impossible to find footwear that is comfortable. Try shoes by several manufacturers. If you still have difficulty finding quality shoes that fit your particular type of foot, consider searching for a certified pedorthist (C.Ped). Kirk Apt, C.Ped, describes the work of a pedorthist:

Even those with no medical conditions, but with common discomfort and general foot fatigue, can find relief by utilizing the expertise of a C.Ped. Specifically, pedorthics is the design, fit, manufacture, and modification of footwear and orthotics to help alleviate problems due to congenital deformity, injury, disease, or overuse. C.Peds function as part of allied health care teams, where a person can go to a medical doctor (family doctor, orthopedist, podiatrist, and so on) and get a diagnosis and a prescription for a conservative, nonsurgical remedy. The patient may then be referred to a C.Ped., who can fill the prescription for therapeutic shoes and/or custom orthotics. Shoes are built around 3-D foot-shaped models called lasts, which are identical mirror images of feet of a given size. Unfortunately, real feet are seldom mirror images of each other. A C.Ped. can help find a shoe built on a last that best matches a person's feet, and then construct a custom orthotic that meets their particular biomechanical needs and interfaces with the shoe in a way that improves its fit and performance. In this way, athletes, active people, and those who work long hours on their feet can be accommodated with footwear designed specifically for their unique feet. In my practice, I work with patients who have a doctor's prescription and with others who want their footwear to fit and perform better. I often work with a physical therapist. Together, we do a pedorthic assessment where we determine the condition of the feet and analyze the gait of a person. Using this information, I can recommend a specific shoe or design and construct a custom orthotic.

Look in the telephone book or ask your orthopedist or podiatrist for references. Information on the Pedorthic Footwear Association can be found under "Medical and Footwear Specialists" in the appendix (see page 351).

Footwear and Insoles

Many people consider footwear as simple, basic equipment that takes little thought. Yet the war against foot problems can be lost over ill-fitting shoes, boots, or socks that cause blisters or insoles that are not right for your activity. Choose your footwear based on which sport you will be doing, the terrain expected, and your level of experience. Find the right shoes or boots and the right socks based on what feels right and fits correctly—not by price. Tom McGinnis, who thru-hiked the Appalachian Trail in 1979, makes a good observation: "Good boots and bad socks can be miserable. Cheap boots and good socks can be a dreamland." This chapter focuses on types of running shoes, sport shoes, hiking boots, custom shoes, sandals, and insoles. Minimalist footwear, such as Vibram FiveFingers, is discussed in the next chapter. Socks play such a large role in preventing problems that they are discussed at length in their own chapter.

Our feet are unique. Yours may look similar to mine, yet they are as different as our fingerprints. Although our feet may fit into the same size and shape of shoe or boot, our feet actually mold into the footwear differently. Corns, bunions, susceptibility to blisters, toe length, the type of arches, and the shape of our feet are just a few of the factors that affect the fit of our footwear. Even how we react to and recover from the stresses of running and hiking is important in choosing shoes and boots.

Only you can determine what type of footwear you need to wear. Certainly runners wear running shoes, but there are many types of running shoes. Hikers and adventure racers have many choices in hiking boots, but many make the choice to wear trail running shoes instead of boots. Many of the top adventure racers wear trail running shoes for their whole event, even on snow and ice and while wearing crampons. Just remember the ifs. If you are used to hiking in trail running shoes, if your ankles are strong, and if the shoes provide the necessary support while wearing a pack, then trail running shoes may be right for you.

Regarding trail shoes, Cathy Corning makes a good point:

> Trail shoes are constructed a bit differently than road shoes. Pronation is an important consideration for road shoes but not for trails. Think about it.

On the road, it's the exact same movement over and over and over, and pronation is a big deal. On the trail, every footfall is completely different with all sorts of soft, hard, and twisted surfaces, and your foot lands differently every time. Pronation is really not a consideration. Trail shoes are far more focused on stability, with your foot sitting lower in the shoe and closer to the ground to help stabilize your foot on uneven surfaces. Even the base of the trail shoe is slightly wider than a road shoe for more stability.

Another important point about trail shoes is how most are made with a mesh upper—to reduce weight and allow heat dispersion. While nice, the mesh creates a different problem. It allows dirt, sand, dust, and trail grit access into the shoes, onto your socks, and then onto your feet. In a long run or race, this can be problematic as it turns into an irritant and leads to hot spots and blisters. It also makes it harder to patch one's feet because the layer has mixed with whatever lubricant has been used to create a hard-to-remove coating. Gaiters can help control this but are not always effective because of how they cover the mesh.

An important consideration in choosing footwear is shoe construction and ventilation. Footwear constructed with Gore-Tex fabric is good at keeping moisture out—but also tends to hold in sweat. In extreme cold, shoes that drain may be a better choice. Footwear made with mesh is lightweight—but the mesh allows grit and dust to get inside the shoe. Your shoes may be lighter and cooler, but the grit can increase friction. Gaiters can help control what gets in your shoes.

Some years ago I spent a trail-running weekend with friends in the Northern California High Sierra. In between the fast hiking and running, while watching my step, I kept an eye on what others had on their feet. Most had good footwear—either trail running shoes or larger, heavier boots. There were some, however, who wore the wrong footwear. They wore running shoes made for roads, or court shoes. These shoes provided no traction on the slippery rocks and no protection from the sharp rocks, and they did not give their feet and ankles the needed support. One friend wore her road shoes and ended the first day with three blisters and very sore feet. I saw several hikers with court shoes and a pack—a very poor combination. Trouble occurs when you end the day with blisters, damaged or black toenails, a turned ankle, or simply very sore feet. You may associate the discomfort and pain with the activity. Instead, the right footwear would have made the hike much more enjoyable. Whether walking, hiking, running, trail running, playing court sports, adventure racing, climbing, or biking, the right footwear can make all the difference.

When shopping for shoes or boots, try on several different pairs from several different companies. This will help you identify those that initially feel good versus those that just don't feel quite right. Knowing how different shoes and boots fit your feet will help in the final selection. When going to buy new shoes, you may have a preferred shoe, sometimes based on magazine ads or on the recommendations of others, but buy only those that fit best. Whichever type of shoe you wear, be sure to train in them. Never wear a new pair in a race. Always wear them before the race to make sure they fit well and there are no problems.

Kevin wrote that he wears a size 7 shoe and has found that the mid- and out-soles are the exact thickness in all shoes regardless of the shoe size—not proportionally thinner. "While shopping, if you pick up a large shoe of a particular model and try bending it, then pick up the smaller size of the same model and try bending that one, you quickly notice how much more rigidity a small foot has to work against. Try repeating that ten times, and you see your arms get tired, not to mention bending it 25,000 times or more over a long day hike! It's not the shoe getting stressed; it's your feet and ankles trying to overcome the rigidity that a smaller, shorter foot has to work harder to overcome. When I am buying new shoes, I pick up each model and bend their size 7 and compare stiffness. I find quite a difference between models, so it helps me in the selection."

John Schumacher, in the *Sacramento Bee* newspaper, wrote about Stacy Dragila, a 2000 gold medalist in the pole vault. She had gone to Athens for the Olympic Trials in 2004 with high expectations—but came home devastated. And yes, it was the shoes. Dragila had provided input for a new shoe design for Nike. When Nike rolled it out before the US Olympic Trials in Sacramento, Dragila decided to make the switch. Her old jumping shoes were a little loose in the heel. The new pair, reinforced to last longer, felt nice and snug at first. As she wore them in the trials, she felt a little Achilles flare-up. "I just attributed it to stress, being at the trials, not sleeping as well as I probably should," said Dragila. "I never thought it was the shoe." By the US Olympic training camp, both Achilles tendons were bothering her. She couldn't do her normal workouts, and during qualifying discovered she couldn't make a full approach on the runway. She tried heights she had easily done before but couldn't make them. "I just knew I was doomed," she says. Doomed, she admits, by her own hand. Or shoe. "When you're a fine-tuned athlete or sports car, you don't change the wheels," she said. "I wish somebody had told me. I don't blame anybody but myself. I shouldn't have tried to break in something new in a crucial time of training. In hindsight, looking back, stay with what you've got."

Socks vary in thickness, and changing socks can change the way your feet fit inside your shoes. When trying on shoes, wear the same socks when trying on shoes that you wear during races. When buying new socks, be sure they will not alter the fit of your shoes. If your new socks make your shoes fit tighter, you may be able to fix this with new, slightly thinner insoles.

TIP: Best Friend to Worst Enemy

Whatever sports shoes you wear, remember to inspect them regularly for problems. Frank Sutman was on the second day of a six-day, 80-mile backpack trip when one boot's outsole split from the midsole to the ball of the foot. He suffered through four days of flapping sole, picking up pebbles, rocks, and sticks and even being tripped up. The moral of his story: Check your boots and shoes before major activities and periodically to keep small problems from becoming major inconveniences. Split outsoles, ripped or torn fabric that lets dirt and rocks into the shoe, cracked heel counters that create folds in the inner heel material, or broken laces retied into a bothersome knot over the top of the foot are all preventable.

Brand Loyalty in Footwear

When athletes talk about footwear, you often hear, "Be loyal and don't jump from brand to brand or style to style." How true is that statement? Let's look at a few different perspectives on the subject.

From the manufacturer's perspective, it makes perfect sense. If buyers are loyal and stay with the manufacturer's shoes, life is perfect. They have an ongoing market that remains faithful and so their shoes will always sell.

From the shoe store's perspective, it makes life easier. They'll keep ordering the same shoes from the same manufacturers. Sure, they'll take chances on new shoes, but if buyers remain loyal to the old shoes, they'll have a harder time convincing athletes to switch brands.

So, that leaves our perspective: the customer. Why would athletes remain loyal to one brand? Let's identify some reasons, keeping in mind that the inverse is true too—when one of the reasons fails, the athlete is often open to a change in shoes.

- The shoes work well for my sport.
- The shoes fit.
- They've never caused problems.
- I hate taking a chance on a new shoe.

Certainly, shoe companies would like us to be loyal. One obvious problem is that companies often seem to disregard the people who buy and wear their shoes. They will change or discontinue shoe styles with no warning. If you've found shoes that work, every spring and fall is tense as you wait to see if your favorite shoes are still being made, or how they have been changed. I know athletes who buy several pairs of shoes once they find a pair that works for their feet. They don't want to take a chance on the shoe companies not honoring their loyalty. I don't blame them.

The Anatomy of Footwear

By understanding the parts of a shoe or boot, you can make informed choices about which running shoe, cross-trainer, or boot is best for your sport—and for your feet. The parts of a shoe are fairly common, regardless of what kind of footwear you are looking for. See the sidebar on the next page.

Tossing Shoes and Boots

There comes a time when shoes and boots need to be thrown out. You may feel a difference in the cushioning of the shoe—they may feel flat or lack the spring they once had. You may experience foot, ankle, or knee pain. The footwear may simply be trashed. Some athletes, especially runners, log the miles they run in each pair of shoes, and then move the worn ones to garden duty. There is no hard-and-fast rule, but many suggest 500–600 miles as the maximum from a pair. How long your shoes will last depends on your technique, running surface, mileage, weight—and the shoe itself. The newer technologies in some shoes can extend their life beyond other shoes. Here are a few tips and reminders to keep in mind when evaluating your shoes:

- Write the purchase date in the tongue of the shoe or on your calendar.

- Exposure to heat and water will shorten the life of shoes.

- Never put your shoes in the dryer—air-dry them.

- Heavier runners should replace shoes more often.

- Buy a second pair, or even three pairs, and rotate shoes in your workouts. This can give you a better feel for worn shoes.

Kevin shared this tip: "I wear New Balance 833s. They wear out fast, before the uppers are even dirty. I couldn't take the idea of tossing them out and ended up with nearly a dozen used pairs. When my knees start to ache, it tells me the shoes are going. I tried this company, Resole America (resole.com), and have been satisfied with the result. The resoled shoes don't last as long as the originals, but for me it's better than tossing them out. Plus because I have five pairs now, I can rotate to make them last longer. When these wear out, I'll send more in to be resoled. The company sends prepaid mailers for the old shoes. Prices are fair and they do all types of shoes, from street shoes, running shoes, hiking boots, work boots, and more."

If your old shoes still have some life in them, consider donating them to one of the companies that sends shoes to Third World countries. The US site soles4souls .org and Canada-based soleresponsibility.org are two organizations that serve as collection points.

Parts of a Shoe

The shoe's **COUNTER** is the part that wraps around the heel of the foot.

The **EYELETS** are the holes the shoelaces run through.

The **COLLAR** is the part at the top that wraps around your ankle.

The **HEEL TAB** is the notch that surrounds the Achilles tendon.

The **HEEL** is the back bottom of the shoe.

The **INSOLE** or **SOCK LINER** is the inner insert on which your foot rests. These are typically interchangeable.

The **MIDSOLE** sits between the shoe's upper and outsole.

The **OUTSOLE** is the shoe's bottom layer.

The shoe's **SHANK** is the part of the sole between the heel and the ball of the foot.

The **TOE BOX** is the tip of the shoe that shapes and protects the toes.

The **UPPER** is the top of the shoe that surrounds the foot.

Running Shoes

There are many sources of information about which shoes may be the best for you. The five main sources are the shoe companies, local running stores, magazines and catalogues, running friends, and the Internet. Recognize the difference in the quality of help available at some chain shoe stores in shopping malls versus stores that specialize in running shoes and equipment. A specialized footwear store usually has personnel who are athletes themselves and can watch you run, look at your old shoes, and recommend specific brands of shoes and styles based on what they see and your answers to their questions.

One might ask why there are so many running shoe brands. Ten years ago, eight major shoe companies dominated the market. Today, there are more than 35 shoe manufacturers. Running's popularity and accessibility have surged, and more people nowadays are embracing fitness. Obstacle races and novelty fun runs draw new people into running. To tap this growing audience, new companies enter the running shoe market, outdoor apparel companies make inroads in the market, and foreign companies also want a piece of the pie. It has led to better shoes and innovative designs and styles. Where it will lead is anyone's guess. Ten years from now, we'll see how many are still here. You have more choices than ever before, which means you need to educate yourself about footwear.

For years, running shoes were all pretty much the same—upper, midsole, and outsole with variations in design and technology. Most shoes were about the same height. Then the minimalist movement caught on and footwear changed. All of a sudden shoes were lighter, with less support and cushioning, and shorter in height thanks to the next-to-nothing components between the foot and the ground.

Then along came the Hoka One One. Super light, very cushioned, with a meta rocker design and low drop geometry, the shoes became popular with runners of all distances. Runners swear by them. Suddenly the oversized running shoe took off, and now other companies are making similar shoes. Brian Metzler, in a Competitor .com article about "8 Hot Running Shoe Trends for 2015" says maximalism is still thriving. In addition to Hoka One One, Altra, Saucony, and Skechers, he suggests that Nike, Adidas, Salomon, Pearl Izumi, and Under Armour will also be introducing maximally cushioned shoes. He quoted a retailer who told him that there are a lot of runners out there who just want a soft, comfortable ride.

I found it interesting that a survey of all finishers in the 2015 Western States 100-Mile Endurance Run found that 34.5% wore Hokas, 19.6% wore Brooks, and 16.5% wore Altras. The remaining 29.4% of shoes were a mix of brands. That means 70.6% of the finishers wore one of three brands. It was pointed out that Hoka was first for the second year in a row, while Altra took second place after not being in the list in 2014.

To understand running shoes, you need to be aware of their construction. The first construction component is the *last*, the form over which a shoe is constructed.

Running Shoe Last Patterns

BOARD lasts have the shoe's upper material glued to the shoe's board, which runs the length of the shoe. This generally produces a fairly rigid and stable shoe.

COMBINATION lasts have the shoe's upper material stitched to either the forefoot (slip-lasted) or the rear foot (board-lasted). This design offers additional stability at either the foot plant or the toe's push off.

SEMICURVED lasts are molded straight toward the rear foot while having some curve toward the forefoot. This mold provides stability and flexibility.

SEMISTRAIGHT lasts are built to curve slightly from the toe to the heel. This provides some flexibility and a high degree of stability.

SLIP last shoes are made with the upper material stitched directly to the midsole without a board. This offers maximum flexibility.

STRAIGHT lasts are built along the shoe's straight arch to provide maximum stability.

Basic Categories of Shoe Construction

NEUTRAL shoes are made for the runner who has good biomechanics and would be categorized as a neutral pronator. These shoes generally have a good blend of flexibility and stability.

FLEXIBILITY shoes are made for runners who are underpronators, who have foot motion toward the outside and need a shoe that offers more shock-absorbing pronation than their body can deliver.

STABILITY shoes offer high stability and cushioning. Midweight or normal-arched runners without motion problems who are looking for good cushioning typically use these shoes. These runners usually overpronate slightly beyond neutral and need a shoe with extra medial support. Most are built on a semicurved last.

MOTION-CONTROL shoes provide the most control, rigidity, and stability. Heavy runners, severe overpronators, flat-footed runners, and orthotic users often choose these shoes. They are typically quite durable shoes, but they are often heavier. Most are built on a straight last and offer the greatest level of medial support.

TRAIL RUNNING shoes usually offer increased toe protection, outsole traction, stability, and durability. Runners who run mainly on trails usually use these shoes.

CUSHIONED shoes are those with the best cushioning. These are typically used by those who do not need extra medial support and by high-arched runners. Most are built on a curved or semicurved last. The new maximum cushioned shoes, like the Hokas, take cushioning to a whole new level.

LIGHTWEIGHT shoes are typically made for fast training or racing. These come with varying degrees of stability and cushioning and can be worn by runners with few or no foot problems. Most are built on a curved or semicurved last.

personal experience

"I did 10 100-mile runs in 1999: Rocky Raccoon, Umstead, Massanutten, Old Dominion, Western States, Vermont, Leadville, Wasatch, Angeles Crest, and Arkansas.

"I really didn't have too much of a problem with my feet that year. The Rocky Raccoon (the first race) is where I had the most trouble. It was 80°F and very humid, and I wore last year's shoes, which were size 11 (my normal size). Because the shoes were a bit worn and [my feet had] some swelling due to the humidity, I had several blisters between my toes. After the run, I drained them with a pin and then pretty much forgot about them.

"I then bought some Asics 2040s and Montrail Vitesse shoes in size 12. I always wear double-layer, blister-free socks. The rest of the [year], I had very few blister problems. The only consistent blister problem was with the Montrails. If I didn't put duct tape on the balls of my feet, they would develop blisters. They also rubbed on the outside of my left big toe. I did not need any tape with the 2040s. Even at the hot and humid Vermont 100, I had little problem with blisters, [and what problems I did have were] mostly as a result of wearing the Montrails. On rare occasions, I would get a small blister on the inside of the big toe on my right foot.

"I never put anything on my feet. I do, however, use Succeed electrolyte caps. This has helped me with stomach distress (I only drink water or, late in the race, Pepsi). I am sure that [the caps] also help with the blistering. I think experience has a lot to do with blisters. The more races I run, the tougher my feet become."

—ultrarunner Jeff Washburn

Buying Running Shoes

Running shoes are changing rapidly. Many major shoe companies roll out new designs twice a year. Shoes now offer midsole air, gel, and tube chambers; springs; recoil plates; Gore-Tex and other membrane fabrics; breathable liners and mesh outer fabrics; more cushioning; and better support and stability. More models have been released for trails as this market has grown many times over.

Before you buy a pair of shoes, run your hands over the inside to check for seams that could cause an irritation and lead to blisters. Look at the stitching and the seam that bonds the upper to the bottom of the shoe. Then pull out the insole and make sure everything is smooth. Once you buy a new pair of shoes, wear them around the house to be sure they fit well and are comfortable. If you sense problems, return the shoes for another style or type. Even the same shoe model that you have worn in the past can have minor design changes in a new release. Wear them for a while until you are sure they fit well.

Shoe designs are always changing. Often our favorite shoes disappear from the shelves and we find ourselves forced to make new choices. Do your homework, study the shoe reviews and the ads, talk to your running friends, and try on various styles. Good stores will let you run in them. Ultrarunner Orin Dahl once found that his favorite shoes were no longer offered. Instead of the old shoes, Nike offered a new type of air shoe. He bought the shoes and began running in them. The new shoes were not as flexible in the forefoot, causing his heel to pull up and out of the shoe. To his dismay, he developed blisters at the back of his heels. He recalls how he turned the shoes over to the Salvation Army and began a search for a different pair. He has no doubt that the shoes were good shoes, but they were just not right for his feet and running style. As you look for shoes, remember that not every pair of shoes is right for your feet.

Sports Shoes

By sports shoes I mean any shoes specific to your particular sport—other than running. These may be soccer, football, baseball, or climbing shoes, or even cross-trainers. Even military boots can be considered in this category—the requirements for getting a good fit are the same.

When shopping for these shoes, apply the same basic principles that you would for other athletic shoes. Try several different brands and styles. Try them on wearing the same socks you will wear during the activity. Lace the shoes up and be sure that they hold your heel, that your toes have wiggle room, and that they feel comfortable.

Many sport-specific shoes such as those for soccer have a simple thin insole with virtually no arch or heel support. These can lead to arch problems, metatarsal pain, blisters, and more. The first thing I do when I find a shoe that fits well is to replace the standard flimsy insoles with a good supporting insole—but do this when buying the shoes to make sure they are big enough to accommodate the insoles.

Climbing shoes are meant to fit close to the skin. These are often worn without socks, so be sure there are no irritating seams that can cause blisters. If you will wear thin socks with the shoes, take them along when shopping for shoes. One problem area in climbing shoes is the tight toe box. If you have Morton's toe, hammertoes, bunions, corns, or other toe problems, be aware of how the tight fit will affect that condition. Understanding any preexisting foot problem will help you make an informed choice of shoes. Each of these conditions is discussed later in this book.

Military boots may not offer much in the way of selection, but you need to be aware of many of the fit issues discussed in the next section about hiking boots. Irritating seams, poor heel fit, thin insoles, toe boxes that are too narrow and too short, and boots that are not correct for the shape of your feet can lead to long-term problems. If given a choice in boots, try on several to get the best fit possible. Again, as with most other shoes, replace the insoles. Then choose a good moisture-wicking sock.

personal experience

"On my feet, I wore a liner sock, SmartWool socks, and Wellco jungle boots with an enhanced cushioned midsole and Vibram-type sole. I coated my feet with Body Glide. This combination had worked very well for me in training, with no blisters, and so I anticipated no problems. During the competition, however, I developed hot spots fairly early on the bottom of my feet. By mile 5, I was pretty sure that some of the hot spots had turned into full-on blisters; my suspicion quickly proved right. At about the 5.75-mile mark, I picked up a trot as the course came off a dike. As I did so, I felt an excruciating pain on the bottom of both heels. I realized two things: my feet were going to hurt a lot, and quitting just wasn't an option. . . . Somehow I did manage to qualify for the new unit.

"As an experienced triathlete, I made some right choices. However, with the combination of a heavier 45-pound pack, gravel roads, liner socks that were too tight, and unseasonable warm and humid weather, my feet were doomed from the start.

"I don't know that anybody teaches foot care to subjects in basic training. A lot of information is passed along through informal instruction in the ranger and infantry communities, but it may not be up-to-date and may not reflect lessons learned from people such as endurance athletes and adventure racers. The sad thing, however, is that if you showed up to a noninfantry (or nonspecial ops) unit on the morning that they'd decided to do a road march, you'd see some frightening equipment choices and personal preparation. There's very little foot-care knowledge in many combat support units. It makes me shudder just to think about it."

—an Army Ranger, describing a 12-mile forced march that was part of the selection process for an elite special operations unit

Hiking Boots

Terry, a dedicated hiker, told me, "After a bazillion miles of backpacking and running, I should know everything about my feet. [Yet] when thinking about another thru-hike next year, I spend more time thinking about my feet than my backpack." We can learn from his insight.

My first pair of hiking boots was all leather, with thick Vibram soles. They laced all the way to my calf and seemed to weigh as much as my loaded backpack. Times have changed and so have hiking boots. They now fit better and are easier on your feet. Running-shoe technology has had a positive influence on hiking boots.

Insoles, molding, padding, and midsole and outsole advances have made many as comfortable as lighter-weight boots. An ad by boot maker Sorel claimed, "Any boot can repel water. Ours will actually suck the sweat off your pinky toes." As technology advances, many boot makers such as Sorel will offer moisture-control systems to wick perspiration away from your feet. Gore-Tex fabrics are commonly built into boots for moisture transfer. Lacing systems are also changing for the better.

Kent Ryhorchuk has the right attitude about hiking footwear:

> When it comes to budget, I would not be stingy on anything related to your feet. Your feet will hurt badly enough without having to deal with blisters and chafing. Bad feet stopped or hobbled many people the year I hiked, mostly due to blisters—even some experienced Appalachian Trail hikers. The shoe-and-socks system I use for footwear is Montrail Vitesse shoes, flat Spenco green insoles, Birkenstock blue footbeds over the Spenco insoles (to control my metatarsal problems), SmartWool low-cut hiker socks, and Fox River X-Static liner socks. It took several years of hiking, trail running, and adventure racing to figure this out, but I went from getting blisters all the time to hardly ever getting blisters at all. The point is that I spent a lot of time on it, not that this system is necessarily right for anybody else. Everybody's feet are different.

Many hikers have been converted to using the newer lightweight boots. These are usually as flexible as running shoes and carry many of the running-shoe benefits of fit and comfort. Because of their flexibility and construction, many of these boots require very little or no break-in time. I completed an 8.5-day, 221-mile ultralight backpack of the John Muir Trail in regular running shoes. Unless you are used to hiking or running trails in running shoes while wearing a backpack, I do not recommend them for backpacking. Since I did the John Muir Trail in 1987, boots have changed. Today, I would consider a trail-running shoe or lightweight boot for the same hike. Newer lightweight boots tend to dry faster and drain better. The typical leather boot can soak up to a pound of water. That means you lift an additional 2,212 pounds to walk 1 mile.

Check out some of the features of new hiking boots at your local store. Many boots offer a combination of features: lighter weight, breathable uppers, high-traction and long-lasting outsoles, improved lacing systems, flexible footbeds, stable and cushioning midsoles, wider toe boxes, and Gore-Tex fabric incorporated into the uppers. Some boot companies have developed what they call their "hiking boot last," which is designed to be snug around the heel and arch, and with a roomy toe box. Using different insoles and different thicknesses of socks and/or number of pairs worn can adjust the fit even more.

Boots fall into three basic categories: lightweight hiking (for trail hiking and light loads), midweight hiking (for on/off trail hiking and light backpacking), and heavyweight hiking (for on/off trail, heavy loads, and multiday trips).

Before you go shopping for boots, determine the type of hiking you will be doing and how much support and protection you will need for the weight you will carry. Then, look at the various features of different boots in each of the three categories. Finally, shop accordingly, but do not rule out a certain type of boot until you try them on your feet. A boot that pinches or rubs in the store will not feel better when you are out on the trail. Rob Langsdorf suggests taking time to really test a new boot before leaving the store:

> I usually wear mine around the store for an hour or more before deciding to take it. It takes time but consumes less time than having to return it or having to spend lots of time treating blisters. Then, break new boots in by wearing them around the house, to work, church, and so on, before going out on the trail. Begin with easy hikes before starting off on a long trip. Only when they feel good on a short hike are they ready for a longer one.
>
> I had a friend who bought a pair of boots but didn't break them in because she felt that wearing them around the house wasn't the feminine thing to do. She ended up with major blisters after 6–7 miles. By the end of our 15-mile weekend backpack, she was ready to throw the new boots away and swear off backpacking—all because she didn't want to look funny wearing her boots in town.

Switchback, a hiker, writes:

> Before you go on a hike, walk a few miles in your hiking footwear without socks. You will be amazed what your feet will tell you about potential hot spots, tight areas, and potential blisters. Listen to your feet when you do this experiment. Remember, each foot is different and will have different things to tell you. Socks not only protect our feet but can also mask problem areas. Then when you are out on your hike walking with your socks and shoes, you will know where potential problems might occur. This is very valuable to you. Why find out about a foot problem after it has developed? Be proactive and not reactive.

Some boots will soften and become more flexible with forceful flexion of the soles and uppers, hand-working a waterproofing solution into the leather, or mechanical flexion of the uppers at a shoe shop. If your boots are too stiff, try one of these three methods.

Rod Dalitz shares a good tip for getting a good fit with hiking boots:

> It's important to shape the heel to fit your foot. Find a heavy-gauge plastic bag and put the boot inside, with the heel immersed in a large pot of boiling water, for a few minutes. (It doesn't do the leather any good to be directly in boiling water!) Make sure the bag doesn't leak. When the boot is hot, the plastic cup in the heel can be molded by gentle hand pressure to a suitable shape.

Ed Acheson made several painful discoveries when he hiked the Pacific Crest Trail. Before he began his trip, he switched to a new pair on a salesperson's recommendation. The boots were too much boot for him and a half size too small—the salesperson told him they were sized larger than most. Ed remembers for the first 20 days having "more blisters than the number of days I had been out." To compensate for the blisters, he changed his gait, which in turn gave him knee problems. Before he could get new boots, he was forced to cross the Mojave in tennis shoes. He suffered for years from problems he attributes to the wrong boots.

And even after you have broken in your boots, be sure they still fit after not wearing them for a while. Wear them for at least one getting-reacquainted walk before going on a major hike. Your feet may have changed, and they may need to get readjusted to the boots before a long hike.

Airing Your Feet

If you are looking for a shoe to wear around camp, an alternative to sandals is lightweight closed-cell foam structure shoes. Sometimes called clogs, these shoes have a soft, pliable feel and provide cushioning to your heels for all-day wear, all the while massaging the bottoms of your feet with their textured footbed to promote circulation. They're warm in winter and cool in summer, with a vented design and antibacterial material to reduce foot odors. They are an especially good way to air your feet after a long day on the trail.

One pair weighs less than 10 ounces! And because they are made from one piece of closed-cell foam, they won't come apart or break down. Choose from an open-back shoe or one with a heel strap. The colors are as wild or sedate as you want. All this for around $30. And they provide better cushioning and support than flip-flops.

I'd toss these on my pack for use as camp shoes without a second thought. They won't add much extra weight. They're easy relief after a day of hiking and wonderful to have waiting outside your tent to slip on when you venture outdoors. They're also great to wear in the communal shower on the road. They're dry in a minute, so you can throw them right into your gym bag.

The most common lines of clogs are Crocs (crocs.com), Oofos (oofos .com), Waldies (waldies.net), and Holey Soles (designit.ca/holeysoles). Vibram FiveFingers are a great lightweight alternative, with a glovelike appearance, stretchy upper, and a Vibram sole (us.vibram.com). There are new lightweight sandals that are also great for this use. Other companies are Bedrock Sandals (bedrocksandals.com) and Luna Sandals (lunasandals .com)—and of course, you can make your own huaraches.

Buying Hiking Boots

Before buying new boots, understand how they are changing. Boot designs are offering waterproof, breathable Gore-Tex liners; thinner leather for better hot-weather hiking; better lug soles for increased traction; lugs that extend up the rounded sides; better insoles; softer uppers for shorter break-in times; snug ankle collars to keep debris out; and more. Boots are being made better, but never buy a pair for their features alone. Buy them because they fit.

Before buying boots, check *Backpacker* and *Outside* magazines (and their websites) for their coverage on hiking boots. These articles evaluate most brands based on fixed standards while identifying their features and costs. Then check out your local backpacking supply store for the brands and styles they carry. Spend as much time as is necessary to get a good fit. Tell the salesperson what type of hiking you will be doing, for how long, and how much weight you plan on carrying. Try on several pairs of boots by different companies. Use your own socks. Walk in the boots. Squat in them. Look for a pair that fits right from the start and grips your heels. Take out the insoles and look at the boot's construction. Find the pair that fits and feels better than the others. Purchase a high-quality boot made for hiking rather than lighter-weight boots sold for general-purpose street wear. These fashion-statement boots will not hold up under the stresses of heavy trail use. Utilize the experience of the personnel of your local camping and backpacking stores to help you make a wise decision, but realize the final decision is yours based on how they feel on your feet.

Remember that the boots you select will each be picked up and put down many times each day. A pound on the foot equals about 6.4 pounds on your back. Hiking 12 miles each day would equate to about 25,000 steps,[8] day after day. Feel the weight of your boot and think about each step. Heavier boots are not always the best. True, they may provide more ankle stabilization, but you could get more benefit from a lightweight boot and proper ankle and foot-strength conditioning before the hike. Ray Jardine, who has hiked the Pacific Crest Trail three times and the Appalachian and Continental Divide Trails each once, estimates that each 3.5 ounces off a pair of boots could add about a mile to a day's hiking progress.[9] A review of one store's boot selection showed weights for a pair of boots ranging from 1 pound 9 ounces all the way to 3 pounds 9 ounces. Selecting boots that weigh 10.5 ounces less than another pair could mean the equivalent of an additional 3 miles hiked per day. An educated choice based on boot features, your personal needs, and the terrain ahead is necessary.

If you are planning a several-week or several-month thru-hike on a multistate trail, you will need to buy boots that are larger than normal to accommodate your feet as they become stronger and enlarge to their normal hiking size. Try on boots that are anywhere from one to two sizes larger than normal, which will allow your feet to fit into them properly. If you need to purchase new boots midway through a long trek, be aware of potential problems of breaking in new boots.

Mara Factor has experienced her feet changing:

> Be wary of buying multiple pairs before you start. Most people's feet change significantly as they hike. The shoes you wear day to day will adjust somewhat and continue to fit your feet. New shoes, the same size as the ones you've been wearing for a while, often do not fit. Longer and/or wider sizes are often required after spending a few hundred miles on the trail. I used to be a woman's size 12 before I started long-distance hiking. Now I'm a men's 13 (I can't find women's 14s or 15s). I may be an extreme example,

but most people do have some change along the way. It may be worthwhile to plan a side trip or two off the trail to go to an experienced outfitter who can remeasure your feet and make sure the next pair will fit properly.

When you do have problems with your feet, and you usually will at some point, you need to look at the boots and evaluate whether you need to replace them with another boot type and/or style. On long hikes, your feet do enlarge and change. Boots wear out. Over a couple of years your feet may also change. Be open to new styles and features in newer type boots and find the pair that best fits you.

If you are always having problems with your boots and a different set of boots does not help, consider trying a pair of trail running shoes. Be aware, however, of the differences. Running shoes do not provide the same degree of ankle support and overall foot protection. While some may prefer the increased ankle mobility of a low running shoe, this choice requires proper strength in the feet, ankles, and legs. My choice to wear running shoes when fast-packing the 221 miles of the John Muir Trail was based on a trial overnight hike with a full backpack and years of running trails. I knew my feet and ankles could handle the stresses of the trail in running shoes, and I did not need heavier boots.

One week into hiking the John Muir Trail, Andrew Ferguson developed a hellacious deep blister on the back of his right foot, 1.5 inches in diameter. By nursing the blister with Spenco 2nd Skin and tape, he hiked for three days in running shoes before reaching civilization and purchasing a new pair of boots. The red heel bothered him for two weeks and took six months to return to normal. Andrew is now a believer in running shoes for hiking. Many people prefer trail running shoes instead of boots for hiking.

Choosing Lightweight Footwear

Our feet need varying degrees of support. Whether you wear a fanny pack, carry a lightweight pack with 10 pounds, or carry a 35-pound pack, the correct footwear is important. If your ankles are weak, you'll benefit from a higher shoe. A good insole will provide support and cushioning, reducing the jarring of your feet. Good outsole tread will provide traction on rocks and on wet trails. Good spacing in the toe box will save your toenails. You can find all these things in a lightweight shoe. Reducing your pack and gear weight will allow you the option of lightweight shoes. Do not make the mistake of choosing lightweight shoes without also considering the weight of your gear and pack. A heavy pack and lightweight shoes can hurt your feet and lead to an uncomfortable outing.

For help in reducing your pack weight and saving your feet, the gurus of lightweight are Ryan Jordan and his team at backpackinglight.com. The book Ryan edited, *Lightweight Backpacking and Camping: A Field Guide to Wilderness Hiking Equipment, Technique, and Style* (Beartooth Mountain Press, 2005) is a must if you are serious about going lightweight. Ryan emphasizes:

> Chapter 1 begins appropriately with the category of equipment that is arguably more important that any piece of gear or apparel a lightweight

backpacker will use: footwear. Lee Van Horn's treatise on footwear includes a comprehensive discussion of lightweight backpacking shoes. Simply put, shoes have such a profound impact on the lightweight backpacking experience because (1) the type of footwear you are able to wear depends in large part on the weight of the pack, and (2) the type of footwear you choose governs the transfer of energy and shock to the rest of your lower torso and spinal joints. Since this book's manuscript was finalized, I've been diving into research about ultralight footwear and experimenting with shoes lighter than anything the market has previously seen. I've been strengthening my feet, hiking in shoes with less support that are more akin to slippers than hiking shoes, and have been making some dramatic discoveries. In particular, I've learned that with proper conditioning, the natural features of the feet (as long as the arch is supported and the heel pad retains its shape for shock absorption) are ideally suited for transferring energy to the rest of your body, and I'm finding that I can walk longer distances in less supportive footwear—with a light pack—than I've ever been able to do before.

Of course, lightening your footwear means you should lighten your load. Get a lighter fanny pack, hydration pack, or backpack. If carrying a pack, lighten its load. Go from a tent to a new ultralight tent or a tarp. Change to one of the lightweight stoves and take advantage of lighter walking or hiking poles. Eliminate gear that you never seem to use but just had to pack. Your feet will feel all these weight savings. A weight loss of a few pounds will feel like heaven. You'll travel farther and your feet will be more comfortable.

Custom Shoes

What happens when you can't find a shoe you like? Your options are limited. Shoe companies are not in the business of making custom shoes. If you have a narrow heel and a wide forefoot, overall narrow or large feet, or have typically struggled to find shoes that fit well, you have probably experienced shoe hell. Most shoes, because they don't fit your feet, lead to blisters, arch problems, tendinitis, squished toes, and more. Rather than finding a shoe that fits your feet, you force your feet to fit into shoes made for the masses.

An excellent choice is to check out the Hersey Custom Shoe Company. They offer shoe models for runners, walkers, race walkers, and hikers. These include trainers and lightweight trainers, high-mileage shoes, racing flats, walking and racewalking shoes, hiking shoes, trail runners, and a high-top for those who need ankle support. Their approach is very simple: "Tell us what you're looking for, and we'll let you know if we can help."

The Hersey staff will work with you to get the shoe you want, based on your unique foot needs. You will answer a set of questions about how often you hike, run, and race, what your usual race distance is, what shoes you have used in the past that have worked and that have not worked, and then a set of questions about your feet (pronate, supinate, abnormal wear, orthotics, shoe breakdown patterns, and so on). You will also send a tracing of your feet based on Hersey's specific instructions. Then choose your model and design options and the shoes will be made to fit your feet and your feet alone.

Do they cost more? Certainly. Are they worth it? If you have hard-to-fit feet, I'd bet they are. If you want a shoe that is solidly made and not an off-the-shelf made in who-knows-where shoe, I'd also bet they will appeal to you. The Hersey Custom Shoe Company can be found at herseycustomshoe.com.

Their custom shoes were named by *Runner's World* as the best in both men's and women's in 1985. This shocked the Hersey staff—but shocked the giant shoe companies even more. *Runner's World* and other publications were pressured to do away with independent judging of shoes. They are a good company that has stood the test of time.

Sandals

Sandals are a nice alternative to shoes and boots. They are becoming more popular as designs improve to provide better traction, foot control, and comfort. Changing from running shoes or hiking boots into an open pair of sandals can be refreshing. When your feet are tired, hot, or sore, sandals can feel like a small piece of heaven on Earth.

Spencer Nelson recommends sandals for some uses:

> I have put in some quality training and raced in them to get a feel for their use. I always wear them with socks (usually SmartWool) and have worn them for flat 5-mile runs to 20 miles on trails to day two of the Tahoe Triple Marathon, which had 13 miles of downhill. They are good for my feet, and I will probably get another pair for the following positive reasons. They are very comfortable and better cushioned than they appear. I don't even notice that they are a sandal after four or five minutes; in other words the straps and open-air feel don't affect me. They are quick to dry on trail runs with water crossings. They keep my feet cool. They feel as good after around 200 miles as they did when I got them. Scree gets in and is easily kicked out . . . honestly! I have not had any problems with stubbing my toes or things of that nature.

Those who prefer the freedom of sandals over constricting shoes may find the Teva or Keen sandals to their liking. Both companies make sandals for cool, comfortable use, providing the cushioning, stability, toe protection, and support of a running shoe in a lightweight, airy sandal.

The minimalist movement has hit the sandals market too. Companies like Xero Shoes, Bedrock Sandals, and Luna Sandals make lightweight, minimalist sandals with simple strap systems. Many runners use these for trail running.

Wearing sandals while running or hiking takes practice. Small pebbles, gravel, leaves, or other debris can easily work their way underfoot. Shaking the foot or a light kick against a rock will usually knock these loose. Be especially careful of sticks on the trail that could inflict a puncture wound to your exposed feet. Try them to make sure the straps don't rub your feet wrong.

SANDAL PRODUCTS

BEDROCK SANDALS are high-quality, minimalist-style sandals. bedrocksandals.com

KEEN FOOTWEAR makes sandals with the protection of a shoe and the comfort of a sandal. The sandals have a toe guard, traction outsole, a wide footbed, and a quick-release drawstring closure. keenfootwear.com

LUNA SANDALS come in a variety of designs and are another minimalist-style sandal, made by Barefoot Ted. lunasandals.com

OOFOS SANDALS and flip-flops are lightweight and made for recovery. Very soft and comfortable; absorb more shock than other foams; support the arch while reducing stress on sore feet, knees, and lower back. Several styles are offered. oofos.com

TEVA SANDALS are for walking, running, and water sports. Many of its designs would work well on trails and roads. teva.com

XERO SHOES, by Steven Sashen, are designed after the huaraches running sandals worn by the Tarahumara Indians, famed for their long-distance running. **UMARA Z-TRAIL** and **AMURI Z-TREK** minimalist packable sandals have zero-drop for natural movement. The company also offers ready-made huaraches and kits to make your own. xeroshoes.com

If you wear sandals without socks, the skin of your feet will eventually toughen into calluses. Check the calluses regularly for cracks that can split through to uncalloused skin and bleed or become infected. If going without socks, a dab of sunscreen on the toes and tops of the foot will protect from bothersome sunburn. Consider wearing socks to protect your heel's protective fat pad and to avoid cracks and fissures in the skin. Some athletes have glued Spenco Hiker insoles onto the sandals, while others use Velcro to secure insoles or foot pads onto the sandal's footbed.

Switchback, a long-distance hiker, recommends several things if you hike with sandals: "[Use] a good insole glued into the sandal footbed, use hiking socks and a foot cream on your feet to keep them from chapping and drying out, and if your heels hurt, use a heel cup under or over the insole to provide a little extra cushion for the heels."

Tired of running shoes that fit him poorly, caused blisters and toenail problems, and seemed to collect dirt, Rob Grant bought a pair of sandals. He used his Tevas in a Sri Chinmoy 24-Hour Run. At 100K both little toes were swollen. The next day he ground down the ridge on the footbeds that fits under the toes. This corrected the problem. After putting 405 miles on the sandals, he reports no noticeable wear on the soles or the straps. Rob found that rubbing petroleum jelly on the inside of the straps helped to soften them. He feels that ankle support in sandals is comparable to that of running shoes.

Skip the Flip-Flops

Flip-flops are almost a classic piece of footwear. In reality, they offer little, if any, support for the foot and ankle. Their spongy sole causes the foot to roll inward even more than usual. This is pronation and can cause problems, which can lead to pain in the heel, arch, forefoot, and toes. Many people wear them so much they become flattened on the side where their heel lands. Wearing them around camp in a multiday event is fine—likewise wearing them around the pool—just not all day.

Insoles

Insoles are funny little things. Most of our boots and walking and running shoes come with removable insoles. Typically, we buy a pair of shoes and wear them until they wear out—without ever thinking about the insoles under our feet. You may

INSOLE PRODUCTS

The replacement insoles listed below are a sampling of what is available to the general public. New models and designs are constantly being introduced. Check your local running, hiking, and footwear stores or check the manufacturers' websites to see what is available. Many of the shoe and boot companies such as Montrail, Birkenstock, Merrell, and Vasque also make insoles. Many drug stores and pharmacies also stock insoles such as those made by Dr. Scholl's. Check the insoles inside your shoes to make sure they fit.

CADENCE INSOLES combines the semirigid orthotic support with the shock-absorbing comfort of an insole. Made with a low-friction top cover. cadence.com

DR. SCHOLL'S makes a complete line of insoles for all types of activities. drscholls.com

ENDURO-SOLE by Montrail ensures a custom fit via thermo-moldable CTX foam over a dynamic molded arch piece. Heat the insoles in an oven, put them into your shoes, and stand on them for 2 minutes to mold them to your feet. montrail.com

FOOTFIX INSOLES are made with a deep heel pocket for stability, a gel heel cushion for minimizing heel pain, and a built-in arch for underfoot support. footfix.com

HAPAD COMF-ORTHOTIC is a full-length or three-quarter–length insole. Many people have had considerable success with these. For more information, see "Orthotic Products" on pages 158–159.

ORTHOLITE insoles feature advanced technology to keep your feet cooler and drier. ortholite.com

ORTHOSOLE offers a **MAX CUSHION** insole that can be customized with your choice of three arch supports and two metatarsal pads for six combinations of support. orthosole.com think insoles are similar, but they differ quite a bit. They range from rigid to flexible, cushioned to hard, no arch to high arches, low to high heel cups, one material to multiple substances, and cheap to expensive, and they come in a multitude of coverings. Newer types can be heated in an oven and then after standing in them, you can mold them to the shape of your feet.

Take the ones out of your shoes. Are they flimsy? Do they easily bend in half? Are they lifeless with little structure to offer support? Are they flattened out? Do they look like squashed cardboard? If so, your shoes came from the "we-cut-corners-on-the-insole" shoe company. Toss the insoles out and get a new pair. The old ones may be contributing to foot problems, including blisters and foot pain.

Insoles, sometimes called footbeds, are designed to provide extra support and/or cushioning during running and hiking. Some models are molded to cradle the heel, support the arch, and cushion the forefoot, while others have only an arch

POWERSTEPS offers a **PINNACLE** insole with a semirigid shell, a deep heel cup, and a strong arch support. powersteps.com

RXSORBO makes an assortment of replacement insoles with Sorbothane visco-elastic polymer inlays in the heel and forefoot for maximum shock absorption and energy return. rxsorbo.com

SHOCKBLOCKERS INSOLES, by Oregon Aero, were originally created for the US military. The two-layer insoles feature a highly shock-absorbing Visco-Kinetic polymer layer and a high-wicking, low-friction fabric. oregonaero.com

SHOCK DOCTOR FOOTBEDS incorporate multiple shock-absorbing, support, and comfort components to create a foot-hugging performance platform. shockdoctor.com

SOF SOLE offers multiple insole designs, including an **AIRR** insole made with a heel air chamber that extends under the arch. Made with a Coolmax top sheet to wick moisture. sofsole.com

SOLE CUSTOM FOOTBEDS use heat-to-fit technology as an excellent, inexpensive alternative to custom orthotics. The footbeds have Poron cushioning, a deep heel cup for stability, and an aggressive arch for support. When you heat the insoles in your oven, put them into your shoes, and stand on them, they mold to your feet. yoursole.com

SPENCO makes several lines of replacement insoles: **POLYSORB, GEL,** and **SPENCO RX.** Products include insoles for stability, cushioning, support, and specialty styles. The **GREENLINE** designs are made from closed-cell neoprene. Sold through stores. spenco.com

SUPERFEET footbeds offer a corrective shape and design with a stabilizer cap that provides excellent support and stability to the bone structure of the foot, allowing the foot muscles to function more efficiently and the body to be correctly aligned. It has designs for specific activities and footwear. superfeet.com support or are flat. Replacement insoles are to be used in place of your shoe's standard insole. Many replacement insoles offer better heel support, shock absorption, energy return, and reduction of friction than the insoles that come with the shoes. Some have a better arch support that will help with flat feet problems. The insoles listed below are typically found in running, camping, and sporting goods stores. Ask to see their product catalogs if their shelf stock is low or if you are looking for a particular type.

There are basically two types of insoles available: foam and viscous polymer. Foam insoles are lightweight and inexpensive, and they retain heat. However, their impact absorption is not as good, and they lose their impact-absorbing properties with use. In general, foam is more suited for runners because of the concern about weight. The viscous polymers, such as those offered by RXSorbo, are a great choice for athletes with sensitive feet or injuries that require protection to the foot's padding. Some insoles offer polymer at the heel and/or forefoot, and the rest is made of foam. This reduces the weight liability of all-polymer insoles.

Superfeet is a good example of an insole made to perform. Many insoles are made to provide shock absorption, support, or alignment. Superfeet are made to do all three. Their deep heel cup design and shape provides the ideal biomechanical support. It is worth trying these before going to a more expensive orthotic.

If you have tried changing socks and other techniques to decrease your chance of blisters and still have problems, try changing insoles. You may find that a particular brand or type of insole may be better at reducing blisters on your feet. This is usually due to the fabric or components of the insole. Replacement insoles may be sized differently. Be sure to check the fit inside your shoes or boots. An insole that is narrow in the forefoot can create problems as the foot overlaps space between the narrow insole and the side of the shoe. Insoles may be different in other areas also. Some may have a higher arch that will put pressure on your foot, creating blisters. Others may have a narrow heel bed and cause friction where your foot rubs against the top edge of the heel cup. Insoles can help reduce the shear associated with friction at the sock and insole interface. When possible, choose an insole that has a smooth or fairly smooth surface. Rough surfaces can adhere to socks, which can lead to shear and blisters.

Finding and using the right insole can make a big difference in the overall fit and comfort of your footwear. But insoles are not made to last forever. Check them for breakdown and replace them when necessary. This will depend on how you run and hike, as well as your mileage.

Replacement insoles are not sold as corrective footbeds. If a particular brand or style of insole is uncomfortable or causes pain, try another type. One brand may fit your feet better than another brand. Some are quite rigid, while others are very cushioned. Try several until you find a pair that is comfortable for your activity. If you purchase insoles and they are too tight in certain areas of your feet, inquire at your local shoe repair shop or a pedorthist about thinning them with a belt sander.

Do not confuse these insoles with an orthotic. Always consult with a pedorthist, orthopedist, or podiatrist if you are having frequent foot problems. Repeated foot pain may be a sign of deeper foot problems that a general-use insole cannot correct. In that case, an orthotic may be necessary to correct an imbalance problem. See the "Orthotics" chapter for more information on the types available and what these can correct.

A study by the American Orthopaedic Foot and Ankle Society found that inexpensive off-the-shelf insoles are more likely to be effective than pricey, custom-made products. According to the society, many foot problems can benefit from the cushioning of a cheap insert more than the repositioning provided by a custom-made insert. Many of these inserts are made from foam, silicone, plastic, wool, or combinations of different materials.

Barefoot and Minimalist Footwear

A few years ago, no one was talking about minimalist footwear. Then *Time* magazine named Vibram FiveFingers one of the best inventions of 2007. A few people got on the bandwagon. In 2009 Christopher McDougall wrote the book *Born to Run* and the issue exploded. McDougall set off to find out why his feet hurt and shared with readers the secrets of the Tarahumara Indians—and a better way to run. Barefoot running and running in minimalist footwear have become much more acceptable, and now the testimonials abound.

Mitch Kern shares his experience with barefoot running: "I've been running for years but my career has always been punctuated by injuries along the way. Like so many others I read McDougall's *Born to Run* and just had to buy a pair of Vibram FiveFingers. From there I transitioned into barefoot running and have been injury free ever since. I feel like I've learned just how to run for the first time. In the past, I was a heel striker/long strider, but now I take a very different approach—faster cadence and on the balls of the feet. I am convinced it is the way to go. People think I'm nuts, but man, oh man, what a difference."

Talk to a few people who are wearing Vibram FiveFingers or who run barefoot and you will discover a culture has developed. This unique line of footwear has five individual toes—for your toes—and with a Vibram outsole, it is akin to going barefoot. People who were previously unable to run now can. Those who had become accustomed to discomfort and pain from bunions, heel pain, and more have discovered relief. It is worth paying attention to.

Daniel Lieberman, a prominent researcher in the barefoot and minimalist movement, has written extensively on the subject. On his website he says, "We do not know how early humans ran, but our research indicates that humans were able to run comfortably and safely when barefoot or in minimal footwear by landing with a flat foot (midfoot strike) or by landing on the ball of the foot before bringing down the heel (forefoot strike)."[10]

Vibram's FiveFingers KSO Trek for trails   Photo credit: Vibram

Running barefoot or in minimalist shoes is different from running in the usual running shoe. Most important, you land differently. Danny Abshire, the cofounder of Newton Running, says you acquire a connection with the ground as you run. You are more agile and run with finesse. Others in the barefoot and minimalist movement echo the same thought.

For purposes of this chapter, minimalist footwear is defined as any footwear that does not have the typical high cushioned heels, stiff soles, and arch support common in today's running shoes. The information and tips in this chapter, generally speaking, apply to someone wearing FiveFingers or other minimalist footwear, or those going barefoot. Many of those wearing minimalist footwear will also forego wearing socks.

And lest you think that going barefoot is only for walking and running, consider the group Barefoot Hikers. Barefoot Chris (his trail name), a member of Barefoot Hikers, recalls the reaction of hikers they encountered while on a weeklong barefoot backpacking trip on the Appalachian Trail. "They told stories of many other barefoot hikers, including at least two that had done the entire trail without shoes."

A quick online search for "barefoot running clubs" finds many cities with these running clubs. There are also clubs dedicated to walking and hiking barefoot.

Shoes vs. Minimalist Footwear

For years, everyone wore shoes, or if we were hikers, boots. We could choose between neutral, flexible, stable, motion-control, cushioned, lightweight, and trail shoes. We might stick to one design or try several. Many athletes went through pair after pair trying to find the perfect shoe for their feet, often in an effort to accommodate injuries. We had choices—as long as it was a shoe the shoe companies offered.

Yes, there were always a few runners who ran barefoot. Many times they received odd looks. Others looked for ultralightweight shoes, which were few and far between. If you wanted to run, shoes were what you needed.

Kevin O'Neall shared his experience with wearing FiveFingers: "I was close to giving up running after 50-plus marathons and two dozen ultras because of chronic heel pain. My feet had developed golf ball–size lumps where the Achilles tendons insert on the heel bone. After a year and a half wearing FiveFingers exclusively, the lumps are 90% gone. There is still heel pain, but it tends to fade while I'm running. At this point I prefer them to running shoes, even though they do make me a slower runner."

Of course, there are many arguments for and against barefoot running. Some claim that barefoot running is better for you. Others argue that barefoot running is dangerous and will lead to more injuries. And still others say that running shoes prevent injuries—or lead to injuries—depending on their point of view. Athletes will point to the few studies available to support their views—whatever they are.

The conspiracy theorists talk about the "big lie" from the shoe companies, which want you to buy their shoes. One ultrarunner, a proponent of the minimalist movement, wrote in an online forum, "They want you to buy heavy, stiff, supportive, motion-control shoes so that all the little muscles, tendons, and bones in your feet get weak, conforming to the brand you run in, so that they can upgrade you to the next model, which will invariably be heavier, stiffer, more supportive, more cushioned, more motion control, more expensive, and wear out faster." Personally, I don't believe that statement. I think there is room for regular shoes and minimalist shoes—and barefoot running. You have to make the choice, and in my view, it should be an educated and informed choice.

Christian Griffith, an ultrarunner, made a valuable comment in an online forum about the barefoot and FiveFingers bandwagon that so many athletes are touting. He wrote, "It's a tool to help strengthen, lengthen, and improve flexibility in the leg muscles with the added benefit of forcing me to run what I view as 'correctly'—meaning upright, with a stable midline, midfoot strike, and gently." Others in the forum agreed, emphasizing it as a way to learn and maintain good running form and to keep that form when moving back to shoes. While some athletes will stick to barefoot or minimalist footwear, many rotate between a combination of trail shoes, road shoes, barefoot, and minimalist footwear.

The Value of "Going Bare"

In the simplest of terms, going barefoot or using minimalist footwear makes your feet do more of the work they were intended to do. The bones, muscles, tendons, and ligaments all work together. You have a lighter gait. Instead of landing on your heels, you land more on the midsole and forefoot. With that comes a better connection between your feet and the ground. Barefoot Ted talks about this connection later in the chapter.

A 2004 study at the Sapporo International Half-Marathon in Japan captured foot strike positions of 283 runners; 75% of the runners landed on their heels,

Running in bare feet requires
a midfoot strike.
Photo credit: Barefoot Ted

24% landed midfoot near the arch, and only 4% landed on their forefoot. The 4% were not the fastest.

When we wear shoes, most of us are heel strikers. Barefoot runners, as well as those in minimalist footwear, tend to strike the ground near or on the ball of the foot. I recently watched a 72-year-old woman—who, because of heel injuries as a child, had been unable to run—show me how she could now run. She was excited and had just finished her first 5K race. FiveFingers had allowed her to run again.

Our body adapts: muscles, tendons, and bones adjust to changes in footwear, our stride, and the way our foot strikes the ground. Many runners who have struggled with chronic injuries have switched to running barefoot or to minimalist footwear and have seen their injuries reduced or eliminated.

The Science on Barefoot Running

Articles in journals have talked about running shoes and barefoot running for some time. Here are a few examples.

- Barefoot running promotes front- and midstrike, which allows the runner to take more "advantage of elastic energy stored in both the Achilles tendon and the longitudinal arch of the foot." This develops more calf and foot muscle strength and avoids "uncomfortable and potentially injurious impact."[11]

- A shoe with any heel height, trainers included, alters the entire body posture.[12]

- "The soles and tips of the toes contain over 200,000 nerve endings" connecting us to the world and helping us balance. The stimulation is a connection from foot to body and foot to brain. This sensory perception is often "denied us because of our thick-layered and inflexible shoes."[13]

- "When running barefoot . . . the runner compensates for the lack of cushioning" by adjusting the foot-landing angle to a more natural mid- to front-foot strike, giving it a softer landing.[14]

- "Humans have engaged in endurance running for millions of years, but the modern running shoe was not invented until the 1970s. For most of human evolutionary history, runners were either barefoot or wore minimal footwear such as sandals or moccasins with smaller heels and little cushioning relative to modern running shoes."[15]

- "The soft materials in modern running shoes allow a contact style [heel strike] that you would not use [if you were] barefoot. The foot no longer gets the proprioceptive cues" that it should, and "a midsole [foot strike] can impair the foot's ability to react to the ground. This can mute or alter feedback the body gets while running."[16]

- Dr. Jack Daniels said, "We found adding 100 grams to the shoe increased the aerobic demand of running by 1%. Now 100 grams is about 3.5274 ounces, so each ounce changes the cost of running about 0.2835%." For each additional ounce, the runner loses "about .83 seconds for a mile."[17]

Function and Form

The barefoot movement has taken the running community by storm. Athletes want to mimic the experience McDougall wrote about in *Born to Run*. Thousands have tried barefoot running, FiveFingers, and whatever new minimalist footwear they have heard others talking about. They want the function and the feeling of venturing out with as little as possible on their feet. They are after the natural movement of going barefoot.

Unfortunately, this barefoot function requires a change in form that many do not consider. You cannot run barefoot, or in the new minimalist shoes, and land on your heels. You will become injured. This new style requires a midfoot or forefoot strike. Newton Running calls it natural running, saying it will help you discover your optimal running form. Newton Running has a YouTube channel with videos on natural running. Danny Abshire is the cofounder of Newton Running, and his book, *Natural Running: The Simple Path to Stronger, Healthier Running* (VeloPress, 2010), is a must-read for anyone wanting to learn more about running better and more efficiently with fewer injuries. The website naturalrunningcenter.com is a good resource for information about learning how to run more naturally.

Think about how we move on our feet. When we walk, we naturally land on our heels first. When we sprint, we land on our toes. Ideally, we need a point in between.

When we run in normal shoes, we land on our heels and roll through to our forefoot and toes. Our heels strike first, in front of our center of gravity. This impact leads to a moment of deceleration, as the heel shock moves upward through the knees and spine. Then we push off with the muscular force of our toes.

When we run barefoot or in minimalist shoes, we naturally land on our midfoot or forefoot. We lean slightly forward, with our center of gravity over where our forefoot strikes. Our stride is shorter with a quicker cadence. We land lightly and quickly lift our foot for the next foot strike. The body should be relaxed rather than tight or tense. This engages our vision, brain, and all the muscles, tendons, bones, and supporting structures of our feet and legs.

It takes time to unlearn old habits and learn the proper technique. Many become injured because they do too much too soon.

Barefoot Precautions

Whether you're going barefoot or wearing minimalist footwear, you need to start slowly. Your muscles need to get used to the new stresses on them. Tendons and ligaments need to be strengthened. Bones need to adapt to the new demands placed on them. Flexibility needs to be developed. None of this happens overnight. You need to ease your way into it. Doing too much too soon could cause damage to all those internal parts. Muscle tears, tendinitis, strained tendons, and stress fractures could result. Long-distance barefoot runner Tellman Knudson suggests starting with five minutes a day running barefoot, then putting your shoes on. After a week, add in another five minutes. Continue this for a few weeks and let your feet be your guide. If you experience swelling, internal pain, or a burning sensation, reduce the amount of time spent barefoot.

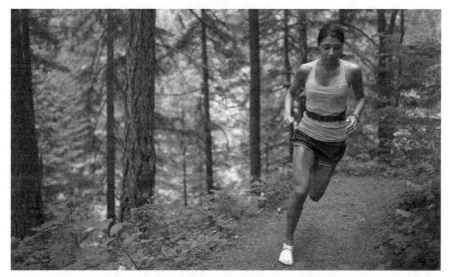

FiveFingers are used by many trail runners.   Photo credit: Vibram

You are also changing from a heel striker to a forefoot striker. Landing on the balls of your feet adds new stresses on your Achilles tendon and calf muscles. Many of those starting out complain of Achilles and calf pain. Starting slowly will give these muscles time to strengthen. Landing on your forefoot or midfoot doesn't mean that your heels don't come down; it just means that they don't touch first. You'll land more in the middle of the foot first and then your foot continues down until the heels touch. The forefoot and midfoot landings provide a natural springing action. You can also investigate Pose and Chi running, which advocate landing more on the forefoot. These two techniques teach athletes to position their bodies during exercises such as running and teach better form and conditioning for reduced injuries (posemethod.com and chirunning.com).

When venturing barefoot onto trails or even on pavement, you should take a few precautions. Start slowly with short barefoot excursions to give your feet time to adjust. Your feet are used to the support and cushioning of shoes, and going without will make a sudden change. Be attentive to the conditions of the path underfoot. Your feet can be cut or punctured by debris on the road or trail. If you want to run barefoot, start by walking.

Walking and running barefoot can be an excellent way to condition your feet in order to prevent blisters when you do wear boots or shoes. Your skin will be tougher and you may develop calluses. Yet, be forewarned: This is no guarantee that you will not get blisters. Remember that when it is raining, the moisture will soften the skin on your feet. That's a good time to switch to one of the minimalist shoes.

Aside from the possibility of cutting your feet on glass or metal, if you have any cuts or open skin on your feet, you run the risk of picking up an infection. Another concern is skin that calluses over. These calluses can split into fissures or cracks in the skin. This opens the inner layers of skin to a greater risk of infection. If you step on something sharp and get a puncture wound, seek medical care. Puncture wounds typically close up, and this seals any debris, germs, or contaminants inside the wound. If you choose to go barefoot, it's smart to take care of your feet. There is no point in getting an infection through carelessness.

After reading about all the possible injuries from going barefoot, you may be worried. Going barefoot may be the goal of many athletes, but in reality, wearing minimalist shoes will provide protection and enhance the barefoot experience. Tellman Knudson likes FiveFingers, especially for people who

- don't want to deal with the pain of running barefoot,

- want to minimize the risk of stepping on something that could hurt their feet,

- run on hot surfaces where their feet would roast without protection,

or

- are in the process of transitioning from running in normal shoes to running barefoot.

Remember that switching to barefoot running or minimalist footwear does not mean that you can't ever run in shoes again. Many athletes employ a combination of going barefoot or wearing minimalist footwear or shoes. Running in minimalist footwear helps runners focus on good form, and for many, it will reduce injuries. If you want or need something more substantial than FiveFingers, consider using one of the minimalist shoes from companies like Inov-8, Nike, Newton, New Balance, Karhu, Merrell, Skora, or Vivobarefoot. These replicate the free and natural flexible motions of your feet better than the usual running shoe.

Avoiding Injuries

Running on any surface in bare feet exposes them to glass, rocks, nails, screws, twigs, wire, and roots—all typical debris in places we like to run. One misplaced step onto a rusty wire or a piece of glass can lead to an infected foot and, if not attended to properly, an even worse outcome. Learn to regularly check your feet for abrasions and cuts. Running on grass or trails offers a softer and more comfortable surface than asphalt or concrete. Wearing at least some degree of foot covering will protect the soles of your feet.

A strip of tape can be put on the ball of the forefoot for protection when running barefoot. Likewise, tape can even be added to the forefoot when wearing FiveFingers to reduce friction. Because the FiveFingers have individual toes, you could wear Injinji toe socks with them if you plan ahead and buy the footwear with room for the socks. That can provide an extra bit of cushioning, toe protection, and padding from any rough inside seams.

Scott Sanders uses FiveFingers and told me, "They are amazing shoes. My ITB [iliotibial band syndrome] and sore knee problems went away almost immediately. I wear them around town all the time, but I really can't run in them. Here are two problems I have had with FiveFingers:

- They offer no protection from roots, rocks, stones, pavement, and concrete. An ultrarunner friend of mine broke her toe wearing them. I banged my foot on a root while training and have been forced to use them on the treadmill and elliptical pretty much exclusively. We have few soft trails to run on in Northern Georgia.

Xero Shoes Z-Trail sandals offer protection and flexibility.   Photo credit: Xero Shoes

■ There is very little cushioning in the bottom of the sole. I tried inserting Dr. Scholl's Gel and regular shoe inserts to give me just a little more cushioning, but it didn't work."

Many athletes, like Scott, are buying FiveFingers and finding that the footwear is fine for walking, but athletes have a hard time running distances they used to run in normal shoes. Minimalist shoes from the companies listed previously are a good choice for athletes who want a shoe designed for running on their midfoot and forefoot—a more natural running form.

Ice can help minimize swelling, especially as you are starting out. The "Cold and Heat Therapy" chapter has information on how to get the most benefits from icing.

When going out to run barefoot, add a few things to a fanny pack. Knudson, known for his efforts to run across America barefoot, suggests including tweezers, moleskin for padding, Gorilla Super Glue to seal wounds and help moleskin stick, duct tape, Band-Aids in case of cuts, and alcohol wipes to disinfect.

Michael Sandler, the author of books on barefoot running, reminds runners to start out slowly. "Start out barefoot and run only a few hundred yards. Work on proper form. Let your skin condition be your guide. If your skin becomes tender, chances are you're overly fatiguing muscles, tendons, ligaments, and even bones. Don't run barefoot two days in a row until your feet are strong (at least three months)."

Barefoot Running Tips

■ Go barefoot whenever possible—help your feet get used to it.

■ Start slowly—give your feet time to strengthen themselves.

■ When your skin gets sore, stop and wear something else.

■ Strengthen your feet and ankles.

■ Let pain be your guide—stop if your arches, top of your foot, or anything else hurts.

■ Watch for abrasions and cuts on your feet and care for them.

■ Be careful of hot and cold surfaces.

■ Rest days are beneficial.

■ Be attentive to roots and rocks, which can cause injury.

■ Stand upright to stay on your toes and be light on your feet.

■ Get over the social implications of going barefoot.

It is imperative that those wanting to try either barefoot running or minimalist footwear understand the importance of starting slowly and letting pain be your guide. Making the change to running barefoot and/or in minimalist footwear can easily lead to months of sore calf muscles, sore Achilles tendons, and various foot and ankle pains that could naturally limit your training. Even stress fractures can occur. Increasingly, many athletes ignore these warning signs and become injured.

Barefoot Ted's Luna sandals   Photo credit: Barefoot Ted

In mid-2010, articles started appearing about the epidemic of barefoot running injuries. Podiatrists and physical therapists reported a surge in injuries that seemed to be related to barefoot and minimalist footwear running. Heel and calf muscle injuries, Achilles tendinosis, and plantar fasciitis can happen when one does too much too soon. The transition from normal running shoes to running either barefoot or in minimalist footwear can take months. Most of us have been heel strikers for years. Changing to a midfoot strike takes retraining our brain, which knows we are used to landing on our heels.

Be careful. Reduce your mileage. Start slowly. If you are older, be prepared for the transition to take even longer. Walk barefoot as much as possible. Let your bones, muscles, tendons, and ligaments get used to being free and unfettered from shoes.

Minimalist Footwear Choices

The choices in footwear when wanting a minimalist-type shoe have multiplied in the past few years. Vibram FiveFingers were once the most commonly used. Some athletes try sandals, whether homemade huaraches or store-bought sandals. Companies like Inov-8, Nike, Newton, New Balance, Karhu, Merrell, Skora, and Vivobarefoot offer excellent minimalist shoes. Remember though that many of these shoes are not sold through running stores.

Remember that just because a shoe is marketed as minimalist doesn't mean that it is designed to accommodate a midfoot or forefoot strike. Some are simply made with less support and structure, and a thinner outsole.

Consider your footwear needs based on the surfaces on which you run, how far you run, your running style, and your history of running injuries. Try the footwear on to make sure it feels right and run a bit—even if it's around the store. Ask the store for pointers and whether you can take the footwear outside for a try.

Vibram FiveFingers

FiveFingers footwear was the brainchild of industrial designer Robert Fliri. He proposed the idea to Marco Bramani, grandson of Vibram founder Vitale Bramani, who invented the first rubber soles used on mountaineering boots in 1936.

Vibram FiveFingers are, simply put, little more than five-toed foot gloves for your feet. There is no arch support and no cushioning. The Vibram outsole is 3, 3.5, or 4 millimeters thick, depending on the style. Your feet and toes can spread out and bend and flex in a natural way, as they were intended to do naturally.

FiveFingers come in many styles. The best designs for running are those where the top of the shoes come up near the ankle. This keeps debris from getting inside and better secures the footwear to the foot. The KSO is one of the standard designs. A more rugged version, the Spyridon MR, is designed for trails and trekking. The Bikila EVO is designed specifically for a more natural running experience with a more natural forefoot strike.

Vibram's FiveFingers Bikila   Photo credit: Vibram

A two-year class action lawsuit against Vibram was settled in 2014 for $3.75 million. The suit contended that Vibram engaged in misleading advertising by claiming certain health benefits by wearing their shoes. Whatever your take on the lawsuit, there are two sides to consider. Yes, people have been injured wearing the shoes—many because they expected to run the same distances as they did in the regular shoes too soon and did not condition their feet to the difference in support from the shoes. However, many people have been helped by the shoes, finding they could run in spite of certain foot conditions that had hindered them in regular shoes. For some people, Vibram FiveFingers are a good shoe and work for their feet.

Getting Fit for FiveFingers

Gillian Robinson of zombierunner.com has fit many pairs of FiveFingers. She recommends them for people with toes that curl downward or upward, toes that overlap, hammertoes, and bunions. She suggests making sure that your toenails are trimmed and filed smooth to avoid poking through the mesh upper. Here are her tips on getting the best fit.

- Get fitted at a store that fits and sells FiveFingers.

- Wear them snugly against the foot, heel back in the shoe, but the toes should not be tight against the ends of the toe pockets.

- Size them to your longest toe (birthdayshoes.com has a section on modifying the second toe for Morton's foot).

- Get the right size: too big and they flop around and cause blisters; too small and your toes can't flatten *and* flex.

The website birthdayshoes.com points out that FiveFingers do not come in American footwear sizing but in European sizing (that is, 34–48, depending on whether they're for men or women), and men and women can wear each other's FiveFingers, but women's are generally narrower.

Inov-8

Inov-8 footwear is worn by many trail runners because of its design, which allows the foot the freedom to move and function as nature intended, without interference from the structure of the shoe. The lightweight Inov-8 shoes protect the foot from the harsh external environment experienced by the off-road runner but maintain the feeling and function of barefoot running.

Newton

Newton running shoes are made to enhance the natural running gait of landing on your midfoot or forefoot. Energy is absorbed and returned back to the runner through their patented Action/Reaction Technology. Runners I have talked to indicate the shoes help them land in a more natural position. For those wanting a minimalist shoe with protection and support that also provides a forefoot running technique, Newton shoes are a good choice.

Newton shoes are made with actuator lugs in the forefoot for energy return.
Photo credit: Newton Running

Vivobarefoot

Shoes by Vivobarefoot were developed specifically to replicate being barefoot. The Evo looks like a normal running shoe. They are lightweight and made with breathable mesh and lightweight micro fiber, and the outsole is 3 millimeters thick. Individuals who cannot wear FiveFingers because of fitting issues may do well in these shoes. The Evos allow for a greater variety of foot anatomy. Other models include the Ultra II, the Trail Freak, and the Hiker. As with FiveFingers, they allow a barefoot running or even hiking experience with some degree of protection.

Other Minimalist Shoes

Because of the growing popularity of minimalist footwear, we can expect more companies to design footwear for this market, such as Merrell, Karhu, and Skora. The websites and blogs listed at the end of this chapter are a good way to stay in touch with changes in the market.

We have to be careful and read reviews from magazines and websites dedicated to the barefoot and minimalist movement (two examples are birthdayshoes.com and barefootrunningshoes.org). Make sure the footwear is made for running, not just casual wear. Because of the growing interest in minimalist footwear, many companies are trying to enter the minimalist shoe marketplace, and those shopping for such shoes need to be informed.

The minimalist movement has hit the sandals market too. Companies like Xero Shoes, Bedrock Sandals, and Luna Sandals make lightweight, minimalist sandals with simple strap systems. Many runners use these for trail running. Refer to "Sandal Products" on page 71 for more about these sandals.

As you might guess, wearing footwear without socks can lead to funky-smelling shoes. Wiping your feet with a premoistened antibacterial wipe is a good start. Kiwi Fresh Force, PediTech, and ZORBX Odor Remover are highly recommended on birthdayshoes.com, which has a great page of tips about keeping your FiveFingers (and any other shoes) stink free. Readers also give washing tips and offer suggestions ranging from powders and sprays to soaks.

Barefoot Ted's tips on page 91 can also be applied to those wearing minimalist footwear. It is about technique and form as well as whether we wear shoes or not.

Another popular barefoot runner, Barefoot Ken Bob Saxton, gave the following quote in an article on barefoot running in *Runner's World* (February 2010): "Barefoot running is actually something that's been tried and tested over millions of years of evolution. Feet have become the engineering marvel that they are because they work. We're just trying to help average runners become more mindful of how they're running and to enjoy it more."

Running barefoot and wearing minimalist footwear can help you get to that point. But remember, start slowly and let pain be your guide.

Barefoot Ted in typical running form   Photo credit: Barefoot Ted

Barefoot Ted's Barefoot Running Goals

So, what are the secrets I share with clients who take my Introduction to Barefoot Running Clinic? First, my aim is to get people to learn how to *feel* what good running feels like. One of the primary feelings becomes an awareness of the texture and hardness of terrain and of impact. This awareness is the beginning.

"To master this awareness, I have clients learn to move on hard surfaces *first*. Not focusing on distance or speed, I have my clients first walk and then trot on hard, fairly smooth surfaces. I work with them to focus on and begin to master three goals: quiet, quick, and in balance.

My Three Goals

1. QUIET Master gentle, quiet, forefoot-centric landings, silent and smooth. Learn to move with no hard edges and no pounding by learning how to have the impact of your landing flow through your forefoot and smoothly spread through the legs. Notice how silent your movement becomes. Imagine the movement of a big cat. Watch dogs trot. Let them be models for a flowing movement that wastes no energy.

2. QUICK Quicken your cadence. Running in bare feet encourages this naturally. Some shoe runners are plodders. You can hear them coming. Lots of wasted energy on poorly timed impact. Quicker cadence ends up making sense when you realize that your ability to absorb and recoil energy through elasticity in your body dissipates quickly and is lost if not used. Learning how to get back in touch with the sweet spot of optimal recoil efficiency is easier when you can feel your feet, a feeling that encourages a landing phase with your foot more in line with your center of gravity. Overstriding is discouraged and nearly impossible when barefoot.

3. IN BALANCE The feeling of balance is a stable, upright posture, balanced head, core engaged, belly button pulled into the spine, no waist bending, and head upright. I think that good running can be judged aesthetically. It should look good, not painful. When you see someone moving or running well, it looks smooth and fluid and graceful and efficient. The opposite looks painful, when someone is hunched and stiff, robotic and plodding. Indeed, efficient running is tall and stable, the upper body acting as the fulcrum from which the legs and arms can move freely with a serious lack of bouncing or swaying of the head.

Ultimately my aim in coaching is to help people perfect what I call a persistent hunt trot . . . a gait not purely about speed, but about smooth, flowing, efficient, sustainable movement, movement that leaves you ready to play another day. Listen to your body. Learn what it is telling you. Then adjust and advance accordingly.

BAREFOOT RUNNING BOOKS

McDougall, Christopher. ***Born to Run: A Hidden Tribe, Superathletes, and the Greatest Race the World Has Never Seen.*** New York: Alfred A. Knopf, 2009.

Robillard, Jason. ***The Barefoot Running Book: A Practical Guide to the Art and Science of Barefoot and Minimalist Shoe Running.*** Allendale, Michigan: Barefoot Running Press, 2010.

Sandler, Michael, and Jessica Lee. ***Barefoot Running: How to Become Healthy, Fit, and Blissful by Getting in Touch with the Earth.*** Boulder: RunBare Publishing, 2010.

Barefoot Ted's Tips to Getting Started

I asked Barefoot Ted to share from his experience. He has been running barefoot longer than most. Here is what he said.

So, you wanna start running barefoot? Firstly, before you begin, you want to evaluate what it is that is leading you to even accept the logic behind the concept of barefoot running. We all know that barefoot running has gotten a lot of attention lately. Much of it is valid and deserves your attention.

Yet, one must still ask: Is this a viable option for me? Before you answer that question, let me explain why I think barefoot or minimal footwear running may not be good for you. It is not good if you are thinking it is some sort of cure-all that only requires taking off your shoes and starting to run injury free without radical changes in the way you may have been thinking of running up to now. If your running strategy has been about very specific time or distance goals, and you have been willing to push through pain to injury, then I would caution you: Your bare feet will not allow you to continue this way.

Barefoot running is not about blocking or pushing through pain, or at least it shouldn't be. Rather it is about *tuning in* to your own body's highly sophisticated set of integrated awareness systems, systems that communicate through feelings and senses that are being collected in real time as you move. From my perspective, learning how to run well means learning how to tap into the feeling of running well, which more often than not requires baring the foot to get the full feel of what happens when you move.

However, even if you decide that barefoot is the route for you, take one step backward and realize that you are most likely in the process of rehabilitating your feet and legs from years of being differently abled, shoed, and cast. Atrophy, loss of range of motion, weakness, neglect—the foot has not been treated well lately. All the padding and support and protection has not led to stronger feet, sadly.

So, the first key is to start slowly, incrementally, and avoid overexuberance; avoid being driven by your ego. The hallmark of my barefoot running philosophy is regaining connectedness, mindfulness, and presence in your running and in your body.

BAREFOOT AND MINIMALIST FOOTWEAR WEBSITES

Note: Including the websites and books with this chapter rather than at the end is a bit of an anomaly, but we decided that it was important to keep these distinct resources with this chapter. For running sandals, check the "Sandals" section in the previous chapter.

KEN BOB'S ORIGINAL BAREFOOTRUNNING.COM by Barefoot Ken Bob is the original barefoot running site. Started in 1997, it offers tips and FAQs and offers a place to have questions about barefoot running answered. barefootrunning.com

BAREFOOT RUNNING UNIVERSITY, founded by barefoot ultramarathon runner Jason Robillard, author of *The Barefoot Running Book,* offers information about running barefoot, a blog, footwear reviews, links, and more. barefootrunninguniversity.com.

BAREFOOTRUNNINGSHOES.ORG is a website with reviews of barefoot running shoes. barefootrunningshoes.org

BAREFOOT TED'S ADVENTURES is the website of Barefoot Ted. It offers tips, a blog, a link to a Google group, his coaching page, and his custom-made huaraches or a do-it-yourself kit. barefootted.com

BIRTHDAYSHOES.COM is a website and blog dedicated to barefoot running shoes, with tips and facts to help your minimalist experience. The "Resource" page offers an FAQ section, design reviews, running and walking tips, and barefoot research. The site also describes how to make modifications and repairs. birthdayshoes.com

DANIEL LIEBERMAN, a Harvard researcher, maintains a website about "Biomechanics of Foot Strikes and Applications to Running Barefoot or in Minimal Footwear." barefootrunning.fas.harvard.edu

INOV-8 FOOTWEAR, the official site of Inov-8 Footwear, has information on its products designed around the natural functions of the foot. inov-8.com

NEWTON RUNNING is the website of the Newton line of running shoes. Good information on the science of natural running and articles on improving your running form. newtonrunning.com

RUNBARE is the website of Michael Sandler and Jessica Lee, authors of *Barefoot Running, Barefoot Walking,* and the *Barefoot Running* movie. runbare.com

SOCIETY FOR BAREFOOT LIVING is a website of resources, facts, and links about living barefoot. barefooters.org

VIVOBAREFOOT's official site covers its extensive line of minimalist shoes. vivobarefoot.com

VIBRAM FIVEFINGERS is the Vibram website for its FiveFingers shoes. us.vibram.com

Socks

Socks perform four basic functions: cushioning, protection, warmth, and absorption of moisture off the skin. Some socks may also offer compression in select areas or in the whole sock. The sock fabric and weave will determine how well they do each. Socks made from synthetic fabrics wick moisture away from the skin and through the sock to its outer surface where it can evaporate.

Mindfulness: The Art of Putting on Your Socks

First, be sure your socks are clean and free of debris. Hold them by the cuff, pull them through the closed fist of the other hand, and then whip them in the air a couple times. Turn them inside out and then repeat. If the socks have a thick seam at the toe, wear them inside out. Next, massage your feet and between the toes, making sure there is absolutely no grit or other debris. Then either roll or bunch the socks up, so the toes can be placed in the toe of the sock. Be sure the seam is across the top of the toes and, if possible, not lapping around the little toe. Now bring the sock up over the rest of the foot and up the leg; use a massaging motion to be sure there are no wrinkles and to detect any rough spots or debris.

Next, remove the insert from your shoe and inspect it. Remove any lint, toe jam, or other debris. Now bang the shoes together sole to sole a couple times and then tap the heel on the ground. Now shake out any debris and reach inside and feel all surfaces for debris or other problems. Replace the inserts and put on your shoes. It sounds complicated, but the whole process takes less than a minute and can prevent many foot problems.

—Rick Schick, ultrarunner and physician's assistant

Tossing Socks

This is a quiz. Of all the socks in your sock drawer, how many should have been tossed out months ago? I'll bet you have at least two or three pairs of socks that should have been aimed at the wastebasket a long time ago. Maybe even more. So how do you know when to toss out a pair of socks? Actually, it's fairly easy. After washing socks, put your hand inside and feel around. Then turn them inside out and check them again. Here are eight tips that indicate socks should be tossed out.

■ Can you see your fingers through the weave of the fabric?

■ Can you see threadbare areas, typically on the heels?

■ Are there holes in the toes, or anywhere else for that matter?

■ Is the inside starting to unravel?

■ Are any areas thinner in cushioning than the rest of the fabric around that area?

■ Is the top cuff around your ankle starting to come apart?

■ Is the toe seam bothersome?

■ Is the top cuff no longer supportive, hanging down your ankle?

■ *Here's an added tip.* Don't check just your old socks. Check them all. I once ran in a fairly new pair of brand-name socks and developed a hot spot on one heel. Taking my shoe off, I discovered the sock was defective and the weave on the heel had separated. I had no more than 60 miles on the sock— but saved it for when I do foot-care clinics as an example of a sock to toss.

When the weather gets colder and you switch to warmer socks, make sure they fit in your shoes. Warmer socks may be thicker socks, with a combination of fabrics and possibly a denser weave. The problem is that thicker socks squeezed into shoes not made for them can cause constriction of blood vessels and impede circulation to the feet. Be sure you can wiggle your toes in the toe box and your heels are not too cramped.

Although I usually inform athletes of their foot-care options and advise them to make the best choices for them, I have three absolutes. The first deals with socks. Serious athletes should avoid 100% cotton socks like the plague and always use moisture-wicking socks. The second absolute is covered in the chapter on gaiters (see page 162) and the third in the chapter on toe problems (see page 298). And yet some athletes prefer common cotton crew socks, while others swear by synthetic socks or synthetic double-layer socks. If cotton crew socks work for you, continue using them. If, however, hot spots and/or blisters plague you, consider trying other types of socks. Some have discovered socks with individual toes and like these because they avoid dirt and grime collecting between the toes and causing friction.

For my first 24-hour track run in 1984, I wore thick cotton socks and used gobs of petroleum jelly on my feet. That was what everyone else seemed to be doing, so that was what I did. It didn't take long for blisters to develop on my heels and toes, which reduced me to a slow walk. Even so, I managed to get in a respectable 103 miles. Without the early foot problems, I am sure I could have done another 10 miles. I learned the hard way what did not work on my feet and set out to find what did work.

Not everyone needs a primer on how to put on your socks, but it is important to know a few tricks. Although it seems like a simple thing, it can make the difference between sore, blistered feet and happy feet.

Clean socks can feel heavenly. Wash your socks inside out to do a thorough job of cleaning the inside fibers and washing off any extra lint. When hiking, wash yesterday's socks and let them dry on the back of your pack. Try to change socks several times during a 100-mile run and once during a 50-mile run. During multiday events, try to change socks several times a day. If clean socks are unavailable from your crew, try to wash the dirty socks so they are clean for later use.

You may be one of a growing number of athletes who wear socks inside out. Rob Langsdorf recommends turning your socks inside out to help prevent blisters: "Most socks have a rib near the toe where the sock is pulled together. The manufacturers put this on the inside of the sock, so it looks nice. Unfortunately it tends to rub the tops and sides of the toes and can cause blisters."

At summer's end, the usefulness of many of your shoes and socks may also be coming to an end. Go through your drawers, and answer the questions on the previous page. If you answer "yes" to any of these eight questions, toss the socks. Socks are relatively inexpensive. Sure, some cost upward of $15–$20, but as with other gear, there comes a time when it is necessary to clean out your drawers. Just remember, when you go shopping for new ones, be sure to get moisture-wicking socks.

Sock Fibers and Construction

Socks come in a variety of fabrics: cotton, cotton blends, synthetics, silk, wool and wool blends, and fleece. An overview of these materials provides insights into their uses. Read the product information on the sock's packaging and try several types to find those that work best for you.

The weave of the sock will vary depending on the material. Socks will range from a loose weave to a dense weave. A loose weave feels coarse and provides less insulation. A dense weave feels softer and generally offers more cushioning. Put your hand inside a sock and stretch the foot portion with your fingers to see the weave. Denser-weave socks will show less space between the fibers.

Double-layer socks can help reduce or eliminate blisters. The two layers moving against each other instead of against the skin reduces skin friction. Most double-layer socks utilize wicking properties to move moisture away from the feet. Before wearing any double-layer sock, align the layers with your hand and then roll the socks onto the foot for the best fit.

More than a few sock companies are making anatomically correct socks for the right and left feet. Some sock companies are making socks designed specifically

Natural, Synthetic, and Combination Materials

COTTON socks provide no wicking or insulating properties, and therefore moisture is retained against the skin. In damp or wet cotton, your feet are generally wet, cold, and more prone to blistering. Do yourself a favor and avoid 100% cotton socks.

COTTON BLENDS containing spandex, nylon, rayon, and acrylic offer a limited advantage over a pure cotton sock.

SYNTHETICS offer protection against blisters caused by moisture, poor fit, hot spots, slippage, and friction. These are made of hydrophobic materials, meaning they don't like moisture or water. Moisture-wicking fabrics such as Capilene, CoolMax, Olefin, and polypropylene wick moisture and perspiration away from the skin to the outer layer of the sock. Synthetic insulators such as Hollofil, Thermax, and ThermaStat help provide insulation. Some of these socks have a single layer, while others have double layers. Most synthetic socks use one of the above fabrics blended with cotton, nylon, spandex, or acrylic.

SILK socks are slick and are generally used as liners. Offering low wicking properties and low heat retention, they do not dry as fast as the newer synthetics.

WOOL wicks while retaining its cushioning. Many sock companies use soft merino wool for durability and comfort. Merino wool can hold up to 30% of its weight in moisture without feeling damp while retaining its ability to generate heat. It also excels in both cold and hot temperatures.

WOOL BLENDS are comfortably warm in winter and cool in summer. Socks made from worsted wool are soft and durable. Merino wool, from sheep with a lighter and softer coat, is less resilient but very soft and comfortable. Wool may also be blended with other fabrics.

FLEECE socks are soft, provide exceptional warmth, and dry faster than wool, but can be looser in shape.

for women. These socks have a more rounded toe and flex-stretch heels designed for a woman's feet. Many companies are making socks with either antibacterial or antimicrobial properties.

Technology is moving faster than we can keep up—even in socks. The following are examples of socks utilizing technology to make them better fitting, better functioning, and longer wearing.

- **DRYMAX** makes socks with a Moisture Removal System, which keeps feet dry with superhydrophobic (water-repelling) fibers. Moisture is lifted off the skin and moved to the outer sock layer. Tests show Drymax socks to be up to 25 times drier than other socks.

- **INJINJI** makes toe socks with a four-point anatomical molding system. These Tetrasoks are constructed without seams. With individual toes to protect each toe, they help those prone to toe blisters. Made with CoolMax or wool, nylon, and spandex, they conform to the shape of your feet and toes.

■ **FARM TO FEET** has developed their Blackburg Water Sock with a combination of nylons and elastic yarns in a unique design that allows water to drain quickly, dries quickly, and provides UV protection. PTFE-coated nylon fibers create a frictionless feel.

■ **SENSORIA FITNESS SMART SOCKS** harness new technology by embedding electronic threads and textile sensors, and pair these with thin anklets on the tops of the socks. These are paired with a smartphone app to capture step count, cadence, and foot strike forces. The full system also has a heart rate monitor for full data capture and a virtual coach in your ear.

■ **ARMASKIN ANTI-BLISTER SOCKS** offer a layer of dermal protection, engineered for extreme endurance athletes. These are thin but tight fitting and are worn under your normal socks. The Si Fusion coating sticks to the skin and prevents any friction generation next to the skin. In addition, the Si Fusion hydrophobic inner layer pushes moisture to the outer layer and is bacteriostatic so the socks can be worn for long periods of time. ArmaSkin's smooth outer fabric reduces friction by allowing the outer sock and shoe to move harmlessly over the foot—preventing blisters. They recommend not using any lubricant inside their socks—other than a small dab between toes as needed.

■ **COMPRESSION SOCKS** go over the calf and stimulate circulation in the muscles, providing support and enhancing stamina. By applying graduated pressure to the lower extremities, starting at the foot and up to the calf, blood is returned more rapidly to the heart and lungs. The patented technology shows a quicker return of oxygenated blood to the legs and reduces fatigue.

■ **BLISTER GUARD** technology utilizes Teflon as a low-friction fiber that prevents hot spots that cause blisters, abrasions, and calluses. The Teflon fibers are woven into the fabric of the sock at the toes, forefoot, and the heels. These socks have undergone strenuous tests, achieving an 80%–100% reduction of blisters, and they are being marketed by various sock companies with combinations of traditional fibers such as acrylic, wool, nylon, and polyester, as well as performance fibers such as CoolMax and spandex. Look for the Blister Guard symbol.

ArmaSkin is a company utilizing cutting-edge technology in its socks. Its anti-blister socks made with a Si Fusion coating fit tight to reduce friction while giving a dermal-like layer of skin protection. The socks are made in Australia, making them harder to find, but their positive features make the search worthwhile. The unique sock design shows how companies are making products that stand out in a crowded field.

Drymax sports socks are a great example of a leading-edge sock company. Its socks' inner Drymax fibers are water hating, while the outer polyester layer is water loving. This combination helps keep the skin dryer than other socks. In addition, it has incorporated friction-free Blister Guard technology, MicroZap antimicrobial technology, Moisture Removal System technology, color sizing marks, seamless design, five sizes for truer fit, and five density levels of protective padding. Its running sock line offers socks for regular, trail, cold-weather, hot-weather, and maximum-protection running. It is constantly tweaking its designs to increase effectiveness. Drymax advises athletes not to use lubricants or powders when wearing its socks.

Buying Socks

Buy socks that fit your feet. The heels, toes, and length should fit snugly without sagging or being stretched too tight. Socks that are too big will bunch up and cause friction and skin irritation. Socks that are too small can cause the toes and joints to rub harder against the socks. Turn the socks inside out and look at the toe seams. Avoid those with bulky seams because they can rub, causing hot spots and blisters. Tube socks have no place in an athlete's sock drawer. After buying socks, be sure to try them on with your shoes or boots to be sure they fit together and are not too tight. Remember also to discard socks when they become threadbare and too thin to provide their advertised benefits. The heels of your socks are a good indication of the amount of padding and loft.

The correct sock is one that fits your foot and fills the inside of the shoe. Being too tight or too thick can constrict circulation and lead to problems, especially in cold weather. Rubbing can lead to hot spots, which lead to blisters. Changing to thinner socks can cause extra movement of the foot inside the shoe, leading to friction, hot spots, and, you guessed it, blisters.

Many stores offer a basket of socks to use when trying on shoes and boots. Avoid these if possible, and instead use your own socks when shopping. This way you will get to feel the fit with your personal socks and avoid picking up a foot fungus from another shopper.

Many people will pick a brand of socks and stick with them. That's fine, but remember, sock manufacturers have made tremendous advances in sock construction. There are many fantastic socks being made, and you owe it to yourself to check them out.

A survey of finishers of the 2015 Western States 100-Mile Endurance Run about sock brands found that 31.5% wore Injinji, 17.6% wore Drymax, 7.6% wore Balega, 7.6% wore SmartWool, and 4.6% wore Swiftwick. The other runners (about 30%) wore a mix of other brands.

Sock designs and the sock market change so fast that company websites are the best source of information for specific lines of socks. Each company introduces new versions of their socks each year. New fabrics and combinations of fabrics make the sock selection ever changing. Your local stores will have displays of many of these socks, or check out the websites listed on pages 104–105 (and there are many more

TIP: Go for the Garter

Sock garters can prevent socks from slipping and getting wrinkled inside of the shoe, which can lead to blisters and hot spots. This is especially true when feet are wet either from rain, stream crossings, or excessive perspiration. It also is more of a problem on trails with steep climbs and descents, although it can also happen when hiking on dry, level surfaces. Making a sock garter can help to prevent the problem.

Go to a craft store or sewing supply center and buy a couple feet of 1.25-inch-width elastic, the kind used in clothing. Be sure to get the ribbed or roll-proof variety. Measure around your leg at the narrowest point, just above the ankle, and then make a loop of the elastic about a half inch shorter. When placed over the sock at that point, the garter should feel snug but not tight.

---

sock manufacturers out there). Investigate your sock options and talk to others about their preferences to determine which socks may be best for your sporting needs.

When you purchase socks, spend a moment reading the washing instructions. With most performance socks, you should not use bleach and fabric softeners as these may break down the fibers.

If you have a hard time finding the socks you want, check out the website thesockcompany.com.

Specialty Socks

The following sections identify specific socks for running and hiking, compression socks, sock liners, and high-technology oversocks. Many of these socks may be used for running, hiking, and adventure racing. Check them out at a store near you to feel them and read their packaging information. The products listing at the end of this chapter notes which companies make socks for each type of sport.

Running Socks

The list of companies making running socks seems endless. Even shoe companies are having socks made under their label. Most are moisture wicking and are offered in road and trail styles, a variety of heights, and a mix of fabric blends. Many runners swear by their favorite sock brand and style. Two innovative companies are Injinji, with its toe socks, and Drymax, with its unique interwoven fiber technologies that make up its moisture-control system.

Hiking Socks

Hiking socks are different from running socks. Hikers most often wear crew or high-top socks. Some wear a wool outer sock with a liner that has wicking properties. Hikers could also try the thinner double-layer wicking socks in a crew style. These wear well, wick moisture away, and are made to reduce the possibility of blisters. Ellsworth V-Channel socks have vapor channels to carry sweat vapors through the channels and off the foot—keeping the foot drier. The channels run from the toes to the heels.

Pacific Crest Trail hiker Matthew Jankowicz used to get blisters, especially on long hikes over 20 miles a day. He tried tape, moleskin, and different kinds of boots. Finally, he switched to wearing three pairs of socks and it worked. He uses one pair of wicking socks over which he wears two pairs of boot socks. Matthew says, "I know some people think I'm crazy, but it works very well for me and I have hiked thousands of miles this way without getting any blisters on my feet."

Another hiker, going by the trail name of Morning Glory, found that wearing a thin liner sock, a Thorlos sock, and finally a wool-blend hiking sock worked well. She bought boots with enough room to accommodate the three pairs of socks. When wearing heavy socks for winter or otherwise, wear a boot a half size larger than normal. If you wear your normal size boot, it compresses the heavy sock and at best you gain little in the way of insulation. In the worst case, it is so tight that it inhibits blood flow to the toes and results in frostbite.

Sock Liners

Sock liners are thin and smooth, and they are usually worn under a heavier insulating or cushioning sock, typically wool. They are lightweight and quick drying. Most liners are made from hydrophobic fibers to wick moisture away from the foot and into the outer sock. A liner will perform in tandem with the outer sock the same way as double-layer socks; friction will occur between the two layers and not against the skin, reducing the chance of blisters. When shopping for liners, look for a style with wicking properties. While many runners are converting to the double-layer socks, some still prefer a two-sock system using liners.

Compression Socks

Compression socks have become popular in the past few years. These unique over-the-calf socks provide graduated compression that stimulates circulation in the foot and ankle with snug compression that tapers off higher up the sock. The improved circulation and reduced fatigue is reported to lead to better performance, reduced swelling, higher VO2 (maximal oxygen consumption) levels, and faster recovery. Some companies make compression calf sleeves.

Many users report a reduction in foot pain, swelling, and aches. Compression socks can also help in reducing postexercise muscle soreness. Delayed onset muscle soreness (DOMS) is a common experience following unaccustomed "eccentric" exercise. In a study, subjects volunteered to perform a single bout of backward downhill walking exercise for 30 minutes. Following this exercise, subjects were required to wear graduated compression stockings for 5 hours per day for three consecutive days on one leg while the second leg had their normal sock. Muscle soreness and neuromuscular measurements on both legs were taken pre- and postwalk, then at 2, 24, 48, and 72 hours postwalking exercise. There was a 28% reduction in DOMS on the leg wearing compression socks 72 hours after exercise. Additionally, the leg wearing the compression socks started to recover contractile properties within 24 hours, but not the other leg. It is theorized that in this study the compression socks might have had the effect of compressing the muscle tissue to such an extent that less structural damage occurred relative to a control condition. Compression socks accelerated the recovery of the muscle force capacity at 24 hours beyond that achieved by the control condition.[18]

Robert Conenello, a podiatrist and past president of the American Academy of Podiatric Sports Medicine, says the theory is that compression socks will increase oxygen delivery and decrease muscle fatigue. He stresses that most of the studies are anecdotal, but if an athlete perceives a benefit, he's all for wearing them.

There are many sock companies making compression socks for athletes. Oxysox was the early entry in this new field. Skins Sport Sox is a spandex compression sock with a stirrup under the foot rather than a whole-foot sock and is worn under other socks. CW-X's compression socks reportedly support the arch and calf and stabilize the ankle. SIGVARIS Athletic Recovery Socks offer graduated compression technology. 2XU's compression socks come in a Run Sock and a Recovery Sock. CEP is a leader in medical compression that makes running socks, graduated socks, and calf sleeves. Zensah also makes compression socks and calf sleeves.

Because of the height, compression socks can be warm when temperatures rise. Be observant for heat rash under the socks, especially at the top and bottom where there might be a constricting band. This is particularly important in extreme heat.

If wearing compression socks in a long race, and you need foot-care help from an aid station or your crew, the tightness of the sock's fit will make their removal difficult. Getting compression socks back on, over taped feet, is even harder. At the finish line of 100-mile runs, I've sometimes been forced to cut these socks off because of their tight fit.

Compression socks are something to try to see if they help your performance, injury prevention, and recovery. There is some debate over their usefulness while running, but many agree they have value for recovery.

High-Technology Oversocks

Oversocks are special high-technology socks that combine waterproof technology and the comfort of traditional socks into a somewhat baggy-looking sock. They were developed for anyone who participates in outdoor activities during which feet are exposed to water. They keep feet dry and comfortable even though the shoes or boots may be soaked and muddy. Even though the socks keep water out, your feet will sweat, creating their own moisture. Two tricks are to wear an inner, moisture-wicking sock and to use an antiperspirant on your feet to reduce the amount of sweat.

Be aware of moisture inside your shoes and socks in extreme cold conditions. Sweat and outside moisture can change to ice inside your socks, leading to frostbite.

National champion ultrarunner Roy Pirrung tested the high-technology oversock SealSkinz for a year in all kinds of weather. Roy recalls his win at the 100K Glacial Trail Run, a grueling race through the wet Kettle Moraine State Forest in

Wisconsin: "It had rained the day before and conditions were sloppy. As other runners stopped every 10 miles to change their wet socks, I just raced ahead. I ended up finishing the race within 25 seconds of the course record and without any blisters." In wet and cold conditions, oversocks can work wonders. Roy found that SealSkinz have helped him to train outside in –25°F weather with a windchill factor of –80°F. His feet "stayed warm, dry, and comfortable."

SealSkinz Hydrostop socks are seamless waterproof socks that use Aqua Dynamic Design (ADD) technology. The socks are made with a hydrophilic membrane so they are waterproof and windproof and they stretch. An inner merino wool blend liner wicks moisture away from the skin while a middle layer of vapor-permeable membrane allows perspiration to escape and prevents water from entering. The outer layer uses nylon for abrasion resistance and durability. Their seamless design gives them a positive edge in preventing blisters. Their socks made with Hydrostop are fully immersible, and their revolutionary in-cuff seal ensures a tight, waterproof fit to keep out everything from water to grit.

Many adventure racers use SealSkinz socks to keep their feet free of blisters; abrasions caused by dirt and grime; and the effects of water immersion during their long, multiday competition. Adventure racer Rebecca Rusch was on Team Montrail at the Primal Quest Adventure race in Telluride, Colorado, where the team used SealSkinz to help them to a second-place finish. Rebecca says, "The only thing I've found for keeping out grit and sand (and leeches) are SealSkinz socks. I've used them in Borneo, Philippines, and Vietnam, and I will use them in Fiji. They're hot in these environments but keep your feet clean and healthy."

Hanz Waterproof socks are very similar to SealSkinz socks. The company offers several designs: Lightweight Waterproof socks in over-the-calf and crew lengths, a calf-length Submerge Waterproof sock, and a crew-length ChillBlocker insulated and waterproof sock. Hanz uses a three-layer construction with a Moisture Vapor Transfer membrane, and its socks are stretch-to-fit and seamless.

Rocky Gore-Tex socks are waterproof, breathable, and designed to be worn over a pair of thin wicking socks. The socks have a Gore-Tex membrane laminated between inner and outer fabric layers. The inner seams are sealed with Gore-Seam tape. The sole and bottom panel are made of a nonstretch Gore-Tex fabric to increase durability and prevent slippage. The upper panels are stretchable Gore-Tex fabric for flexibility and conformity to the foot's shape. A spandex cuff helps the socks stay up.

Several other sock companies offer waterproof socks. Dexshell and Showers Pass each have a line of waterproof socks in crew and over-the-ankle styles.

eZeefit makes full-foot booties out of an ultrathin fabric like neoprene but super thin and supple. They insulate even when wet, and prevent rubbing and friction.

Seirus Stormsocks rely on closed-cell insulation to provide warmth for winter activities. They are made from four-way stretch neoprene with breathable macroporous technology to prevent moisture buildup while sealing in body heat. These socks have a nylon fabric on either side of the neoprene that allows moisture to pass through. The regular Stormsock has an outer layer of Lycra and an inner membrane of high-technology Weather Shield that stops wind and water, and it is lined with Polartec fleece. The Hyperlite Stormsock is fleece lined. Both socks have seams that are not sealed.

Whatever type of oversock you are wearing, it is recommended to test whether water will get inside the socks through the top cuff. Simply stand in a bucket that has enough water to cover the top of the sock. If the cuff is loose fitting, water may get inside. Once water has gone down the leg into the sock, the wicking process slows or stops, depending on the amount of water in the sock. Over time, the body's heat combined with the wicking action of the liner may dry the inside of the socks, but this depends on both the amount of water inside the sock and the degree of activity. Roy Pirrung recommends wearing tights over the cuffs to provide a covering seal.

Try any type of oversocks before a competitive event. You may find that they do not work on your feet. Some athletes roll the tops down when not going through water to ventilate the feet. Oversocks work best when used with a CoolMax or other wicking material sock liner. This further enhances moisture dispersion as well as comfort. Care must be taken when pulling the socks on or off to avoid tearing the inner membrane. A torn membrane will allow water to penetrate at the tear site.

Going Sockless

In 1973 a running magazine advertised "new, lean, and luxurious—the first sockless athletic shoe." After three years of development, Bare Foot Gear offered the "original sockless shoe" with prime leather inside and out, no staples or nails, no seams or ridges, and no textiles to touch your foot, just unpainted and unsealed leather. Cupping the foot only at the heel and instep, it offered a large space up front for flexion and good air circulation. It claimed that with a drier foot, friction is minimized. Looking at the ad today, we might find humor in the ad's claim: "Most men prefer no socks because of the sheer maleness of the feel."

Some people prefer not to wear socks in their shoes. Matt Mahoney found that for him, the best way to prevent blisters was to train for them. Walking barefoot and sometimes running barefoot on grass, dirt, or sand toughened the skin on his feet. He does not wear socks with shoes but rotates between several brands of shoes to develop calluses at every spot that could rub. Matt found that socks caused his feet to slide around inside his shoes, and he couldn't grip the trail on steep hills. When he finds spots rubbing, he uses tape, petroleum jelly, or a blister pad.

Running in shoes without socks takes time and careful monitoring of your feet to avoid problems. Matt has conditioned his feet by walking a mile barefoot on roads every day. He estimates that he runs 15% of the time barefoot on grass and dirt and the other 85% in shoes without socks. He has strengthened the small muscles and tendons in his feet. The skin on the bottom of his feet has toughened to provide some

TIP: New Life for Old Bags

An alternative to oversocks is to put on a pair of thick socks and then a soft plastic bag over the feet, finally adding a thin outer sock. The inner socks, in the plastic bags, will get damp from body sweat and heat, but will stay reasonably comfortable compared to totally wet feet. The plastic bags that bread or newspapers come in work well, but check them first for leaks by blowing in them and squeezing them lightly while holding them closed.

SOCK PRODUCTS

In addition to the sock companies listed below, many shoe and boot companies, and even some insole companies, also offer their own brands of socks.

ACORN FLEECE SOCKS (hiking socks) acorn.com

ARMASKIN ANTI-BLISTER SOCKS (endurance socks for running and hiking) armaskin.com

BALEGA INTERNATIONAL (running and trail running socks) balega.com

BAYSIX (running socks) baysixusa.com

BRIDGEDALE (running and hiking socks) bridgedale.com

CEP (compression socks) cepcompression.com

CW-X (compression socks) cw-x.com

DAHLGREN (hiking socks) dahlgrenfootwear.com

DARN TOUGH VERMONT (running and hiking socks) darntough.com

DEFEET (running socks) defeet.com

DEXSHELL WATERPROOF SOCKS (oversocks) always-outside.com

DRYMAX SPORTS (running and hiking socks) drymaxsports.com

ELLSWORTH V-CHANNEL SOCKS (hiking socks) ellsworthandcompany.com

EZEEFIT (oversocks) ezeefitsports.com

FARM TO FEET (sports socks with merino wool) farmtofeet.com

FEETURES (running and hiking socks) feeturesrunning.com

FITSOK (running socks) fitsok.com

FOX RIVER (running, hiking, and liner socks) foxsox.com

HANZ WATERPROOF SOCKS (oversocks) hanzusa.com

HILLY (running socks from Britain) hillysocks.com

ICEBREAKER (running and hiking socks) icebreaker.com

INJINJI (running and hiking socks) injinji.com

LORPEN (running and hiking socks) lorpen.com

degree of protection for running barefoot. If trying to go without socks, check your shoes for rough seams or ridges that can cut into your feet. Like Matt, use tape or a lubricant on areas that rub. Matt strongly believes that we need to "learn to run in simple shoes, sandals, or barefoot as people have done for thousands of years before Nike." Barefoot running and hiking is becoming more accepted. See the "Barefoot and Minimalist Footwear" chapter for more on this trend.

OXYSOCKS (compression socks) revelsports.com/oxysox.asp

PATAGONIA (hiking socks) patagonia.com

POINTÉ (wool socks) point6.com

POWERSOX (running socks) powersox.com

PROSOK are made with bamboo (running and hiking socks) prosok.com

REI socks (all types of socks for the outdoors) rei.com

ROCKY GORE-TEX WATERPROOF SOCKS (oversocks) rockyboots.com

SAVE OUR SOLES (running socks) sossocks.com

SEALSKINZ SOCKS (oversocks) sealskinz.com

SEIRUS STORMSOCKS (oversocks) seirus.com

SENSORIA FITNESS SMART SOCKS (socks with sensors) sensoriafitness.com

SHOWERS PASS CROSSPOINT WATERPROOF SOCKS (oversocks) showerspass.com

SIGVARIS ATHLETIC RECOVERY SOCKS (compression socks) sigvaris.com

SKINS (compression socks) skins.net

SMARTKNITACTIVE SOCKS (running socks) smartknitactive.com

SMARTWOOL (running, hiking, and liner socks) smartwool.com

SOF SOLE (running socks) sofsole.com

SWIFTWICK SOCKS (running and hiking socks) swiftwick.com

TEKO SOCKS (running and hiking socks) tekoforlife.com

THORLOS (running and hiking socks) thorlo.com

2XU (compression socks) 2xu.com

WIGWAM (running, hiking, and liner socks) wigwam.com

WRIGHTSOCK (running socks) wrightsock.com

X-SOCKS (running and hiking socks) x-socks.com

ZENSAH (compression socks and sleeves) zensah.com

Part Three

Prevention

Making Prevention Work

The Sixth Law of Running Injuries:
Treat the cause, not the effect. Because each running injury
has a cause, it follows that the injury can never be cured
until the causative factors are eliminated.
—Tim Noakes, MD, Lore of Running[19]

Tim Noakes's sixth law of running injuries must be heeded—any running injury can be cured only after the cause is found and eliminated. All of us who run, hike, or adventure race at some point have problems with our feet or sustain foot injuries. The prevention chapters are numerous and lengthy because many factors contribute to foot problems and injuries, and for every factor, there is a preventive measure that can reduce or eliminate it. Prevention is the key to saving your feet. Dave Scott, a good friend and ultrarunner, put the foot problem in proper perspective: "When you don't take care of your feet during a long run or race, each step becomes a reminder of your ignorance."

It's very easy to relinquish our responsibility for preparedness and let someone else dictate what we should do. We tend to listen to those whom we look up to and to those who are more experienced. In many ways this is OK, and it is often the way it should be. However, only you can determine what works for your feet.

Knowing your prevention options is important. But you also need to know what *your* feet need and how to do it before you have to do it. I have patched thousands feet at ultras and adventure races and have found that most athletes have a fairly good knowledge base of what they should be doing. They know it's smart to wear the right kind of socks and to have footwear that fits well. Many have also made foot-care kits for their crews. I would guess that about 30%–40% are well versed in what their feet need and how to do it. The other 60%–70% just wing it. They've read about foot care, but somehow it falls lower on the priority list than does training, finding foods they can tolerate, locating the right flashlight for night running, and other choices. So they start their race and manage well for a while—until problems develop.

Ultrarunner Gillian Robinson shares a story from one of her long races that illustrates what all athletes need to learn:

> I sat for a shoe change and foot fix-up. I wasn't exactly sure what to do with my feet. I had taped the balls of my feet and my big toes. The big-toe taping wasn't working out so well. On the left, it had rubbed the next toe to cause a big ugly blister that had to be lanced. On the right, maybe the taping was too tight, because the big toenail was bruised at the base. I put 2nd Skin on the left toe and taped it up with Micropore tape. For the right toe, I just cut off the existing tape and hoped for the best. I sprayed my feet with Desenex to cool them down and dry them out, and then smeared them all over with a lubricant. I changed to new socks and different shoes. I felt a lot better. My toes didn't feel perfect, but better.

To have and keep healthy feet, you have to know what works for them in the sports in which you participate. You also have to know what to do when what worked no longer works—in other words, a fallback plan with the equipment to implement it and the knowledge to use it.

Hard-Won Lessons

- Understand the concept of shear and how it causes blisters, and then how friction, heat, and moisture factor in.
- Learn what lubricant works, but have a container of powder handy.
- Learn what socks work, but have one or two extra pairs of other types.
- Learn how to tape your toes, heels, and every other part of your feet just in case blisters form.
- Learn how to tape like a pro, and then practice taping, and then practice some more. Then start over until your taping is perfect.
- Learn how to lance blisters and patch over them.
- Learn what happens to your feet when you don't change wet socks. Your feet become macerated and feel as though one humongous blister is covering the bottom of each foot.
- Learn that something simple, such as properly trimming and filing your toenails, can prevent toe blisters and even black toenails.

The bottom line is that if you don't consciously learn what works for your feet, you will learn the hard way. Prevention is *proactive*. Time spent being proactive in preventing problems will pay off in the long run. Taking a proactive approach will mean that you spend less time being *reactive* to problems when you have neither the time to spare nor readily available materials.

The key to making prevention work is to find what works for you in the environment where you will use it. In other words, try the fix in the context in which it will be used. When you are trying to find what works for you on trails, running

Tried-and-True Foot Care

The four keys to winning any extreme sport are having a strong mental attitude, working as a team rather than as an individual, keeping hydrated, and having a great foot-care regimen. After every race my team and I are generally the only ones without bloody, blistered feet. Everyone wants to know my secret, so here it is!

■ Spray feet with compound tincture of benzoin spray. This provides a tough protective layer where blisters usually form. Be careful not to apply too much or in the creases of the feet as it will crack and dry the skin.

■ Put a thin layer of Hydropel around the feet over the compound tincture of benzoin. Note: Hydropel is no longer available so consider one of the following: SportSlick, Trail Toes, ChafeX, or RunGoo.

■ It is essential to keep feet comfortable and dry, so I put on a pair of liner socks (I recommend Wigwam) followed by a pair of SealSkinz waterproof socks. SealSkinz come in a variety of styles, but I recommend either the insulated socks (for colder conditions), over-the-calf socks, or their sock with in-cuff seal to keep water out even when feet are submerged!

■ Wear a pair of boots or running shoes that are very lightweight but stable enough to handle rigorous terrain (every ounce counts in racing). When wearing running shoes, choose a lightweight model that allows water to squeeze out as you run.

■ Add a pair of gaiters to further prevent grit, dirt, and small rocks from getting in the boots, which will help prevent unnecessary friction and abrasions.

■ Use a pair of adjustable walking poles (I use Leki poles) to help distribute weight throughout the body every step of the way. Poles are great for balance on the downhills and help prevent feet from taking a pounding.

—Cathy Sassin, globe-trotting adventure racer

---

on roads will not typically provide the same results as actually running on trails. Walking around town wearing a backpack and your hiking boots is not the same as hiking on a rocky trail with uneven terrain. It may help to break in your boots but will not give the same feeling as a rough, rocky trail. I made my own gaiters for trail running after determining that the dirt getting into my shoes was causing hot spots and blisters. Getting out on the roads or trails will help you determine whether your footwear fits and if there are problems to correct. That's being proactive.

Mike Palmer has spent years finding what works for his feet: "This can be one hell of a frustrating process—you may have an overwhelming urge to throw in the towel and take up playing chess instead. One runner will swear on his mother's grave that such and such a thing solved his problem, but his solution won't work at all for you." It cannot be overstressed; you must find what works for your feet. Taking the time to learn what works for your feet is the key to being proactive.

Cathy Sassin knows what her feet need. One of the top adventure racers in the United States, she has trekked across the sands of Utah and South Africa, the volcanoes of Ecuador, and the glaciers of British Columbia and Patagonia. She has bushwhacked through Maine, gone spelunking through Borneo, paddled and ridden through New Zealand and Australia, and raced across New England. Cathy sums up the method behind her success on the facing page.

Blister Prevention:
The New Paradigm

The one problem with our feet that we experience most often—which drives us crazy, costs us time, and, in some cases, leads to unfulfilled dreams—is blisters. Although the rest of the book deals with all aspects of foot care, the prevalent theme is keeping our feet healthy by preventing dreaded blisters.

This new edition will change the way you think about blister formation. In the past, and for as far back as I can remember, it was friction, heat, and moisture that combined in one form or another to cause blisters. It was thought that excessive pressure caused the friction, heat, and moisture. The three factors are still relevant, but there is more to learn. The new and important word is "shear."

This chapter takes a new look at blister prevention. We'll start with how blisters form, followed by a look at shear and its relation to five factors in blister formation. Finally, we'll look at 13 components that can be used in blister prevention and how everything fits together. For those who want to delve deeper, a short history of blister studies is included at the end of the chapter.

The complete picture of
5 Blister Formation Factors and
13 Blister Prevention Components

Blister Formation

To talk about blister prevention, we need to look at how blisters form. Blisters are the result of shear trauma to the skin. When running, every step is "repetitive loading" as the foot moves through the foot strike. The whole of the body's weight is put on the skin and inner tissues, onto the bones and joints, up the leg, into the knees and hips, and into the pelvis and spine. For now, let's focus on the foot. The skin can take a lot of repetitions without a problem, but once skin and tissue damage reaches a painful level, the trauma is escalating rapidly.

Repetitive loading has two components. The first is a vertical loading to the surface of the skin; by itself it is relatively harmless. The second is a repetitive friction loading parallel to the surface of the skin. The two combine to create shear stresses within the skin. When these shear stresses exceed a certain level, micro tears begin to form within the third layer of tissue. As more repetition occurs, more micro tears appear and existing tears grow. These tears in the tissue form a cleft parallel to the skin's surface. The cleft fills with serous fluid and a blister has formed—caused by shear stressors. This typically occurs in the stratum spinosum, the inner fourth layer of the epidermis that is the least resistant to shear.

If the blister is deep or traumatically stressed by continued running or hiking, the serous fluid may contain blood. When the serous fluid lifts the outer layer of epidermis, oxygen and nutrition to this layer is cut off and it becomes dead skin. This outer layer is easily burst. The fluid then drains and the skin loses its natural protective barrier. The underlying skin is raw and sensitive. At this point, the blister is most susceptible to infection.

Rebecca Rushton, an Australian podiatrist and the author of *The Blister Prone Athlete's Guide to Preventing Foot Blisters,* has studied extensively about blister formation. She has identified four requirements for shear that cause foot blisters to form:[20]

1. Skin resilience: The skin on our feet is, by its very nature, susceptible to blister formation. Repeated gradual exposure to shear can improve the skin's ability to withstand shear stress. Often times the skin is stressed by a sudden increase, or an increase over many days. Examples include increasing one's mileage too quickly and doing more than normal in a multiday event.

2. Moving bone: Bones within the foot move throughout the foot strike. The more they move relative to the skin's surface, the higher the shear stress created, and the more likely you are to develop a blister. An example is the movement of the heel bone underneath the skin as it moves up and down in the shoe's heel counter.

3. Repetition: It's the repetitions throughout the foot strike that increase the odds of a blister forming. Studies show that runners in a multiday event blister more as the race progresses.

4. Friction and normal force: The levels of friction and pressure determine the amount of shear that impacts the skin.

It's worth talking about how blisters will deroof—when the top layer of skin is torn off the top of the blister. Consider a back-of-the-heel blister. A blister has formed because the heel bone has moved up and down while the outer skin has remained fixed inside the sock and shoe. The shear stressors, as described previously, have caused the blister. With repeated levels of movement against the skin on the back of the heel, the skin can be rubbed over and over. This is what causes abrasions. When the forces that cause blisters combine with forces that cause abrasion, the skin is stretched past normal levels and is torn off.

In reality, some people are more blister-prone than others, irrespective of the amount of training and preparation. In spite of having done everything right, the shear strength of their skin is going to be lower than others—no matter what they do. They are simply blister-prone. For others, some of this has to do with the training that they do in preparation for races. It's quite common at races to see lead runners come through aid stations without any blister problems. They typically have conditioned their feet through extensive training. But as the race progresses, the middle- and back-of-the-pack runners enter aid stations with a lot of blister problems. They typically have put fewer miles on their feet and, in some cases, have made poor choices about footwear and foot care.

Understanding Shear

In the chapter "Taping for Blisters," I tell the story of a runner at Badwater whose feet I patched. In short, he had run 90 miles of the 135-mile race, on pavement, in extreme heat. He had Elastikon tape on both balls of the feet. His feet were hurting to the point of quitting. I replaced the Elastikon tape with smoother kinesiology tape, which allowed movement between the tape and his sock, greatly reducing the shear movement between the layers of skin and the bones of his feet. I also added a large ENGO Blister Prevention Patch on each insole under the ball of each foot. By reducing the shear level, the runner was able to finish the race with less pain.

Try to picture the following: As your foot moves through its foot strike, the bones of the foot move against the layers of underlying skin—then you apply a tape that is not smooth to the skin, pull on a sock, and finally put your foot inside a shoe. The tape sticks to the skin. As you run, the foot naturally moves a bit inside your shoes. However, the sock cannot move freely against the coarseness of the tape. The sock and tape move as one, which stresses the outer layer of skin against the inner layers. The only movement is the shearing effect between the layers of skin.

That experience was the first time I made the connection to shear, although I didn't know it by that name. All I knew was the stickiness at the sock–shoe interface, the tape–sock interface, and the tape–skin interface—and one, or all three, had created this major problem for the runner. I never forgot the story. His skin was stuck to the Elastikon tape, the coarse tape didn't move against his sock, and the sock didn't move against the shoe's insole. With the smoother kinesiology tape and the new slipperiness between the tape and the sock, the coefficient of friction was reduced, and in turn shear was reduced.

Shear is a new concept for most athletes, especially as it relates to blisters. Shear is defined as a strain in the structure of a substance when its layers are laterally shifted in relation to each other. Applying the definition to the above example, shear happened between the layers of skin as the bones of the foot moved through the foot strike.

The internal layers of skin are connected. But those connections can break under the stress of shear and the cavity fills with fluid—and you have a blister.

To understand shear, try this. Place the tip of your index finger against the skin on the back of your hand. Keep it stuck to the same bit of skin while you move it back and forth while. See how your skin stretches? The skin on your hand has moved against the underlying bones. That is shear that causes blisters.

Note that nothing has rubbed against the skin. Your finger did not rub the skin.

J. Martin Carlson, the founder of Tamarack Habilitation Technologies, has championed shear as the cause of blisters. Tamarack has a long history of providing innovative orthotic-prosthetic componentry and materials. Their focus on friction management, especially for amputees, has won them many awards and much recognition. This knowledge in turn led to the creation of a new product that can be applied to footwear to reduce high friction levels and, in turn, the shear that leads to blister formation: ENGO Blister Prevention Patches.

Shear in Action

After watching a video on Tamarack's website, I understood more about shear in action. The video showed a cutaway on the heel area of a shoe, showing the sock and foot inside moving through a foot strike motion. In one video, the cutaway showed a sock and foot on an insole where there were high levels of friction. The sock and foot were distorted as they were held against the insole. It was as if they were stuck together. In another video, the sock and foot were on an insole with an ENGO patch underneath. No distortion occurred as the sock and foot moved easily through the foot strike, over the slippery surface of the ENGO patch.

It's important to grasp how shear happens. As described above, shear results in distortion occurring between the skin and soft tissues underneath. This shear distortion is what causes blisters. The bones in our feet move back and forth as they move through each foot strike. When the skin at the bottom of the foot is stuck by high friction (stickiness) to the sock and shoe, the middle tissues are distorted. When this is repeated over and over, traumatic levels are reached and a blister forms. This distortion can happen anywhere on the foot: in an up-and-down motion in the heel, the sides of the foot, and between toes; in a side-to-side motion at the ball of the foot, under the heels, and at the bottom of the toes; and in rotation as the foot moves through its foot strike. As we walk, run, and pivot in our shoes, the surface of our skin incurs a shearing force.

Certain amounts of shear are normal, and our feet can deal with a lot. However, with repeated traumatic levels of shear, blisters will develop. How much is too much? It varies from person to person, and, as described in "Blister Formation" on page 113, some people are simply more blister-prone than others.

Understanding the Five Factors in Blister Formation

For years, we thought blister formation was caused by heat, moisture, and friction. So, ever since the first edition, the image used to show this was a triangle with

A view of the factors in blister formation

heat, moisture, and friction at its three sides. Everyone thought the three factors combined to make the skin more susceptible to blisters. That's what was promoted in articles, running forums, and general discussion. It seemed to make sense.

Then we discovered shear, as you read in the previous section. Shear encircles everything. The image shows a series of four concentric circles where shear is outside as the base on which everything else rests. The next circle contains the five factors that contribute to shear: skin resilience, bone movement, pressure, friction, and moisture. Inside and above them are two additional circles: the first with the five major components of blister prevention and the innermost circle with the remaining eight minor components, which I will explain later. For now, we'll look at the five factors that contribute to shear.

Skin Resilience

Our skin is very resilient. However, repeated stressors to the skin, over time, can cause breakdown. The healing process can't keep up with the ongoing trauma. This is why well-fitting shoes are important. Skin that is thin (like on the top of our feet) will abrade before it blisters, whereas thicker skin (like on the soles of our feet) is more likely to blister. We can make the skin on our feet more resilient by progressively increasing distance over time. This gradual increase of the frequency and magnitude of forces applied to the skin helps change the characteristics of the skin. Reducing calluses and using moisturizers also contributes to skin resiliency.

Bone Movement

As the bones in our feet move back and forth and up and down through the foot strike, and the overlaying skin remains stationary, the soft tissue layers in between stretch in a shearing motion. The more movement, relative to the skin surface, the more chance you'll blister. When that happens, there is stretching and distortion between the inner tissues under the bone. Shoe fit is an important component in controlling bone movement. Changing your biomechanics is another way to work at reducing blister formation.

Pressure

Pressure is vertical force exerted against an object or surface. In this case pressure is the normal force of the foot through the foot strike. The heel comes down, the foot rolls forward onto the forefoot and off the toes. At all of these transitions, there is pressure downward, forward, and most likely side to side. Optimizing the fit of your footwear, correcting any biomechanical issues with an orthotic, and adding cushioning or padding can reduce pressure.

Friction

Mention the word friction to athletes and they most commonly think of rubbing. For instance, "My heel rubbed inside my shoe and created a blister." It may help to know that the dictionary gives two definitions for friction. The one most people think about is the action of two surfaces rubbing against each other. Rubbing can cause abrasions to one or both surfaces, but not a blister. Forget about this definition as we talk about blisters. Let's look at the second definition.

Scientifically, friction is defined as the force that resists one surface sliding against another. It's easiest to view friction in one of two ways. When two surfaces slide easily against each other, we have a slippery connection—and low friction. When two surfaces resist movement against each other, we have a sticky connection—and high friction. Friction is required for shear to reach traumatic levels.

Rebecca Rushton says it well: "There is high friction in your shoe. Surfaces are resisting movement against each other. When your skin is moist, your skin grips your sock; your sock grips your shoe. All three surfaces grip together so your foot doesn't move around in your shoe. But with every step you take, your foot bones are moving under the skin. And while the skin is stuck the bones are moving back and forth. Everything in between is pulled and stretched. This pulling and stretching is what causes blisters. We call it shear."

There is good friction and bad friction. High friction, as Rebecca described, is when things grip together. From this comes traction, which we need for the mechanical efficiency of our gait. Most friction is good, but when high friction causes blisters, it's bad friction, and has to be managed—but only in that specific location. ENGO patches are an example of targeted management of friction. Now let's look at the forces affecting friction, specifically the coefficient of friction.

The Coefficient of Friction

The coefficient of friction (COF) describes the relationship between the force of friction and the normal force between two objects at which sliding is initiated. It is a number that represents the slipperiness or stickiness between two surfaces and is generally below 1.0. Within the shoe, the COF between the foot, sock, and insole can range from 0.5 to 0.9. In contrast the COF between a sock and a polished floor is around 0.2. The lower the number, the better the effectiveness in preventing blister formation.

Here's an example. A runner may have damp feet, creating a moist condition. The COF in his case might be a 0.7. By moving away from the moist condition to either very dry feet or very wet feet, he might reduce his COF to 0.5. If his blister-causing threshold is 0.6, getting to 0.5 will reduce his chance of blistering. Moist skin is higher friction than dry or very wet skin, meaning it's more susceptible to blistering.

Understanding the COF of materials is beneficial to knowing how shear starts and what we can do to reduce blistering. Managing the moisture on the skin, using different socks systems, and using ENGO patches are the easiest ways to reduce the COF. The COF of an ENGO patch is about 0.16 equally against a dry or wet sock, effectively reducing friction by 80%. Compare that to the COF of moleskin against a dry sock of 0.6 and a wet sock of 0.86. Again, the lower the number, the better the result.

Moisture

Moisture is the last factor. Increased moisture leads to an increase in friction. Beyond that, moisture does not cause blisters in any other way. Generally speaking, a lower COF is achieved with dry socks compared to wet. Some degree of moisture control can be gained with moisture-wicking socks, antiperspirants, powders, and some special lubricants. Our feet have approximately 250,000 sweat glands that can produce continuous moisture, without factoring in sweat produced though an increase in body temperature as we engage in physical activity. When active, most athletes have feet that are always damp from moisture. Moisture can also occur from stream crossings, rain, and puddles, as well as from pouring water over our heads to cool us down, which runs down our legs into our shoes.

Other Factors

There are three additional factors worth mentioning, but they are not important enough to warrant lengthy explanations or inclusion on the chart. The first is heat. Heat is not a factor in blister formation, but many athletes equate heat to causing blisters. Heat produces moisture as the feet sweat, leading to a higher COF and an increase in friction levels. But heat does not cause blisters in any other way.

The second is repetition. We can minimize the chance of blisters by reducing repetitions. This can be done by shortening the length of your activity, reducing the level of intensity, and changing the frequency of your activity. But not many athletes will stop running or hiking—so there's little point in talking about reducing repetitions.

The third factor is shear absorption. The less shear absorption in your footwear, the more pressure and friction your skin has to absorb—and that means more chance of blisters. Most of this is covered in cushioning components like socks and insoles as they work to reduce pressure and absorb shear.

The Power of ENGO

Tamarack Habilitation Technologies, a company dedicated to the prevention and relief of skin breakdown for individuals with prosthetic limbs and ortho-pedic braces, created ENGO Blister Prevention Patches in 2004. The patches are designed to prevent blisters and reduce pain from existing blisters. These patches are one of the best products to help athletes that have been released in many years.

ENGO low-friction patches are applied to your shoe, insole, or orthotic—not your skin. The patches are made with three layers: a low-friction outer surface made of polytetrafluoroethylene (PTFE), a fabric backing, and an adhesive. Patches range from small and large ovals to a large rectangle to a shaped strip for heels—and each can be cut to size. These thin patches can greatly reduce friction in targeted locations within your footwear by giving a slick, slippery surface to the area of your footwear or insole where friction is a problem. Socks slide over the patch, reducing the usual drag, which allows the foot's skin and the sock to glide with the underneath bone through the foot strike, reducing shear distortions in that area.

ENGO offers multiple advantages over other blister prevention and treat-ment products:

■ Reduction in friction levels

■ Targeted protection at the specific problem area to reduce friction

■ Durable and can last for months

■ Cost-effective based on its small size and durability

■ Well tolerated because it is placed on and in footwear

■ Takes up virtually no space so it doesn't change the fit of the shoe

ENGO patches can work in footwear to reduce shear, prevent blisters, and provide relief almost anywhere on the foot: the bottom and sides of the heel,

ENGO patches are applied to footwear.

ball of the foot, side of the foot, and arch areas. Patches should be applied to dry and clean footwear, which makes them perfect for proactive prevention.

Sometimes when shoes are wet, patches are applied to dry socks. The section "Overlapping Toes" in chapter 24 describes how ENGO patches can be used to help with this common problem. The patches have many uses, including on bike seats, paddles, tool handles, and more.

Tamarack is always developing new products, for instance, a thin low-friction tape that could be useful for athletes. The best way to connect with Tamarack is through the ENGO website, goengo.com.

The Components of Prevention

Blister prevention takes place through a combination of 13 components. Five are the most major components: fit, socks, ENGO patches, lubricants, and powders. Eight others are minor but still important components: skin-toughening agents, taping, insoles and orthotics, skin care and hydration, antiperspirants for the feet, gaiters, lacing, and changes of socks and shoes.

Within our shoes many things are happening, and everything is related in some way. Where something touches another, we have what we'll call an interface. The basic interfaces are between the skin and sock, the sock and the insole, and the sock and the inside of the shoe. When you put tape on the skin, it adds two more, between the skin and tape, and the tape and the sock. Adding an ENGO patch adds two more. Since the tape and the ENGO patch are stuck to the skin and shoe respectively, the only interfaces we are concerned with are the tape and the sock, and the ENGO patch and the sock. The interface with the lowest COF determines or limits the magnitude of friction. If the tape loosens on the skin, another damaging interface is added.

The Five Major Components

We'll start with the top circle comprised of fit, socks, ENGO patches, lubricants, and powders—the first line of defense against blisters. It's important to remember that these five components and the eight from the next circle all work in some way to reduce shear distortion. They may increase skin resilience; reduce bone movement, pressure, friction, and moisture; absorb shear; or reduce the number of repetitions. Remember that the more you use shear-reducing or shear-absorbing materials in your shoes, the more you are taking that stressor off the skin.

■ **FIT** comes first. You need to start with properly fitting shoes with a quality insole. No matter how well you tape, how good your socks are, or how good any other component is, if the shoes fit incorrectly, you will have problems. If your footwear is too loose, your feet will slide around, creating shear. If your footwear is too tight in certain areas, your feet will experience excessive pressure. Wearing too-loose or too-tight footwear will change the biomechanics of your foot strike, which in turn will affect your gait and throw off your whole stride and balance.

G = Gaiters	I = Insoles and Orthotics
T = Taping	L = Lacing
N = Nutrition and Hydration	A = Antiperspirants
C = Shoe and Sock Changes	S = Skin Tougheners and Adherents

The 13 components of defense against blisters

■ **SOCKS** come in either single- or double-layer construction. Some single-layer socks, particularly those without wicking properties, allow friction to develop between the feet and the socks, which in turn can create blisters. Double-layer socks allow the sock layers to move against each other, which reduces friction between the feet and the socks. Socks can also wick moisture away from the skin. Injinji toe socks give each toe its own sock.

■ **ENGO BLISTER PREVENTION PATCHES** are effective at reducing shear distortion by reducing friction at the skin and sock–shoe interface. The patches are an alternative to taping.

■ **LUBRICANTS** create a shield to reduce friction and protect skin that is in contact with socks during motion. This lubricant shield also reduces chafing.

■ **POWDERS** reduce friction by reducing moisture on the skin, which in turn reduces friction between the feet and the socks.

The Eight Minor Components

Now, imagine another circle made up of eight components that play a strong supporting role in prevention—the second level of defense against blisters. This innermost circle is made up of skin-toughening agents, taping, insoles and orthotics, skin care and proper hydration, antiperspirants for the feet, gaiters, lacing, and frequent sock and shoe changes. Each can contribute to the prevention of blisters and other problems. You could argue that these outer components should be identified as major components, and to some extent you may be right—some components may be more important for your feet than for mine. The trick is to determine what we each need to keep our feet healthy under the stresses of our particular sport. Let's look at each component.

■ **SKIN-TOUGHENING AGENTS** form a coating to protect and toughen the skin. These products also help tape and blister patches adhere better to the skin and lead to a reduction in perspiration.

■ **TAPING** provides a barrier between the skin and socks so friction is reduced. Proper taping adds an extra layer of skin (the tape) to the foot to prevent hot spots and blisters. Taping can also be a treatment if hot spots and blisters develop. ENGO patches can be an alternative to taping or complement taping. Toe caps are silicone gel devices that go over the toes and absorb shear.

■ **INSOLES AND ORTHOTICS** help maintain the foot in a functionally neutral position so arch and pressure problems are relieved. Some also have absorption qualities. Small pads for the feet may also help correct foot imbalances and pressure points. They can be bought over the counter or be custom made for your feet.

■ **SKIN CARE** for the feet includes creams and lotions to smooth and soften dry and callused feet. This also includes good toenail care. Proper hydration can help reduce swelling of the feet so the occurrence of hot spots and blisters is reduced. These all contribute to skin resiliency.

■ **ANTIPERSPIRANTS** for the feet help those with excessively sweaty feet by reducing the moisture that makes the feet more prone to blisters. It's another help in skin resiliency.

■ **GAITERS** provide protection against sand, dirt, rocks, and grit. These irritants cause friction, hot spots, and blisters as shoes and socks become dirty.

■ **SHOELACES** and boot laces often cause friction or pressure problems. Adjusting laces can relieve this friction and pressure and make footwear more comfortable.

■ **FREQUENT CHANGES OF SOCKS AND SHOES** help keep the feet in good condition. Wet or moist socks can cause problems. Changing the socks also gives an opportunity to reapply either powder or lubricant and deal with any hot spots before they become blisters. Sometimes shoes are also changed as they become overly dirty or wet.

Finding the Right Combination

Each athlete needs to find a prevention strategy that works for him or her. One may use a lubricant, another may use Zeasorb powder, and yet another may pre-tape his or her feet. Each may use one of many types and styles of socks. There are many combinations. Remember, the goal of all these components is to reduce shear stress by bone movement, pressure, friction, and moisture; increasing skin resiliency; and absorbing shear. A look at the image will show how the 5 Blister Formation Factors and the 13 Blister Prevention Components are related.

A high-level view of the factors in blister formation and components in blister prevention (see page 121 for legend)

Try any of the suggestions in this book and find those that work for you. Some will and some won't. That's OK, because it's a process. You are gathering information that will help you now, and file away other information that may help you later. Here are two examples of runners using blister prevention components in combination.

Ultrarunner Dave Scott claimed his feet are often "as soft as a baby's bottom" after the 100-mile Western States Endurance Run. Dave found that he rarely had foot problems. He trimmed his toenails, used a small amount of petroleum jelly, and regularly changed his shoes and socks. That is what worked for him.

Ultrarunner Tim Twietmeyer has won the grueling 100-mile Western States Endurance Run five times while accumulating 25 silver belt buckles for finishes less than 24 hours. Over the years, in addition to running ultras, he has enjoyed fast-packing in the California High Sierra. He has found the differences interesting.

A week before running a 100-mile trail ultra, Tim trimmed his toenails as short as possible. The morning of the run he coated his feet with lanolin to reduce friction, provide warmth if running in snow or through water, and make his skin more resilient to getting wrinkled. Then he pulled on a pair of Thorlos Ultrathin socks. His strategy is "that the more sock you wear, the more moisture close to the foot. The more moisture, the more blisters and skin problems." He usually wore the same pair of shoes and socks the entire way. Tim acknowledges, "My feet don't usually have problems, and when they do, I'm close enough to the end to gut it out."

Tim found that fast-packing affected his feet differently. When he hiked the John Muir Trail in 1992 (doing 210 miles in five days and 10 hours), his feet were trashed more than ever before. His group of five experienced ultrarunners averaged 14 hours per day on the rough trail. Tim remembers, "We covered the ground so fast that my feet swelled and I almost couldn't get my shoes on the last day." He used the same strategy of using lanolin and thin socks. Instead of running shoes, he chose lightweight hiking boots. Foot repair became the group's daily ritual as the 40-mile days took their toll. They realized that "an important strategy for keeping our feet from getting any worse was to get that first piece of duct tape on in just the right spot and make it stick. If we did that, our feet held up pretty well." By the end of the fifth day, the last piece of duct tape had been used on their feet. Tim's cardinal rule for fast-packing is to "keep your feet dry." That can be hard to do when fighting afternoon thunderstorms, but when your feet are wet too long, it's only a matter of time before they blister. Whether running ultras or fast-packing, Tim knows the importance of keeping his feet healthy, and he has experimented to find what works well for him.

Both Dave and Tim used a combination of components: skin care, socks, lubricants, taping, toenail care, and changes of shoes and socks in an effort to prevent blisters. Determine what foot problems you normally experience, study this book, and then begin the task of finding what works best for your feet.

We need to understand the importance of other elements that contribute to prevention. Proper strength training and conditioning will help make the foot and ankle stronger and more resistant to sprains and strains. Everything you put on or around your foot becomes related to how well your foot functions. Keep in mind that whatever you do, the aim should be to reduce shear, moisture, bone movement, pressure, and friction, and to increase skin resiliency.

A Short History of Blister Studies

There are relatively few current studies on blister prevention and treatments. In reality, there has been little progress in blister management in recent decades—so blisters remain a common injury for athletes—often with a lot of misunderstanding. Many studies come from the military because of how foot problems can negatively affect soldiers. The rise in popularity of multiday stage races has increased the number of studies coming from those races. Here are three examples of findings from recent studies.

In paper number three (see page 126), it was reported that blisters were the most commonly encountered medical problem, occurring in 17%–40% of participants at continuous ultramarathons and 33%–74% during multistage ultramarathons. It was also noted that they are most likely to occur during the middle of multistage races. The authors said blister care would likely be the most frequent use of medical resources during ultraendurance foot races.

In paper number four (see page 126), paper tape was applied prerace to one foot of 136 participants in a multiday stage race in an effort to see whether the tape would result in a reduction in blisters. Ninety of the 136 completed the study with data collected, and 100% developed blisters, taped or not.

Finally in paper number five (see page 126), a study of 50 runners in a 219-kilometer multistage race found that after day one, 34% had blistered, by day two 54%, by day three 74%, and after the fourth day of running, 76% of the participants had blistered feet. Of the runners who blistered, 82% had multiple blisters. Blister locations were toes, 65%; the ball of the foot, 16%; heel, 14%; and sole, 5%. Not surprisingly, the authors noted that blisters were more painful toward the end of the race. The only predictive marker they found for reduced blister incidence was previous ultramarathon experience (in men). As background, the paper states that blister incidence, localization, pain scores, and risk factors in field conditions are poorly understood.

With the help of Dr. Andy Pasternak, I put together a study at the 2015 Tahoe Rim Endurance Runs, where a team of medical personnel tracked what we saw on runners' feet and what treatment action we provided, along with pre- and postrace surveys. Because we saw many of the runners multiple times at the same aid station, we hope the resulting data will be helpful. We hope to have the study completed in 2016.

So you can see everyone knows that blisters happen and how multiple blisters are common. What is understudied is how the different factors of blister prevention and treatments play into what athletes and medical teams should be doing to reduce the numbers. There are numerous ways to prevent blisters, just as there are numerous ways to treat blisters.

Here are several quotes that are relevant to blisters.

"Little insight or research into the prevention or treatment of the most common foot injury in sport has been produced in the past 30 years. Physicians, coaches and athletic trainers continue to advocate the use of petrolatum jelly and skin powders to prevent blisters while the scientific literature suggests these measures may actually increase the chance of blistering on the feet."

—Doug Richie, 2010

"The research literature clearly indicates that the shear (friction) component of the contact loading is the direct culprit. Pressure is not the direct cause of repetitive loading skin trauma (hot spots, blisters, abrasions, and ulcers). Pressure is a factor that enables the friction/shear to reach traumatic levels."

—J. Martin Carlson, CPO, MS (Engr.)

"Few things applied to the feet will stay intact for more than one hour of vigorous activity. Therefore, measures that focus on footwear may be more efficacious."

—Richie, 2010

In her *Blister Prevention Report: What Every Podiatrist Should Know About Blister Prevention*, Rebecca Rushton lists 36 resources and references for suggested reading.[21] Below are 16 of the studies, plus 5 new studies for those who want to dig deeper into blister research. The 21 are listed in chronological order with the most current at the top. Many of the studies are available through PubMed.gov for a fee.

1. Hashmi, Farina, Suzanne Kirkham, Christopher Nester, and Sharon Lam, "The effect of topical anti blister products on the risk of friction blister formation on the foot," *Journal of Tissue Viability* (2016).

2. Kelly, Rhonda Alice, "The Incidence and Prevention of Foot Problems Among Male Phase One British Army Recruits at an Army Training Regiment," *Journal of the Royal Army Medical Corps* 161, no. S1 (2015): 156–59.

3. Hoffman, Martin D., Andy Pasternak, Ian R. Rogers, Morteza Khodaee, John C. Hill, David A. Townes, Bernd Volker Scheer, Brian J. Krabak, Patrick Basset, and Grant S. Lipman, "Medical Services at Ultra-Endurance Foot Races in Remote Environments: Medical Issues and Consensus Guidelines," *Sports Medicine* 44, no. 8 (2014): 1055–69.

4. Lipman, Grant S., Mark A. Ellis, Erica J. Lewis, Brandee L. Waite, John Lissoway, Garrett K. Chan, and Brian J. Krabak, "A Prospective Randomized Blister Prevention Trial Assessing Paper Tape in Endurance Distances (Pre-Taped)," *Wilderness and Environmental Medicine* 25, no. 4 (2014): 457–61.

5. Scheer, Bernd Volker, Dejan Reljic, Andrew Murray, and Ricardo Jose Soures Costa, "The Enemy of the Feet: Blisters in Ultraendurance Runners," *Journal of the American Podiatric Medical Association* 104, no. 5 (2014): 473-78.

6. Scherer, Paul, "The Case for Friction Management," *Podiatry Management* 31, no. 7 (2012): 111–16.

7. Richie, Doug, "How to Manage Friction Blisters," *Podiatry Today* 23, no. 6 (2010): 42–48.

8. Yavuz, Metin, and Brian L. Davis, "Plantar Shear Stress Distribution in Athletic Individuals with Frictional Foot Blisters," *Journal of the American Podiatric Medical Association* 100, no. 2 (2010): 116–20.

9. Carlson, J. Martin, "The Role of Friction in Repetitive Loading Soft Tissue Damage" (Blaine, MN: Tamarack Habilitation Technologies, 2009), tamarackhti .com/assets/pdf/The_Role_of_Friction_in_Repetitive_Loading_Soft_Tissue _Damage_Oct_2012.pdf.

10. Payette, Mark, and John Lampe, "ENGO as a Means to Prevent and Treat Friction Blisters" (Blaine, MN: Tamarack Habilitation Technologies, 2009), tamarackhti.com/assets/pdf/ENGOPatches_WP-52209.pdf.

11. Hanna, T., and J. M. Carlson, "Freedom From Friction," *OrthoKinetic Review* 4, no. 2 (2004): 34–35.

12. Carlson, J. Martin, "The Friction Factor," *OrthoKinetic Review* 1, no. 7 (2001): 1–3.

13. Knapik, Joseph J., Katy Reynolds, and John Barson, "Influence of an Antiperspirant on Foot Blister Incidence During Cross-Country Hiking," *Journal of the American Academy of Dermatology* 39, no. 2 (1998): 202–6.

14. Knapik, J. J., M. P. Hamlet, K. J. Thompson, and B. H. Jones, "Influence of Boot-Sock Systems on Frequency and Severity of Foot Blisters," *Military Medicine* 161, no. 10 (1996): 594–98.

15. Bergeron, B. P., "A Guide to Blister Management," *Physician and Sportsmedicine* 23, no. 2 (1995): 37–46.

16. Knapik, Joseph J., Katy L. Reynolds, Kathryn L. Duplantis, and Bruce H. Jones, "Friction Blisters: Pathophysiology, Prevention, and Treatment," *Sports Medicine* 20, no. 3 (1995): 136–47.

17. Herring, K. M., and D. H. Richie, "Friction Blisters and Sock Fiber Composition: A Double-Blind Study," *Journal of the American Podiatric Medical Association* 80, no. 2 (1990): 63–71.

18. Akers, W. A., and M. B. Sulzberger, "The Friction Blister," *Military Medicine* 137 (1972): 1–7.

19. Sulzberger, Marion B., Thomas A. Cortese, Leonard Fishman, Hugh S. Wiley, and Paul S. Peyakovich, "Studies on Blisters Produced by Friction," *Journal of Investigative Dermatology* 47, no. 5 (1966): 456–65.

20. Naylor, P., "Experimental Friction Blisters," *British Journal of Dermatology* 67, no. 10 (1955): 327–42.

21. Naylor, P., "The Skin Surface and Friction," *British Journal of Dermatology.* 67, no. 7 (1955): 239–48.

10

Compounds for the Feet

There are four basic compounds you can put on your feet. Some athletes will use only one, while others may use two, or at times, all four. The most commonly applied compound is lubricant, typically used to make the feet slippery to reduce friction. Powder is used more and more frequently as athletes learn how dry feet are subject to far less friction. Skin-toughening agents and tape adherents are used by many involved in ultras and extreme sports. A small percentage of athletes use an antiperspirant to control excessive sweating of their feet.

One of the best ways of preventing hot spots and blisters is by using either powder or a lubricant on your feet. Both work well, but one may be better suited to your feet. If you have been using a lubricant on your feet and still get blisters, first try one of the newer, state-of-the-art lubricants. Lubricants will soften the skin, and for some, this makes the feet more sensitive to the stresses of walking, running, and hiking. In some cases, you might even feel the weave of the socks as an irritant. The softened skin can lead to painful feet and, in some cases, even blisters. If the blisters continue, try powder. Some skin will respond better to being dry, and powders that prevent moisture buildup on the skin are a good choice. For other athletes, lubricants are a better choice. If you have continued problems, try several of each.

As socks become more technical at transporting moisture away from the skin, athletes need to be aware of sock makers' advice. Make sure you read the instructions on the packaging. As an example, sock company Drymax recommends not using powders or lubricants with their socks because of the tendency to clog the Drymax fibers, inhibiting their ability to properly move moisture away from the skin, and not to put their socks in the dryer.

Powders

Athletes who find their feet become too soft and tender with lubricants can use powders as an alternative foot treatment. For these athletes, powder works better or as well as a lubricant.

POWDER PRODUCTS

ANTI MONKEY BUTT POWDER contains Calamine to help control moisture and stay satin-smooth. antimonkeybutt.com

BLISTERSHIELD POWDER made by TwoToms helps prevent hot spots, blisters, and calluses. Containing micronized wax and cornstarch, the very slick powder reduces friction and heat buildup. BlisterShield repels water by allowing vapor (perspiration) to pass through it, and it keeps moisture off your skin. To use the powder, just shake one teaspoon in each sock, distributing it evenly without bunching all of it at your toes. Add some extra in the heel after you put your sock on. 2toms.com

BROMI-TALC is made by Gordon Laboratories as a triple-action foot powder containing potassium alum, an astringent that retards perspiration, and bentonite, an absorption agent that absorbs 18 times its own weight in moisture. **BROMI-TALC PLUS** powder contains additional properties to control excessive foot odor. Both powders are available through your local drugstore or pharmacy.

GOLD BOND is a medicated body powder that contains active ingredient zinc oxide as a skin protector and menthol to cool and relieve itching. Use the extra-strength powder for maximum benefits in absorbing excessive moisture. Gold Bond can be found in your local drugstore and pharmacy. goldbond.com

ODOR-EATERS FOOT POWDER is 25 times more absorbent than talc and also destroys foot odor. It's also available in a medicated powder. It can be found in most drugstores and pharmacies. odor-eaters.com

ZEASORB is a superabsorbent powder, absorbing six times its weight in moisture. Zeasorb contains talc, a highly absorbent polymer-carbohydrate acrylic copolymer, and microporous cellulose. This powder works without caking. The talc provides softness and lubrication to reduce friction and heat buildup. **ZEASORB-AF** (which contains 2% miconazole nitrate) provides broad antifungal therapy and moisture control. **ZEASORB-AF LOTION/POWDER** is a unique product for patients who need an antifungal lotion. Zeasorb can be found in your local drugstore or pharmacy. zeasorb.com

There are powders and then there are powders. Cornstarch and talcum powder have been used for years as foot powders, but times and powders have changed. Having tried a super-absorbent powder, I would never again use a plain powder. Powders can be effective in reducing moisture on the feet, which, in turn, reduces friction and prevents blisters. Their effectiveness depends on their ability to absorb moisture while not caking into clumps, which can cause skin irritations and blisters. When using powders, remember to reapply the powder at regular intervals or after the feet have been exposed to water. If you have problems with athlete's foot or other skin problems, use an antifungal medicated powder.

After lightly powdering your feet, massage the powder between the toes. Next, roll your socks on to the level of the heel and put some powder in the socks. Then squeeze off the top of the sock and shake the sock to distribute the powder inside.

Lubricants

Two of the old-time tried-and-true lubricants are lanolin and Vaseline (petroleum jelly). However, these are greasy, can cake up on socks, and tend to attract grit particles that can become an irritant and themselves cause blisters.

Technology has led to formulas such as BodyGlide, BlisterShield Roll-On, and Sportslick. Many of these are petroleum-free, waterproof, nonsticky, and hypoallergenic. Many athletes use Bag Balm or Udder Balm, while athletes whose feet are

L U B R I C A N T   P R O D U C T S

ANDREW LOVY'S FORMULA was developed over several years and described in an article "New Blister Formula Revealed! Free!"[22] It helped him solve his blister and friction problems. Take vitamin A and D ointment, petroleum jelly, and Desitin ointment, and mix together equal amounts. To this add vitamin E cream and aloe vera cream (the thickness can be varied by the amount of these two ingredients). The result is a salve. For a thinner mixture, use vitamin E and aloe vera ointments instead of the creams. Andrew recommends applying a thin layer the evening before your run to clean skin where friction occurs. In the morning, before you run, apply a more generous amount to friction areas. Add more to problem areas as necessary during the run.

AQUAPHOR HEALING OINTMENT is a petroleum-based ointment that can be used as a lubricant on the feet and other body parts. As a healing ointment, Aquaphor can be used after events to return your feet to like-new condition. It can be found in most drugstores. aquaphorus.com

AVON SILICONE GLOVE is a silicone cream for hands, but it works equally well on feet. Its nongreasy and nonsticky formula lubricates and softens while protecting against dryness and irritants. avon.com

BAG BALM comes in a green tin that has become familiar to many athletes. Bag Balm is made and advertised for use on cow udders, but it has found acceptance in sports circles. Consisting of a combination of lanolin, petrolatum, 8-hydroxy, and quinoline sulfate, it has proven healing properties. It can be used on cracked, callused, or sore skin, or simply as a lubricant for your feet or other body areas. It is usually found in drugstores, pet and feed stores, tack shops, and hardware stores. bagbalm.com

BODYGLIDE products are petroleum-free lubricants that protect against friction and skin irritation. These products come in a glide-on applicator similar to a deodorant stick. These are hypoallergenic, waterproof, nonsticky, nongreasy (so they will not clog pores), and long lasting and include **BODY ORIGINAL ANTI CHAFE ANTI BLISTER BALM, FOOT ANTI BLISTER BALM, SKIN ANTI CHAFING CREAM,** and **FOR HER ANTI CHAFING MOISTURIZING BALM.** bodyglide.com

BRAVE SOLDIER'S FRICTION ZONE creates a water- and sweat-resistant shield that even under grueling conditions delivers long-lasting skin protection and superior antichafing properties. Its occlusive silicone/botanical barrier protects and conditions skin for hours, while the antibacterial formula helps prevent minor skin irritations. bravesoldier.com exposed to extended periods of moisture often prefer one of the newer formulas like Trail Toes or RunGoo, or even Desitin, that are water repelling and sweat resistant. Other athletes make their own special formulas. In a pinch, lip balm can be used as a lubricant.

Newer lubricants are being developed that utilize state-of-the-art ingredients to make them even more effective. The newest lubricants that have caught my attention are Trail Toes, ChafeX, and RunGoo. Trail Toes is advertised as a

(continued on page 132)

CHAFEX is a unique product that bonds onto the skin to form a protective layer of a permeable, flexible film that allows moisture out but not back in. It resists removal by wear, abrasion, perspiration, and cleansing. chafex.com

CHRIS KOCH'S SECRET FORMULA is made by an adventure racer. He suggests mixing a container of petroleum jelly, a tube of antibacterial ointment, and a tube of antifungal cream in a double boiler. Blend the ingredients and put the mixture in a small plastic jar, squeeze tube, or similar container. Chris has used this formula during multiday adventure races with good success. He usually uses it with a thin liner sock and a heavier outer sock.

DESITIN MAXIMUM STRENGTH ORIGINAL PASTE has the highest level of zinc oxide available—40%—to help seal out wetness. It can be found in most drugstores or pharmacies.

LANOLIN CREAM contains lanolin hydrous, a natural topical skin emollient that lubricates, protects, and sooths. It can be found in most drugstores or pharmacies.

RUNGOO works as a lubricant while providing exceptional moisture control. Its consistency is a thick white cream that should be applied liberally to your feet. footkinetics.com

SKIN LUBE is a lubricating ointment with a high melting point, which gives it longer-lasting protection against blisters and chafing than petroleum jelly. Its main ingredients are petrolatum, zinc stearate, and silicone. Colorless and nonstaining, it can be used on any friction-prone area of the body. cramersportsmed.com

SPORTSHIELD adds a smooth, thin, invisible coating to the skin that will not rub off. This coating eliminates or greatly minimizes the friction that causes blisters, chafing, and irritation. A silicone-based product, it is nonstaining, nontoxic, and nongreasy. Use it anywhere you chafe. Available in roll-on and towelettes. 2toms.com

SPORTSLICK, created by a sports physician, is a multipurpose lubricant made for athletes. The gel is easily applied to the toes, feet, inner thighs, underarms, nipples, and lips. SportSlick prevents blisters and chafing with antifriction polymers, silicone, and petrolatum that create a silky feel. It also enriches the skin with vitamins E and C, soybean oil, the antibacterial agent Triclosan, and the antifungal agent Tolnaftate (1%). SportSlick is available in two sizes. sportslick.com

(continued on page 132)

L U B R I C A N T   P R O D U C T S   *(continued)*

SPORTWAX provides relief from friction and skin irritation. It is made with a natural beeswax-based formula, and it is hypoallergenic and waterproof. Available in a twist-up stick in two sizes. sportwax.com

SQUIRREL'S NUT BUTTER is an all-natural antichafe and restorative skin salve that is also useful as a lubricant. squirrelsnutbutter.com

TRAIL TOES calls its product a phenomenal ultraextreme, antifriction foot and body cream. It has been tested and endorsed by runners through many multi-day stage races around the world in extreme conditions. trailtoes.com

TRISLIDE was developed for triathletes. It is an antifriction/antichafing continuous-spray skin lubricant. It sprays on evenly and leaves a silky feeling that allows skin to breathe. Waterproof and sweatproof, it works on all areas of the body, including feet. Trislide is available in a 4-ounce canister. trislide.com

UDDER BALM has a lemon fragrance, is nongreasy, and is quickly absorbed by the skin. Similar to Bag Balm, Udder Balm was first made for cow udders. With ingredients including lanolin, aloe vera gel, and vitamins A, D, and E, this cream is ideal for relief from rough and cracked skin, and also for corns, cracked cuticles, and sunburn. Udder Balm is available in 4-ounce tubes and a 1-pound jar. udderbalm.com

VASELINE is the old-time standard with 100% pure petroleum jelly. Vaseline is available in most drugstores. vaseline.us

(continued from page 131)

phenomenal ultraextreme, antifriction foot and body cream. It has dedicated users who swear by the product after using it in multiday races in extreme conditions. ChafeX was made to form a protective layer on the skin that lets perspiration out but won't let moisture wick back onto the skin. It dries into a permeable, flexible film that resists removal by abrasion, perspiration, or cleansing. ChafeX is more of a skin protectant than a lubricant. It bonds with the skin and is ablative—not easily washed or abraded away. RunGoo is a product similar in appearance to Desitin. It's thick and should be applied to your feet liberally. It works to effectively control moisture and has a loyal fan base.

Ultrarunner Robert Boeder used Andrew Lovy's formula (see page 130) on his feet in 1994 when he completed the Grand Slam of trail ultrarunning, running four 100-mile runs in 14 weeks. Robert comments, "The idea is that these lotional charms will have the desired magical effect and blisters will not arise from my feet during the race."[23] This formula worked well for him. Since that time he switched to Bag Balm and then back to petroleum jelly, mainly because of its availability. Ultrarunner Jim Benike found success using Udder Balm on his feet and then wearing socks to bed. He used Udder Balm more as a skin softener and conditioner than as a lubricant. Udder creams may go by different names (for example, Bag Balm, Udder Balm, Dr. Naylor's Udder Balm, and Aunt Irma's Udder Balm).

J. Martin Carlson, the creator of the ENGO Blister Prevention Patches, makes an interesting point when describing how lubricants work with our skin cells. Our skin is constantly producing new cells that migrate to the surface and exfoliate. Within an hour or two after the application of a lubricant, the exfoliating cell flakes mix with perspiration and the lubricant. This mix acts more like glue than a lubricant. Most often, athletes will apply more lubricant, which can cause issues as it spreads out on the foot to areas that don't need it. Carlson also says many lubricants hydrate the epidermis, the outer layer of skin, by acting as a partial moisture barrier.

Carlson's point is supported by studies showing that lubricants may initially reduce friction, but over long periods of time they may actually increase it. After 1 hour the friction levels returned to their baseline factor, and after 3 hours the friction levels were 35% above the baseline. As the lubricants are absorbed into the skin and into the socks, friction returns and increases.[24] Based on this study, we should learn to reapply lubricants at frequent intervals, but clean off the old coating.

Use lubricants on your feet, hands, underarms, inner thighs, and nipples—anywhere you chafe. The important thing to remember about lubricants is to clean off the old coating before applying the new one. This is especially true during trail runs and hiking, when dust and dirt buildup can foul the lubricant with grit. Wipe off the old stuff with a cleansing towelette or an alcohol wipe.

Many athletes apply a lubricant the night before a long event. After applying the lube of your choice, put on socks. In the morning, your skin is soft and supple. With Desitin, this method will help the skin resist pruning when exposed to moisture. A clean way to coat your feet is to put a large amount of your lube into a large zip-top bag, then put one foot at a time into the bag. Massage the lube onto the foot from outside the bag.

As always, try any new product before using it in a competitive event or taking it on a long hike. It is foolhardy to buy something and count on it in competition or on a six-day hike without trying it first. It may not work for you. Try any lubricant on a small patch of skin to be sure you are not allergic to the ingredients.

Skin-Toughening Agents and Tape Adherents

Some athletes toughen the skin of their feet to prevent blisters. Often athletes think that toughened skin or calluses will always prevent blisters. For some it does. Others have found themselves with blisters under the calluses or toughened skin. These blisters are very difficult to treat. You still must use other blister prevention products such as moisture-wicking socks, lubricants, or powders.

If you wish to try the skin-toughening approach, begin by spending time walking barefoot on various surfaces. Sandals, worn without socks, can build calluses, but be careful that the calluses do not become too thick or rough. As

SKIN-TOUGHENING AGENTS AND ADHERENTS

COMPOUND TINCTURE OF BENZOIN is available in liquid, swabs, or squeeze vials. Commonly used as a tape or bandage adherent, it is sometimes used as a skin toughener. After applying the tincture, let it dry for about two minutes before applying tape. Compound tincture of benzoin leaves an orange-brownish color on the skin. Avoid getting the tincture into any cuts, abrasions, or open blisters—it can burn! Usually available in liquid form at drugstores, pharmacies, or medical supply stores. medco-athletics.com

CRAMER TUF-SKIN has been used for years by athletic trainers as a taping base. It is ideal for pretaping and skin toughening. Its main ingredients are isopropyl alcohol, isobutane, resin, and benzoin. cramersportsmed.com

MASTISOL is a clear, nonirritating liquid adhesive that is not water soluble and is routinely used in hospitals for dressing wounds. It is advertised as stickier than compound tincture of benzoin. medco-athletics.com

MUELLER TUFFNER CLEAR SPRAY is used as a base for athletic taping, but it is also identified as a skin toughener. Its main ingredients are acetone; 1,1,1–trichloroethane isopropanol; resin; and compound tincture of benzoin. Look for this product at sporting goods stores. muellersportsmed.com

NEW-SKIN LIQUID BANDAGE comes in either an antiseptic spray or liquid that is useful as a skin protectant or toughener to prevent hot spots and blisters. It dries rapidly to form a tough protective cover that is antiseptic, flexible, and waterproof, while letting the skin breathe. A second coating is recommended for additional protection. Keep toes bent when applying and drying. Its main ingredients are pyroxylin solution, acetone ACS, oil of cloves, and 8-hydroxyquinoline. Look for New-Skin at drugstores or online. newskinproducts.com

PERFORMSTIK TAPE ADHERENT is a spray tape adherent made specifically for use with kinesiology tapes. performtex.com and theratape.com

RUBBING ALCOHOL was the preference of renowned walker Colin Fletcher as a skin toughener.[25] Use it on your toes, soles, and heels several times daily. He recommended almost hourly applications of rubbing alcohol followed by foot powder while walking and hiking with sore feet. Available in drugstores.

SKIN-PREP PROTECTIVE WIPES BY SMITH & NEPHEW are individually packaged wipes that help tapes stick to the skin. These are easy to carry in a small foot-care kit. Available through online stores.

TUF-FOOT is made from nature's healing balsams and other ingredients. Dr. Andrew Bonn created this unique and original compound in 1935. Made exclusively for feet, either human or animal, Tuf-Foot is guaranteed to toughen soft, tender, or sore feet by working on the tissues. This protects against bruises, blisters, and foot soreness. Recommended use is daily until feet are in good condition and then twice weekly. tuffoot.com the skin is irritated through exposure to rough surfaces, it thickens and calluses develop. Remember to keep calluses and roughened skin surfaces smooth by using creams, a pumice stone, or a foot file (see "Skin Care" on page 172 and "Skin Disorders" on page 326).

You can use several products to toughen your skin or choose the tea and Betadine soak (see sidebar below). After applying the last coat of the toughening agent, apply a light coating of either one of the lubricants or powders to cut the stickiness. Skipping this step may cause your socks to stick to your feet.

You can use several of the tape adherent products to help tape or moleskin better stick to your feet. Without the adherent, most tapes and blister products will begin to peel off after an hour or two. After applying a blister patch or taping your feet, apply a light coating of powder over any dry sprayed area to counteract the adhesive.

Allow the compound tincture of benzoin or any sticky tape adherent to dry before applying any tape. Generally 1–2 minutes' drying time is sufficient. Wet benzoin is very sticky and slippery. Tape and blister-care products can move around on the foot and fold over on themselves, creating problems. Socks can become stuck to your feet and toes can stick together if you do not allow enough time for the benzoin to dry.

Tom Gets Tough—Why Shouldn't You?

TOM CRAWFORD'S TEA AND BETADINE SKIN TOUGHENER was developed by an ultrarunner who has completed numerous ultras, including the challenging Death Valley to Mount Whitney, both one-way and as an out-and-back run. Tom's method begins with mixing 10 tea bags and 1 cup of Betadine into a half-gallon of water. For one week, dip your feet 20 times over the course of a day, letting them air-dry between dips. The second week, add 1 cup of salt to the water, tea, and Betadine mixture. Then for one week, soak your feet for 20 minutes at a time, several times daily. Betadine can be found in drugstores and medical supply stores.

Richard Benyo recalled how he used Tom's method to prepare his feet for the Death Valley 300. "Each night I'd pour the solution into a plastic foot bath and keep my soles and toes in the solution for 15 minutes; then I'd alternately raise one foot out of the brew for three minutes, allowing it to dry, then lower it and bring the other foot out. I'd do that for a half hour. Then I'd let them dry and I'd go to bed with orange soles. When I showered the next morning, it would wash off. But little by little, it made my feet more resistant to blisters."[26] Even with this preparation, Richard sometimes found his feet susceptible to blisters.

FOOT ANTIPERSPIRANT PRODUCTS

Antiperspirants that can work on your feet are available in drugstores. Check the shelves at your local store and try one or two. **CERTAIN DRI FEET, GILLETTE CLINICAL STRENGTH ANTIPERSPIRANT,** and **BAN ROLL-ON** are all worth trying. **DRYSOL SOLUTION** and **XERAC AC** are prescription-strength antiperspirants that, when applied according to instructions, virtually eliminate all perspiration.

BROMI-LOTION is a unique antiperspirant formulated as a soothing lotion, rather than as a spray or roll-on. Made by Gordon Laboratories, it is available only by special order through your local drugstore, pharmacy, or podiatrist.

BROMI-TALC PLUS is an antiperspirant powder from Gordon Laboratories containing a deodorizing powder, sodium potassium, aluminosilicate, bentonite, and talc to eliminate odor instantly and help reduce sweating of the feet. See "Powder Products," page 129.

CERTAIN DRI FEET is available in either **MOISTURE CONTROL PADS** or **MICROSPONGE POWDER** with 12% aluminum chloride, the active ingredient used in prescription antiperspirants. Because Certain Dri is water based (instead of alcohol based, like its prescription competitors), it is available without a doctor's prescription at drugstores nationwide. certaindri.com

DRYSOL SOLUTION is made with 20% aluminum chloride hexahydrate, a strong antiperspirant for excessive perspiration. Available through a prescription from your doctor.

DRYZ INSOLES help the feet stay dryer and cooler while eliminating odor. See "Insole Products," pages 72–73.

FOOT SOLUTION by Onox is a spray solution made to control excessive moisture and foot odor. A combination of mineral salts decreases excessive sweat and foot odor symptoms. The spray also helps reduce blistering and itching while repelling athlete's foot fungus. Ingredients include zinc chloride, deionized water, sodium chloride, sodium nitrate, boric acid, and sodium silicofluoride. Be aware that the salt solution will sting if you have cuts or breaks in your skin. footsmart.com

GOLD BOND is a medicated body powder. Use the extra-strength powder for maximum benefits in absorbing excessive moisture. See "Powder Products," page 129.

ODOR-EATERS FOOT POWDER is 25 times more absorbent than talc and also destroys foot odor. It can be found in most drugstores and pharmacies. odor-eaters.com

ZEASORB is a superabsorbent powder, absorbing six times its weight in moisture and four times more than plain talcum powder. See "Powder Products," page 129.

Antiperspirants for the Feet

According to the American Podiatric Medical Association, our feet have approximately 250,000 sweat glands and produce as much as a pint of moisture each day. An increase in body temperature will increase the perspiration level. Some people experience excessive perspiration of their feet. Hyperhidrosis is a medical term meaning excessive moisture. This moisture often increases the chance of blisters. Individuals with this condition may find that applying an antiperspirant to the feet reduces the amount of perspiration, which in turn prevents the formation of blisters. David Zuniga is one runner who has found that the use of an antiperspirant has helped his feet. He started using an antiperspirant on the recommendation of his podiatrist and finds his feet stay "dry as a bone."

Aside from antiperspirants, problems associated with excessive moisture can often be reduced by wearing moisture-wicking socks, changing socks frequently, and changing shoes if the moisture is particularly excessive.

Certain Dri and Gillette Clinical Strength antiperspirants offer perspiration control that will also work on feet that sweat excessively. If something stronger is needed, ask your physician for a more powerful solution, such as Drysol Solution, available by prescription.

To save your shoes from faster than normal deterioration from the excess moisture, here are a few tips. Stuff newspaper into your wet shoes to dry them out overnight. Sprinkle a bit of baking soda powder into each shoe after using them. Remove the insoles and shake the shoes to get the powder evenly distributed. The baking soda will also help control the harsh smells that are common with heavy sweating inside shoes. Rotate between two pairs of shoes to give them a chance to dry out. Use one of these odor control products: Penguin's Fresh Twist Shoe Deodorizers or Sof Sole's Sneaker Balls.

Blisters and Antiperspirants

Ultrarunner Mike Palmer has worked at resolving blister problems related to sweaty feet. He wears sandals as much as he can to keep his feet dry during the day. A couple of weeks before an ultra of 50 miles or more, he uses alcohol at night to dry his feet. He has also found coating his feet with compound tincture of benzoin dries the skin and provides a protective coating. As much as possible, he wears sandals to prevent perspiration buildup and toughen the skin. Then before the run he uses an absorbent foot powder and puts dispensers of this powder in his drop bags for every point where he will make a sock change. Mike also recommends frequent sock changes during long races. Even though this is time consuming, it's better than trying to run on hot spots and blistered feet. For Mike, the moisture promotes blistering. Since using benzoin, the maceration (the whitish, flaky condition of moist skin) has been eliminated and blistering is not so frequent or extensive.

In an interesting study, cadets attending the US Military Academy were separated into two groups that used either an antiperspirant or placebo preparation. Each group was asked to apply their preparation for five consecutive nights before completing a 21-kilometer hike. After the hike, only 21% of the cadets who reported using the antiperspirant preparation for at least three nights before the hike were diagnosed with foot blisters. The placebo group reported a 48% incidence of foot blisters. Joseph Knapik, ScD, the lead author of the study that appeared in the August 1998 issue of the *Journal of the American Academy of Dermatology*, reported, "Blisters are usually minor problems, but they can cause great discomfort for the patient. Typically they only require simple first aid and a short period of limited activity. It is possible, however, for them to lead to more serious problems such as local or systemic infections."

Researchers theorized that reduced sweating might reduce friction and consequently lower the occurrence of blisters. The cadets applied the preparation to completely dry feet, up the ankle to the top of the boot line. Before the hike, each cadet was examined for existing foot conditions. Immediately after the hike, the feet of each cadet were inspected for blisters using the same criteria as the prehike examination. Researchers found that sweat reduction was a key mechanism for the reduction of blisters.

While the antiperspirant was found to be very effective in reducing blisters, some side effects did occur. "Itching and rashes occurred in 57% of the antiperspirant group, but only 6% of the placebo group," Dr. Knapik noted. "This suggests that a large portion of the population may have problems with the antiperspirant used in the study. However, reducing the amount of the active compound or applying the antiperspirant every other night, rather than every night as the cadets did, may reduce the irritation."

Taping for Blisters

If your feet are prone to blistering, taping may be a lifesaver. After 12 hours of a 72-hour run, my Vaseline-coated feet were almost too sore to run on, and I had a blister between two toes. Nancy Crawford, an experienced running friend, taught me how to prepare my feet for taping and use duct tape to both fix the blister and tape the tender balls of my feet, which would likely blister in the hours ahead. I completed the next 60 hours without a foot problem!

While you may consider taping an extreme, consider the benefits of taping if you are highly susceptible to blisters. You can tape before your event as a proactive preventive measure or in a reactive mode after hot spots or blisters develop. Tape can be applied to more than feet. Rich Lewis finds that applying duct tape to his socks over where he typically develops hot spots or blisters, particularly in new shoes, is a good prevention measure. Others use duct tape inside their shoes or boots to cover irritating seams in their footwear.

Ultrarunner Gillian Robinson usually tapes her big toes because the skin underneath the toe almost always rubs. For a long ultra (100 miles) she tapes more extensively—all of her toes, the balls of her feet, and the arches. She typically does not have heel trouble. Don Lundell usually follows a specific regimen for short ultras: taping the places where he gets blisters (left foot: heel and inside of the foot behind the big toe).

Keep in mind that the overall goal of taping is prevention. While taping is a great skill to learn, you need to be sure the shoes you wear are the best fit possible for your feet. With shoes that fit well, your taping needs will hopefully be minimal.

I recommend that runners first train in the conditions for the race intended. Once a runner has trained in this environment, it becomes evident what areas of the feet are prone to problems and they can then be pretaped. Just as training for the distance is vitally important, so is trying the technique of taping in training prior to the race.

Taping is useful for prerun preparation as well as for fixing newly developed problem spots. If you typically blister on the balls of your feet, consider taping

Preventive taping over the Achilles tendon, heel, and side of the foot

before the run when you have the time to do it right rather than at an aid station when you need every minute of time. Practice taping to learn how best to apply the tape to meet your particular needs. Determine how much time is needed to do a complete application. If you are going to have crew support for an event, teach them how to do the taping. It is usually easier to tape the night before an event than wait until the morning when time is rushed and you may do a hurried job.

If you are bothered by blisters and have found that powders and/or lubricants do not work, try the different tapes to find a tape and taping method that work for you. In the chapter on foot-care kits (page 341), you will find a list of taping materials to carry during your runs and hikes.

Beginning on page 146 are three methods of taping the feet. The first, developed by Badwater Blister Queen Denise Jones, uses a combination of Kinesio Tex and Hypafix tapes. It is the method I use. The second method, devised by Suzi Cope, uses Johnson & Johnson Elastikon tape. The third uses duct tape. Following a description of each of these methods are descriptions of how to tape different parts of the feet. Remember, any tape that moves or shifts is worse than no tape at all.

Tapes

There are many types of tape available to try. Duct tape was the standard for years, but kinesiology tapes, Leukotape, and Micropore have become popular with ultra-runners and adventure racers. Hypafix, EnduraSports, and EnduraFix tapes can be used as well. Elastikon is not a good choice because of its coarseness. Athletic white tape is not well suited for taping feet because of its lack of quality adhesive. While you might find other tapes, the ones below are the most commonly used and have withstood the test of time. They can be found at or ordered through most medical supply stores or ordered online.

Types of Tape

The following tapes are available online or through drugstores unless otherwise noted. Several of the most reliable online sources are theratape.com and medco-athletics.com.

Kinesiology Tapes

Kinesiology tapes are ribbed and stretch longitudinally with a paper backing that is removed when applying. Designed for muscle taping, they come in 1-, 2-, and 3- and 4-inch widths and in a variety of colors, depending on the company. This tape is very smooth, soft, breathable, and water resistant. It can stay on for three to four days and leaves no tape residue when removed. theratape.com

Zinc Oxide–Based Tapes

ENDURASPORTS (optp.com) and LEUKOTAPE P are breathable tapes in one width, 1.5 inches. They have a specially formulated zinc oxide heat-sensitive adhesive that is triggered to ensure secure adhesion—even with perspiration, water, or cold weather. They can leave tape residue on the skin when removed.

Woven Tapes

ENDURAFIX (optp.com), HYPAFIX, and OMNIFIX tapes are a 2-inch, thin, soft, and breathable tape, with a removable backing. It works well on toes, over hot spots, on heels, and for anchoring tape between the toes.

Paper Tape

MICROPORE is a soft paper tape made by 3M that comes in 0.5-inch and 1-inch widths. It's often used for toes.

Tapes Generally Not Recommended

DUCT TAPE is a 2-inch-wide, very sticky silver tape with a fabric core that has excellent adhesive qualities. It does not breathe but is very strong and tough. Buy high-quality duct tape, which is available at any hardware store.

ELASTIKON is a thick, stretchy, breathable tape that comes in 1-, 2-, 3-, and 4-inch widths. It is thicker than most tapes and requires an edging tape such as Micropore. It has excellent adhesive qualities but leaves serious tape residue when removed. Because of its rough surface, it is not recommended.

WHITE ATHLETIC TAPE is generally a 2-inch tape found in sporting goods stores. While great for wrapping ankles, for our purposes it does not stick well.

While there are many other types of tapes, the ones mentioned individually above have stood the test of time.

The best tape depends on what your objective is. If you want to save money, duct tape is cheap. But duct tape does not mold well around the curves of heels, sides of the feet, and toes. Leukotape and EnduraSports tapes are also sticky but come in only one width, don't shape well to the curves of the feet, and leave tape residue on the skin; however, many athletes love these tapes because of their superb adhesive. Hypafix and EnduraFix are thin and are especially good on toes and between toes. Micropore's use is limited to toes. That leaves kinesiology tape.

Kinesiology tape is my tape of choice for 90% of my taping jobs. The other 10% is done with HypaFix, EnduraFix, Leukotape, and Endura Sports tapes, which are great, fairly inexpensive tapes to use on any part of the foot. I recommend these for general use when cost and ease of application is a concern. I have become a proponent of the "less is better" theory. Kinesiology tapes are thin, easily applied, and stick exceptionally well. The thicker the tape, the more it is felt. If it doesn't lie smooth, it can be uncomfortable. If you add 2nd Skin or any other patch under a thick tape, you stand the chance of it being uncomfortable. This can change the runner's gait, potentially leading to other problems.

Smooth Versus Coarse Tape

Some tapes are smoother than others. Try to picture the following: Your skin's outer layer typically moves against the inner layers—then you apply a tape that is not smooth to the skin, pull on a sock, and finally put your foot inside a shoe. The tape sticks to the skin. As you run, the foot naturally moves inside your shoes. However, the sock cannot move freely against the coarseness of the tape. This forces the tape to move with the sock, which doesn't move well against the shoe, and stresses the outer later of skin against the inner layers. The only movement is between the layers of skin. The result is very sore feet. Others may not agree, but I have seen too many runners with sore feet, many at the point of not being able to run anymore, and the common denominator has been tape that is not smooth. A story will illustrate this.

At Badwater 2008 I removed tape from the bottoms of a runner's feet and repatched them. He had run 90 miles and had another 40 to go. Over and over he told me, "My feet hurt. I can't run. I can't walk." The balls of each foot were hurting him so badly that he wanted to quit. As I carefully removed the Elastikon tape I discovered he had a small hard-cored callus on the ball of each foot. I put a small Spenco gel patch over the hard core of each callus and used two 2-inch strips of Kinesio Tex tape across the ball of the foot, from the toe crease to mid-foot. I also added a large ENGO patch on each insole under the ball of each foot. He went on to earn a 48-hour finisher's buckle. The smooth Kinesio Tex tape worked where the Elastikon did not. His skin was stuck to the Elastikon tape; the coarse tape didn't move against his sock, and the sock didn't move against the shoe's insole. There was shear between the layers of skin as the bones of the foot moved through the foot strike. The takeaway from the story is to try to use smooth or fairly smooth tape.

Beware of Tape Residue

Some tapes will leave a sticky adhesive residue when removed. This is not a factor in most cases, but when using tape in a 100-mile or multiday event, it becomes an issue. The residue is usually very sticky, often in clumps, and hard to remove without tape remover or nail polish remover. Applying new tape over the old residue is challenging. Some tapes will leave more residue the longer they are on the skin. Kinesiology tapes and the woven tape do not leave a residue.

Kinesiology Tape

I have to be honest and say how much I love kinesiology tapes. After years of using duct tape, Elastikon, and Leukotape, and trying to get it on smooth with no creases, and dealing with tape reside when retaping, kinesiology tape solved all those problems. Many people remember the colored tape from seeing it on athlete's shoulders, legs, and arms during sporting events shows on television.

The tape molds well to the contours of the foot, going around toes and heels better than any other tape. This molding to contour ability allows me to tape any part of a foot. It has a heat-activated adhesive that bonds especially well on the skin. I like how I can cut the tape into the shape needed without having it stick to my hands or the scissors. You can also precut tape into commonly used sizes and shapes. Kinesiology tape is sometimes referred to as myofascial tape.

Kinesiology tapes are made with an elastic polymer and cotton fabric, are very thin and very porous, and have a heat-activated medical-grade acrylic adhesive, which bonds with the skin. The tape comes in 1-, 2-, and 3-inch widths and in a variety of colors (RockTape makes a 4-inch width). It is commonly used in physical therapy. Because it has a paper backing, pieces can be measured and precut. It is best applied to clean, oil-free, dry skin, preferably an hour before being exposed to moisture. The more body heat in the taped area, the faster the bonding.

Types of Kinesiology Tape

There are a number of companies that make kinesiology tapes. Kinesio Tex was the first to offer the tape. Over the years, others have evolved: RockTape, StrengthTape, KT Tape, Kinetic Pro Tape by PerformTex, SpiderTape, and several lesser-known players. My choice is based on what I want the tape to do. First and foremost, it has to stick well under adverse, often wet conditions. Secondly, it has to be high quality and mold or shape to any part of the foot. Its surface must be as smooth as possible and it needs to hold up to heat and cold conditions. To help me, I use the people at Theratape.com, who carry most every kinesiology tape made. They let me know when new tapes are coming out and what their research has shown them about the tapes. The tapes are sold in rolls about 15–16 feet long and in bulk rolls of about 115 feet at a substantial savings over single rolls. Although precut strips are offered, I don't find them useful for working on feet.

StrengthTape and RockTape H2O are my favorites because they hold up well under wet conditions. Kinetic Pro Tape by PerformTex shows good promise too. Color is cosmetic only. I like to have two colors on hand when working an event so I can tell which has held up the best when I see people more than once.

The Theratape.com website has information on kinesiology tapes in general, taping instruction, videos on taping, FAQs on the different tapes, and more. It also offers a professional discount that people can apply for. Those interested in learning more about using the tape therapeutically for injuries and rehabilitation can find information on the website too. theratape.com

Getting the Best Stick

There are three phases to getting the best use out of kinesiology tape.

- Phase 1 is skin preparation. The skin must be clean and completely dry. Then apply a tape adherent and let it become tacky to touch.

- Phase 2 is tape application and wearing the tape. Round all corners; don't touch the adhesive side; go easy on the stretch; all strips must end on skin, not on another piece of tape; and activate the adhesive. You can also apply a strip of tape adherent at the edges of the tape and skin. If possible, apply tape the night before your event. Bunch up your socks and roll them on and off to avoid pulling the tape loose. If any ends start to come loose, trim the edges with scissors.

- Phase 3 is removing the tape. Work slowly and carefully, from the sides to the center. Hold the skin with one hand and loosen the tape with the other hand.

Kinesiology tape is designed for therapeutic use to help athletes recover from injuries. To help in recovery, the tape stretches in length. I won't go into all the details here, but remember to lay the tape on skin without stretch. In patching feet with the tape, there is no need to stretch the tape.

I use high-quality scissors that make clean cuts, and I occasionally clean the blades with alcohol wipes. Theratape.com also offers scissors with special coatings to prevent adhesive buildup. Cheap scissors can affect the adhesive at the ends of the tape and keep it from sticking effectively.

It's important to activate the adhesive after applying the tape. All it takes is a brisk 20- to 30-second rub from the center to the ends with your fingers to warm the adhesive. This helps it bond with the skin.

Why Use Kinesiology Tape

Denise Jones says of kinesiology tape, "This tape has superior sticking power, breathability, and stretch." She has used the tape at the Badwater Ultramarathon in the extreme heat of Death Valley in the summer. Here's why she likes the tape.

- Kinesiology tape has a paper backing, which is peeled off before applying and prevents it from sticking to itself in extreme heat.

- It's much easier to work with.
- The tape is latex free.
- It has a much smoother texture and is far easier to apply.
- It's very sticky, has a nice longitudinal stretch, and is resilient.
- It can be used on the toes.
- It can be cut and shaped to any part of the foot.
- It works in heat and cold conditions.

Working the Tape

There are three important steps to know about working with any tape. The first, skin preparation, is important to provide a base for the tape to adhere to. The second, tape application, is important to reduce problems later. And third, knowing how to remove the tape will save your skin.

Skin Preparation

Athletes who decide to try taping should purchase a tape adherent that provides a taping base to hold the tape to the skin (see "Skin-Toughening Agents and Tape Adherents," page 133). The best adherents are compound tincture of benzoin in a liquid or swabs (6-inch single-tipped Q-tips are great if applying the liquid benzoin), PerformTex's PerformStik Tape Adherent, Cramer's Tuf-Skin spray, or Mueller's Tuffner Clear Spray.

Preparation involves several steps. Before taping, clean the feet of their natural oils, dust, and dirt. This is vital to getting a good stick with the tape. If you have used any lubricant on your feet, wipe it off with a towel first. Rubbing alcohol works well to clean the feet, and it dries quickly. For fanny pack use, buy alcohol wipes in small disposable packets. Next, apply the tape adherent to the areas needing tape and let it dry so it becomes tacky. Then apply the tape based on your specific needs or problems.

Tape Application

When applying the tape, keep it as smooth as possible. Ridges in the tape can cut into the skin and lead to irritation that can cause blisters. If the tape must be overlapped, be sure the overlapping edge of the tape is in the same direction as the force of motion. For example, if taping the ball of the foot, the force is toward the rear of the foot, so the most forward piece of tape should overlap over the piece toward the back. If taping the heel, the force is toward the rear and up the back of the heel, so the tape on the bottom of the heel should overlap the piece higher up on the back of the heel. This will keep the tape from catching on the sock and peeling up. The less overlap the better. Applying the tape too tightly may cause circulation problems. If, after application, the skin becomes discolored, cool, or numb, loosen the tape. If there is any indication of skin irritation (itching, redness, or rash), discontinue use of the tape immediately.

Apply a small dab of antibiotic ointment, zinc oxide, or lubricant over any existing blisters where the outer skin has pulled loose from the inner skin. This keeps the adhesive from attacking the sensitive area and protects the blistered skin when the tape is removed. Do not use gauze because it is too abrasive.

After the foot is taped, several finishing touches should be made. Apply a thin layer of tape adherent over the edges of the tape. This reinforces the tape's status as part of your foot by allowing the taped surface to slip easily across friction points without snagging. Then apply a sprinkling of powder to any sticky areas that are not taped to counteract any adhesive left uncovered. Jane Moorhead saw a podiatrist using a votive candle and, after taping, rubbing it over the edges of the tape. The small amount of wax reduces friction and helps prevent curling. This is less messy than using a lubricant.

You may be able to tape all areas of your feet yourself. If you have problems reaching the outer edges of your feet, your heels, or any other awkward area, find someone to help with the taping.

As important as taping the feet is, all those benefits can be lost if the athlete is not careful in putting on or taking off his or her socks. The socks should be rolled on and off. All the time and value of a good tape job can be ruined when changing socks too fast. The use of a shoehorn is recommended to keep additional fiction off the heel as it is lowered into the shoe.

Removing the Tape

When removing the tape, work slowly and carefully. You do not want to pull off a layer of skin or a toenail with the tape. Work from the sides to the center, using the fingers of one hand to hold the skin tight or taut while pulling the tape with the other hand. Ultrarunner Suzi Cope suggests using baby oil and gentle massage to roll off the tape and excessive adhesive. You can use fingernail polish remover to get rid of any leftover adhesive on your skin or toenails. After a race, Will Brown gets in the shower with the tape still on. After it's wet, he lifts one side of the tape up so more water can get in. After a few minutes, it's easy to remove. Nik Weber has found that ethyl rubbing alcohol removes tape the best, but warns it will sting until it evaporates when applied to open wounds. But it still hurts less than lifting the blister skin up with the tape. He says, "I use a long cotton swab with a wooden stick and soak through the tape if it is porous like Elastikon, then use the soaked cotton swab to peel the edges of the tape loose. You sort of push at the tape–skin interface with the cotton swab until the tape releases."

Three Taping Techniques

Denise Jones's Taping Techniques

Denise Jones has taped feet in one of the most grueling environments—the extreme heat of California's Death Valley for the Badwater Ultramarathon. Her method uses kinesiology tape with compound tincture of benzoin or Mastisol as an adherent and HypaFix to anchor tape between toes. She also uses foot powder.

Denise and I are constantly discussing tapes and taping techniques and have fine-tuned these techniques. When I tape feet, I use these same techniques.

To prepare feet for taping, Denise insists that you have to file down any calluses with a pedicure file so that if a blister develops, it can be treated. If thick calluses are allowed to remain, they can prove next to impossible to get underneath to drain blisters, and those blisters become larger and more painful. Before taping, also make sure toenails are trimmed square and filed so no rough edges remain.

Kinesiology tape can be easily applied. It is very sticky, smooth, and stretchy; and it breathes. Applied well, it forms a bond with the skin. Denise uses the following taping method:

> When I use kinesiology tape on the larger areas of the foot, it's imperative that compound tincture of benzoin is first swabbed onto the area where the tape will be applied. This sticks the tape to the foot. Allow the tincture to become tacky, and then tape as flatly and neatly as possible. After taping, I reapply tincture around the edges of the tape to help seal the tape.
>
> If the ends of the toes blister, then I tape over the top of the toe first, then around the toe to encase it like a glove. I make sure that all areas of the toe are secure with no gaps and no ridges. If a corner is bulky, I cut it off and secure it with more tincture. If one toe is taped and the toe next to it is not, I make sure the tape is absolutely smooth so that the rubbing that occurs in running will not blister the untaped toe. After taping, I use foot powder to keep feet dry within the socks.

If taping over a blister, Denise first uses foot powder to dry the feet before taping, and then she cleans the feet with an alcohol wipe. She cuts a hole in each blister for draining, and then applies either zinc oxide or antibiotic ointment. This allows the runner to continue with little pain. It's the fluid in the blister that causes the pain.

Finally, Denise recommends pretaping the night before a race and wearing socks to bed to help the tape conform to the foot. If anything comes unstuck during the night, it can then be restuck the next morning.

Suzi Cope's Taping Techniques

Suzi Cope, an ultrarunner, developed this taping technique while completing the Grand Slam of trail ultrarunning, five 100-mile runs in one summer, with only a couple of small tape blisters. Suzi's technique involves taping the bottom of each foot up to the heel and around the sides of the foot and each toe. She recommends taping the night before an event, after taking a shower. She has often had the tape on up to 36 hours without a problem. River and stream crossings are not a problem because the tape dries as fast as socks and shoes. Suzi stresses this technique will not work for everybody. Individual footprint and running style can affect the taping.

Suzi used Elastikon tape but kinesiology tapes are a better choice. Do not stretch the tape; simply form it to the foot and press firmly. All points where the tape folds or is pinched together should be folded like gift wrap and cut flush with the skin. This is truly preventive maintenance, creating a sock-type effect.

Determine your specific hot spot or blister problems and try taping as needed. When cutting the tape flush with the skin, be careful not to cut the skin. Suzi's technique uses three steps to tape the whole foot. First she tapes the bottom of the foot, and then the sides, followed by the toes. If you only have problems on the ball of the foot, the heel, or the toes, use the appropriate taping strategy.

Duct Tape Techniques

Athletes who have found other tapes won't hold, especially in wet conditions, often use duct tape. I have seen duct tape stay on for days. Its adhesive is one of the best around! For some athletes, the silver duct tape is a staple of their foot-care kit.

Many runners have successfully used Gary Cantrell's article "From the South: The Amazing Miracle of Duct Tape"[27] to learn how to prevent and also to treat blisters. Gary's basic principle is to cover the spot that's injured with a patch, and in some cases then anchor the edges and corners of that patch. The powerful adhesive of duct tape holds it close and true to the outline of your skin and the tough plastic outer tape reinforced with fabric can withstand almost unlimited friction. The friction points on your skin will then have what amounts to an additional layer of skin—the duct tape.

Remember a few general duct tape rules. Choose a good quality duct tape with a visible fabric core, not a cheap plastic imitation. Many hardware stores carry several different types of duct tape. The standard grade is typically 9 millimeters thick, while the contractor and professional grades are generally 10 millimeters. Duct tape is available only in a 2-inch width. Although the tape is sometimes available in a variety of colors, the common silver tape works the best.

Apply the tape over the danger spots where blisters frequently occur. Don't apply tape where it is not needed. Use only a single thickness, because additional layers become too hard and unyielding. When the tape is applied, that part of the foot should be flexed to its maximum extension. Cut the ends of the tape so they are rounded. If your feet are hairy, shave the parts where the tape will be applied.

Generally speaking, with duct tape do not tape all the way around toes or the foot because of possible circulation problems. If, after applying tape, the skin or portion of the foot farthest from the body becomes discolored, cool, or numb, loosen the tape.

Taping the Feet

A good tape job is an art. It takes practice. It also cannot be rushed. Doing it the night before an event when you have time can result in a better tape job than doing it at an aid station, when you are anxious to get back in the race. Denise Jones warns:

> If taping isn't done properly, it's almost worse than no taping. I've tried so hard to get the message out there, but often when I see the job of taping that is done, it's less than adequate and is sometimes even a setup

for blistering; for example, when the tape is too close to the toe junction on the balls of the feet, blisters can develop between the toes once the feet swell.

So practice early, and practice often. Develop taping skills with each part of your foot. And then practice on your friends and with your teammates. Taking 10–20 minutes to patch a blister and tape feet during a race may seem hard to do. However, it can get you back on your feet and able to run more efficiently.

Remember when applying tape to the bottoms of your feet or heels to grasp the toes of the foot and pull back to stretch the skin to its fullest. Otherwise as you run or walk, the shear forces will loosen the tape and may cause additional blisters.

All the images showing the techniques on the following pages are done with kinesiology tape. It is my tape of choice, along with an occasional strip of HypaFix, for all my taping jobs.

The taping methods described on the following pages can be done directly over blisters if you apply a dab of antibiotic ointment or zinc oxide, or a Spenco 2nd Skin patch over the top of the drained blister. If the blister's roof is torn off, a dab of zinc oxide will help dry the skin and protect the new skin from the tape.

Ball of the Foot

Taping the ball of the foot can be tricky. You may find it easier to make a card template in the shape of your foot, from the ball of the foot to the base of the toes. Then cut the tape according to the template. This makes trimming easier, if needed at all, especially if you are taping your own feet.

Kinesiology tapes are stretchy and will shape to follow the crease where the toes meet the ball of the foot. Other tapes have to be cut to fit this curved area.

Shape a piece of tape at the toe crease and up the side of the foot. To tape the ball of the foot, cut a long strip of full-width tape and lay it on the ball of the foot, with the forward edge following the shape of the forefoot as it transitions into the toes. Pull the ends of the tape up, cutting them an inch up on either side of the foot. Cut or shape the tape at the forward edge of the ball of the foot so it does not contact or cut into the crease at the base of the toes or the toes themselves. Be sure to apply the extra figure eight tape between the toes to anchor the forward edge of the tape. See the section "Between the Toe and Foot" later in this chapter.

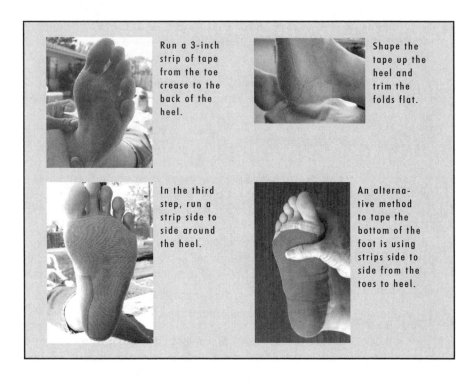

Run a 3-inch strip of tape from the toe crease to the back of the heel.

Shape the tape up the heel and trim the folds flat.

In the third step, run a strip side to side around the heel.

An alternative method to tape the bottom of the foot is using strips side to side from the toes to heel.

Bottom of the Foot

Taping the bottom of the foot from the ball of the foot to the heel can be done with one piece of 3-inch tape. Apply the tape from just behind the bend of the toe base, centering the tape on the bottom of the foot from front to back. Have equal edges on the inside and outside of the foot. Trim the front edge to follow the contour of the toe base, avoiding the crease. Form the tape to the foot's arch. Bring the back edge up the heel and fold over on each side, like a gift wrap, making a dart. Cut the fold flush with the foot, leaving two edges just meeting in a V pattern. Then tape the sides of the foot as described below. Be sure to add two figure eight pieces of tape according to instructions in the section "Between the Toe and Foot" on page 152. A second method of taping is to run strips of tape side to side from the base of the toes back to the heel. This usually requires three to four overlapping strips.

Sides of the Foot

Once the tape is affixed to the bottom of the foot, apply tape to the sides of the foot. Apply a 1- or 2-inch piece around the foot from one side, around the back of the heel to the other side. Slightly overlap the edge of the bottom of the foot tape. Trim the edges to avoid rubbing at the toe crease and anklebone. This also provides protection to the sides and back of your heel. This strip can be done independently from the strip on the bottom of the foot.

If you find the bottom edge of the tape catching on your socks, put this layer on before taping the bottom of the foot. Then tape the bottom of the foot so that tape overlaps the side of the foot tape. This method keeps the overlapping tape in the direction of the force of motion. You can also add an optional strip across the ball of the foot for added protection.

Sides and Bottom of the Heel

Many times, feet blister at the area where the insole meets the inside of the shoe. The side of the heel can be taped by either running a piece of tape around the back of the heel or under the heel from side to side. Start with a strip of 2-inch tape, applied side to side around the back of the heel. Try and keep the top edge under the anklebone and end just forward of the anklebone. To tape the bottom of the heel, place a strip of 2- or 3-inch tape under the heel, anchoring it to the tape running around the sides. If you are taping only the back part and/or the bottom back of the heel, pinch the folds and trim them with scissors. If you need two pieces on the bottom, apply the forward piece first and the back piece last. If you have a roll of 3-inch tape, an alternative method is to use one strip going side to side, under the heel.

Run a strip of tape side to side around the back of the heel.

Then run a strip under the heel side to side.

The Toes

Toe taping can be done with kinesiology, Micropore, or one of the woven tapes. Even though Micropore is paper tape, it sticks well and is strong, even when the foot gets wet. The best method of taping toes is a two-piece tape job. First, apply a strip of tape over the top of the toe, going over the toenail and around the tip to the bottom of the toe, even with the end on top. Pinch the folds and trim with scissors. Wrap another strip around the toe, from one side to the other, over the tip of the toe. Then pinch any folds and trim with scissors. This puts a smooth section of tape against the neighboring toe—not the edges, had you reversed the order of the pieces applied. Sometimes it's easier to wrap a strip of tape around the circumference of the toe than side to side. If using a nonstretchy tape, be careful not to wrap the toe too

This shows the two strips of tape: top to bottom and side to side.

The side-to-side tape won't curl when rubbing on neighboring toes.

tightly. Never extend the tape far enough down that it will dig into the tender skin between the toes. If taping for toenail pain, you can apply a piece of Spenco 2nd Skin over the nail and tape directly over that. This provides a bit of cushion to the nail. Cut the width of the tape to best fit the toe being taped.

A proper taping on toes or larger areas should appear like an extra layer of skin on the foot—no lumps or bumps. If any folds bunch anywhere, pinch them together and cut the excess flush with small scissors. Sometimes tincture needs to be applied again to keep corners and edges down.

Between the Toe and Foot

This important method comes in handy for those hard-to-tape areas at the base of your toes or between the toes. Cut a figure eight from a piece of tape and, spreading the toes, anchor the bottom of the figure eight on the ball of the foot, pull the top of the figure eight between the toes and anchor it on the top of the foot. A soft tape such as Hypafix, EnduraFix, Omnifix, or Kinesio Tex works best. This figure eight taping is also important to use when taping

A simple piece of tape cut in a figure eight runs between the toes.

the ball of the foot. Use two figure eights, one between the big and second toes, and another between the third and fourth toes. The figure eight anchors the forward edge of tape on the bottom of the foot and keeps it from curling as the foot moves through its stride.

Other Areas of the Foot

Any part of the foot can be taped. For instance, a blister in the crease of the big toe can be covered by running a strip of tape from the top base of the toe, in between the big and second toe, and under and around to the outside of the toe. The strip will be thinner at the top and wider as it runs under the toe. The arch can easily be taped side to side, under the foot with one or two 2-inch strips or one 3-inch strip.

Taping Alternatives

Toe pads and caps made from gel are an alternative to taping toes. ENGO patches work well to relieve friction when applied to footwear. Another alternative to taping is a blister prevention method that uses compound tincture of benzoin, or a similar benzoin-based product, and a lubricant. Marv Skagerberg used a benzoin and lubricant combination that worked for him for the last 78 of 86 days of the 1985 cross-country Trans America race. Averaging 43 miles per day through 12 states, Marv did not get a single blister.

1. Clean the feet thoroughly, and dry them completely.

2. Coat the feet, heels, soles, and toes with compound tincture of benzoin.

3. Let the feet dry for 3 minutes, keeping the toes spread. The feet will still be quite sticky.

4. Apply your choice of lubricant.

5. Reapply the lubricant and change socks every 4–6 hours.

TAPING ALTERNATIVE PRODUCTS

BUNGA TOE PADS and **TOE CAPS** are made from a medical-grade polymer material. bungapads.com

BUNHEAD GEL products are made of a nonsilicone polymer, formulated with medical grade mineral oils to cushion and protect those areas of the foot prone to friction trauma. They are washable, supple, comforting, hypoallergenic, and nontoxic. Styles include **JELLY TIPS, JELLY TOES, THE BIG TIP,** and **CLEARSTRETCH TIPS.** Locate a retailer through its website, capezio.com.

ENGO PATCHES are low-friction patches uniquely applied to blister-prone areas of footwear, insoles, socks, and athletic equipment—not skin—for easier, longer-lasting, blister-free protection. Ultra-thin patches leave footwear volume virtually unaltered. Strong, latex-free adhesive prevents migration and movement, even through moisture and sweat. Scientific and field tests show ENGO's slippery blue surface significantly reduces rubbing, providing immediate relief. Several sizes are available: small ovals for toes; large ovals for the ball of foot, arch, and heel areas; rectangles for custom trimming; and a back-of-the-heel patch. goengo.com

PEDIFIX VISCO-GEL TOE CAPS can be used over toes to prevent blisters. pedifix.com

PRO-TEC'S TOE PROTECTORS, made from custom-grade silicone, are soft and stretchable and designed to fit all toes. pro-tecathletics.com

Orthotics

Orthotics are custom-made or over-the-counter insoles that replace the generic, removable insoles in store-bought shoes and boots. Their purpose is to cure lower extremity ailments. Many runners wear an orthotic device in one or both shoes to help maintain the foot in a functionally correct position. Orthotics may be prescribed for the treatment of plantar fasciitis, tendinitis, knee pain, shin splints, lower-back pain, Morton's neuromas, and other conditions. Orthotics can correct gait irregularities and provide support for flat feet and pronation problems. They can also relieve pressure by providing support behind a problem area such as a callous, neuroma, or metatarsal injury. Malalignment problems such as leg-length inequality can also be corrected. Typically prescribed by a podiatrist or orthopedist, orthotics are medical devices made from cast impressions of your feet. A properly fit orthotic will control arch and pressure-point problems. A custom-made orthotic will position the foot in the ideal position in every stage of motion—whether walking, running, or pivoting.

Orthotics can help reduce the shear associated with friction at the sock–orthotic interface. When possible, choose an orthotic that has a smooth or fairly smooth surface. Rough surfaces can adhere to socks, which can lead to shear and blisters.

Signs that you may need an orthotic can include repeated overuse strains or injuries, excessive fatigue in your legs and feet, or genetic structural problems (over- or underpronation, bunions, differences in leg length, arch problems, and so on). Other signs are your shoes showing different wear patterns or wearing out more quickly than usual. The need for orthotics may begin with pain in your feet, repeated blistering in the same place on your feet from pressure, or even problems in your knees or hips as your gait is changed due to biomechanical stresses. Doug Mitchell says, "I had substantial pain in the ball/metatarsal area many years ago. I was doing about 60 miles a week and heavy lifting too, including very heavy calf raises. It turned out that I had a minor structural problem in the foot that created a lot of stress on the ball of my feet. After a while, I went to see a podiatrist, which resulted in my first orthotics. They solved the problem." Doug uses his orthotics almost exclusively in his running and athletic footwear. Check with your health care plan to determine if it covers orthotics.

An added benefit of orthotics is the way they support the body's natural movements. This reduces the demands placed on the muscles when the body is out of alignment. The result is less work by the muscles, which translates to less fatigue, fewer injuries, and higher performance.

If possible, visit a pedorthist, podiatrist, or orthopedist for a complete foot-strike and gait analysis to determine the right orthotic for your feet. Remember several key points:

- Inquire about soft, semirigid, and rigid designs.

- Fiber-reinforced orthotics are typically stronger than other types.

- Make sure that your shoes will accommodate the orthotics. This may depend on the depth of the uppers and the design of the shoe's inside.

- Determine whether your orthotics are to be used alone or with your shoe's stock insole.

- If possible, have a padded layer of material added to the top of the orthotic or use a flat Spenco insole on top of the orthotics for cushioning.

- If you change the model of shoes you wear, have the orthotics adjusted to fit the new shoes.

- Ascertain whether the orthotics are for short- or long-term use. This will depend on your reason for needing them.

- The clinician might recommend specific shoes for your foot type.

Typical Orthotic Modifications and Alterations

- Extra-deep heel seat for more rear-foot control
- Extra heel cushioning
- Soft forefoot extensions at the end of toes
- Metatarsal pads, either soft or pressed into the shell, which can take pressure off neuromas and metatarsal pain
- Morton's extension for a short first metatarsal/long second
- Extra varus (roll out)/valgus (roll in) forefoot or rear foot posting, which inverts or everts the foot more
- Cutouts in the extension for relieving pressure

Bob Williams shares an important point about having orthotics made:

The foot can change over time, just like other parts of the body. Particularly prone to change are our arches because they will drop as we age. Then the foot elongates and you may be forced to get larger or longer shoes.

Orthotics can make the difference in simply allowing one to be able to run again. However, when I first started noticing some sagging arches and had orthotics made, it wasn't until I was on my third different pair that I found comfort. If you do choose to get orthotics, make sure that you have a satisfaction guaranteed arrangement with the podiatrist.

It is worth trying a pair of inexpensive inserts before spending the extra money on much more expensive custom-made inserts or even orthotics. Researchers at Hadassah University Hospital in Israel found that made-to-order inserts were no better than generics at helping solve Israeli soldiers' foot and gait problems. Author Charles Milgrom, MD, said semirigid insoles were the most comfortable.

Another study, by the American Orthopaedic Foot and Ankle Society, found that inexpensive off-the-shelf insoles are more likely to be effective than pricey, custom-made products. According to the society, many foot problems can benefit from the cushioning of a cheap insert more than the repositioning provided by a custom-made insert. Many of these inserts are made from foam, silicone, plastic, wool, or combinations of different materials.

Custom-Made Orthotics

Custom-made orthotics may be soft, semirigid, or rigid, and are made specifically for your feet. Materials may include felt pads, cork, foam, viscoelastic, silicone, closed-cell rubber or closed-cell polyethylene, fiberglass, carbon fiber, or leather. Orthotics can be made in various lengths and include metatarsal pads or heel wedges. They are made to work in partnership with your boots and shoes. Poor-quality boots and shoes may alter the corrective action of an orthotic.

In the article "The Ideal Running Orthosis: A Philosophy of Design,"[28] the authors build a case for the ideal orthotic. They recommend a custom fit in either semirigid or semiflexible design, lightweight, yet inexpensive, with a covering to decrease shear while giving control to both the forefoot and hindfoot, all while retaining memory in its shape and being adjustable at a later time. It also needs to be transferable to most of the client's shoes. They place orthotics in two categories of design: corrective and accommodative. A *corrective* orthotic should attempt, with a rigid design, to correct the foot's position so that its abnormal anatomy will mold to the corrected position. An *accommodative* orthotic should attempt to relieve areas of high stress or reposition the foot to better deal with its stress, usually with a soft or semiflexible design. The most common type of orthotic is semiflexible.

Getting Orthotics

Orthotics can be ordered and cast by many professionals: physical therapists, trainers, physician's assistants, pedorthists, orthopedic techs, chiropractors, and podiatrists, to name a few. Given a choice, I would recommend a pedorthist or sports podiatrist to do the ordering and casting. In reality, pedorthists are the only professionals trained in the actual fabrication of custom foot orthotics. Other health care professionals have to order from a supplier. Finding the professional who has the patience to listen to your history is important. There are some other professionals who do a fine job diagnosing and casting for orthotics, but feet are not their primary interest.

All Orthotics Are Not Alike

Custom-molded orthotics are devices made from an actual mold or cast of the foot. There are two media to cast in, foam and plaster splints. Foam is neater but is inaccurate. Impressions are usually taken with the patient seated. Once the material is compressed, it cannot be changed. Too much pressure in one area and the casting is flawed. Plaster splints allow for the foot to be manipulated into the correct position while the material is still soft. The cast then hardens over the next two to four minutes. Impressions are either taken with the patient sitting with the legs straight out to the caster or lying prone (stomach down) with feet dangling off the end of a table. This author prefers the latter.

The majority of orthotics that are used for sports are made from white polypropylene or any one of the many varieties of carbon fiber. Carbon-fiber orthotics may be flexible or ultrarigid. If adjustments such as raising or lowering the arch or removing a high spot are needed, the carbon-fiber varieties are easily adjusted by heating with a heat gun and then manipulating. They hold their adjustment much better than the polypropylenes that have a lot more memory. These devices tend to go back to their original shape after attempted heat adjustments. Permanent adjustments have to be made by the maker of the orthotic.

The stiffness of the orthotic is an important feature. The more flexible devices provide less control but can be more comfortable. These are ideal when an accommodative forefoot or metatarsal pad is used. Though if control is what is needed to prevent excess movement such as overpronation or over-supination, then a rigid device will normally be well tolerated. I can't even begin to count the number of times I have replaced another doctor's flexible orthotics with a pair of semirigid or rigid ones with great success.

—podiatrist Tim Jantz

Whoever makes your orthotics needs to ask the right questions and order the right tests to make the correct diagnosis about which type of corrective orthotic is necessary. The typical process includes a detailed injury history; complete lower-extremity biomechanical examination, including a gait analysis; and a check of your shoes or boots. The aim is to identify the cause of your injury and try to prevent its continuation or recurrence. *Patient compliance in wearing the orthotic is the dominant issue in resolving foot problems.* Modifications to the orthotics may be necessary to ensure a proper fit—if the orthotic is uncomfortable, chances are that

O R T H O T I C   P R O D U C T S

Many custom-made orthotics are available, and your pedorthist, podiatrist, or orthopedist will help select the correct one for your feet. The product lines of custom-made orthotics and insoles are constantly changing.

The insoles listed below are proven alternatives to the more costly custom orthotics. Your podiatrist or pedorthist can show you other types.

ARCHCRAFTERS CUSTOMCOMFORT INSOLES are computer machined to the exact shape of your foot. Placing your feet into a specially designed "foot printer" captures the imprint of your feet. A scanned image of your feet is then made from the imprint and is used to make your custom insoles. archcrafters.com

ARCH FLEX SYSTEM is made by Swedish running shoe manufacturer Icebug and offers a deep heel cup with low-, medium-, and high-arch support. icebug.com/int/icebug-insoles

CURREXSOLE offers insoles for all types of sports. These are engineered in Germany with multiple profiles based on your foot type. currexsole.com

DR. SCHOLL'S makes a line of pain relief orthotics for foot, knee, and back pain. drscholls.com

EXOSOLS ORTHOTICS are custom-made by using the SOLS Custom Fit app to snap six photos of your feet. sols.com

EZ ORTHOTICS are a lightweight, thin-profile, fluid dynamic orthotic. Silicone fluid is sealed into a polyurethane pouch with a viscosity matching that of the foot's fat pad. Gel flows precisely with each stride from heel strike to push off. It provides cushioning and correction at the forefoot and metatarsal heads. ez-orthotics.com

HAPAD ORTHOTICS are either full-length or three-quarter–length insoles. Both are made from Hapad featherweight wool. The coiled, springlike wool fibers provide firm and resilient support while offering arch, metatarsal, and heel cushioning. Multiple types of insoles are offered. hapad.com

you won't wear it. Once you are using orthotics without any pain, continue to use the orthotics as long as they work for your feet. Some injuries that require orthotics will be relieved after a short period of time; other gait, support, and foot-function problems will require long-term use.

Technology has evolved to offer athletes foot scanning that typically identifies your arch type, foot size, and pressure points. Then the ideal orthotic is selected for your feet. Several companies offer this technology: Aetrex offers their iStep system and Spenco their Custom Fit system, with both then using that to select the best insole from their line. ArchCrafters scans your feet to create a custom-made orthotic—not an off-the-shelf orthotic. Other companies offer a box filled with

INSOLES AND BEYOND offers a wide range of insoles for all types of foot conditions and foot pain. insolesandbeyond.com

LYNCO BIOMECHANICAL SPORTS ORTHOTICS, made by Aetrex, offer a ready-made, triple-density orthotic system that comes in enough variations to accommodate 90% of foot disorders. They offer three versions for athletes: a **CUSTOMIZABLE SERIES,** a **SPORTS SERIES,** and a **MEMORY FOAM SERIES.** Each model comes with a cupped heel or a medial posted heel, and with or without a metatarsal pad. Aetrex also offers iStep scanning of your feet to help select the best orthotic for you. aetrex.com

POWERSTEPS INSOLES, by Dr. Les Appel, offer a unique four-phase design to relieve heel and arch pain. With a heel cradle and platform, a strong prescription-like arch support, an antibacterial top fabric, and a double-layer cushion casing, they provide optimal arch and heel support and stability. They also offer a heat-moldable maximum cushioning insole. powersteps.com

SOLE CUSTOM FOOTBEDS, which use heat-to-fit technology, offer an excellent, inexpensive alternative to custom orthotics. They come in regular and ultra-cushioning versions. The footbeds have Poron cushioning, a deep heel cup for stability, and an aggressive arch for support. When you heat the insoles in your oven, put them into your shoes, and stand on them, they mold to your feet. yoursole.com

SOFTSTRIDE ORTHOTICS use a viscoelastic polymer to mimic the qualities of soft body tissue and redistribute pressure and impact. Styles are designed for heels, the forefoot, and insoles. brownmed.com

SPENCO ARCH SUPPORTS are offered in several designs ready made for your foot size. They offer foot scanning to help select the best insole for your feet. spenco.com

moldable foam that you stand in to capture the uniqueness of your feet for custom insoles. ExoSOLS custom orthotics are made using its app and an iPhone; you take pictures of your feet to get the exact measurements for proper biomechanical alignment to reduce pressure.

Mail-order orthotics need to be checked out thoroughly and purchased only through reputable companies. Adjustments to mail-order orthotics can be difficult. Arch supports sold in sporting goods stores and drugstores should not be mistaken for orthotics. The Hapad, Lynco, and Spenco orthotics identified above are just three of many low-cost orthotics that can be helpful as an alternative to custom orthotics and quick-fix drugstore remedies.

Over-the-Counter Orthotics

Not everyone needs a custom orthotic, and it may be worth your while to try one or two over-the-counter insoles. They may work. Some of these insoles are designed for specific foot problems. Ultrarunner and podiatrist Tim Jantz explains:

> Store-bought orthotics are just that—they are purchased at a store such as Walmart, Kmart, Osco, Walgreens, or running specialty stores. These devices I refer to as arch supports. They support the arch, which can provide relief of mild arch strain and heel pain to name a few. But they don't address the biomechanical problems that often are the cause of many maladies. They are simple, soft, and flexible. After all, they are made to fit every foot type that is a size 8 or 10 or 12. Some examples are Sof Sole and Dr. Scholl's DynaStep. These types of devices consist of soft to firm foam, and some even have a thin layer of carbon fiber for more support. They range in price from $5 to $35.

Nick Williams tells how he "had tried hard orthotics, soft orthotics, Spenco orthotics, and just about anything else to keep my feet from hurting." Then an orthopedic surgeon told him about Hapads and gave him a pair. They have kept him pain free for five years and are flexible on trails. Nick swears by Hapads and via e-mail told ultrarunner Ed Furtaw about them. Ed wore custom-made orthotics for 10 years but since has used the Hapad's Comf-Orthotic three-quarter–length insoles without heel pain. He says, "They are definitely more comfortable than wearing orthotics." Ed added Hapad Scaphoid Pads for extra arch support. Ed's wife then switched from custom orthotics to the Comf-Orthotic. After an area on one arch got a little sore, they peeled away some of the wool material to make it fit better. Ed believes, "With something such as Hapads, a person can take more responsibility for their own orthotic adjustments, which would be very difficult or impossible with custom-molded rigid orthotics." An orthopedist told me that if he had only one product to offer his patients, he would choose Hapads!

Using Your Orthotics

Ask your pedorthist, podiatrist, or orthopedist what you need to do to help the orthotics work. You should receive complete instructions on the use and care of your orthotics. He or she might give you a detailed treatment schedule of stretching and strengthening exercises and advice on shoe or boot selection. You may also be advised to wear the orthotics for several hours a day and gradually work your way up to longer periods.

If your foot seems to slip on your orthotic, ask about changing the surface material. A thin layer of Spenco insole material or your favorite insole material can usually be glued to the orthotic using rubber cement. The use of Spenco's Slip-In Insoles can add needed cushioning to your orthotics. Check with the maker of your orthotic before adding anything to the surface because doing so can change your gait and affect the purpose of the orthotic.

If you have orthotics that are three-quarter length, basically stopping at the ball of the foot, you need to use a thin insole, similar to the green Spenco flat insoles, under the orthotic. Usually running or hiking on the exposed bottom of the shoe is uncomfortable. Ask the maker of your orthotic how to add cushion under the forefoot and toes.

Once you have your orthotics, you need to put them into your shoes. Full- and partial-length orthotics are meant to replace your current insoles. Partial-length insoles, ending just behind the ball of the foot, may be more comfortable with a thin, flat insole over the top or underneath to avoid less of a drop-off at the end of the orthotic.

It is not unusual for orthotics to require a tune-up every few years. If you start having foot pain or other problems, contact whoever made them and ask about having them checked. Sometimes all that needs fixing is a resurfacing of the top fabric.

13

Gaiters

I usually tell athletes of their foot-care options and advise them to make the best choice—however, I have three absolutes. The first: You should always use moisture-wicking socks. The second: You need properly trimmed toenails. The third: If you are going out on trails, you need to wear gaiters.

A few years ago when I was working an aid station at a 50K trail run, I was amazed at how few runners wore gaiters. One thing was certain—all had muddy shoes and many had muddy socks. And I don't mean a few drops of mud. I mean the gooey, down your shoes and between your toes type of mud. The mud hardens and causes friction and hot spots, and blisters form. The pace slows, good running form dissolves, your biomechanics alter your stride, and the downhill spiral begins.

Gaiters have been proven to be functional trail gear that all dedicated trail runners and adventure racers should use on trails. Hikers wearing low-top boots could also benefit from using gaiters. Forming a barrier around the leg and the top of the shoe, gaiters keep rocks, dust, and waterborne grit from getting into socks or between the socks and shoe. Gaiters can mean the difference between finishing a trail run or long hike with feet in good shape or feet plagued with hot spots and blisters. Some gaiters slip over the foot, while others close on the side or in the front with Velcro.

My infatuation with gaiters began in 1989. Before my third Western States 100-Mile Endurance Run, I knew I had to do something extra to help my feet. Because I was prone to blisters and the trail was known for its dust and rocks, I decided to make a pair of gaiters out of socks. While I realize the gaiters alone did not make the whole difference, I did lower my personal best time by 1.5 hours. The bottom line was that my feet were protected from the dust, grit, and rocks of the trail, and I had minimal problems.

Lisa de Speville, an adventure racer and ultrarunner from South Africa, says, "Interestingly, too many people still don't seem to get this gaiter thing. To us it is soooooo obvious. In addition to reducing the amount of grit in your shoes and thus friction and blister-forming opportunities, I find that the life of my socks is substantially increased. You can run through rivers and not get a tea-spoon of sand in your shoes. I advise people to have the Velcro stitched—not glued—onto their shoes. Sand and grit is sneaky and it can lift even the strongest superglue, especially if the event is over a few days." Lisa makes gaiters and does custom orders.

John Wood has tried a number of gaiters and has learned a few tricks. He comments:

> The ones that strap under the shoe are a nuisance if you need to change shoes or socks in a 100-mile race. First of all, you are likely to be a bit stiff at the later stages of the race, so unless you have a pit crew, trying to loosen the strap and get it refastened is liable to put you into a cramp, let alone cost you a bunch of time. Also, the strap under the shoe can get chewed through and break if you are running on trails with sharp rocks. The gaiters that have a Velcro fastener in the back are very easy to loosen and pull back so you can change socks or shoes. The disadvantage is that you have to affix the Velcro to the back of all shoes that you plan on wearing. The self-stick Velcro is pretty worthless. Instead, get the nonadhesive Velcro at a fabric store and some Liquid Nails glue or Gorilla Glue to stick the back of the Velcro to your shoe. To help hold the Velcro while the glue is drying, just tape it down. Some people use Super Glue, but I have even had that come off.

Whether you are an adventure racer, a simple short-distance trail runner, a hiker, or an ultrarunner, you owe it to yourself to cover your socks and shoes with gaiters.

Making Your Own Gaiters

You can find any number of gaiters at your local stores. But sometimes, homemade ones work just as well or even better. Homemade gaiters can be easily made by anyone willing to try.

Ultrarunner Raymond Zirblis wore women's knee-highs over his shoes during the Marathon des Sables. The nylons stretched well, covered the whole shoe and up the leg, and kept sand and pebbles out, but the mesh was too open to keep dust out. They tore and wore away, but they stayed on all day. Ray used a fresh pair each day, reporting that while not perfect, they worked better than most of the gaiters he saw there during the six days of the desert run. Cathy Tibbetts-Witkes has also run the Marathon des Sables, and after much experimenting, she, too, designed her own gaiters.

Kent Holder tells of using the arms off an old nylon jacket with elastic sleeves. He cuts the sleeves off about 6 inches up the sleeve from the cuff. He simply

Lisa's homemade gaiters provide sand protection.

GAITER PRODUCTS

DIRTY GIRL GAITERS are made by ultrarunner Chrissy Weiss and are popular for their groovy colors and patterns. Her design is a soft, comfortable, four-way stretch spandex unisex gaiter that attaches to the front shoelace with a hook and secures to the back of the shoe with a self-adhesive Velcro strip—thus avoiding the strap under the shoe. dirtygirlgaiters.com

EASTERN MOUNTAIN SPORTS offers a variety of gaiters in different heights. All use a strap under the shoe's arch. ems.com

EQUINOX makes a line of gaiters, which can be used by hikers and adventure racers. Styles include mini- to mid- and high-gaiters featuring a strap under the shoe's arch. equinoxltd.com

The **INOV-8 RACE ULTRA GAITER** is designed for total debris control and fastens securely against the shoe. inov-8.com

JOE TRAILMAN GAITERS are made without the usual strap under the shoe. They attach to the shoelaces closest to the front of the shoe via a hook and to the rear with a Velcro tab. The tension of the four-way stretch material holds the gaiter in place. The gaiters are offered in small and regular to fit all types of shoes. This style slips on your foot before putting on your shoes, which also makes it easy to change shoes or socks. joetrailmangaiters.com

LISA DE SPEVILLE'S CUSTOM GAITERS are offered in different types and heights. She makes **AR ADVENTURE GAITERS, AR MINI GAITERS,** and **AR DESERT GAITERS.** adventurelisa.blogspot.com

MONTBELL SPATS are made for rugged wear. They have a hook that attaches to your shoelace up front, and a stretch cord runs underneath your shoe to keep

pulls the arms, elastic end first, onto his legs over his socks. The loose nylon covers the top of the shoes, and Kent reports that it keeps all of the usual trail debris from entering the shoe. With this type of gaiter, there are no straps, so changing your shoes and socks is a breeze. Rodney Hammons has found another way to get a gaiter effect. He wears a pair of knee-high–type nylons under his Ultimax socks and then pulls the nylons down over the socks and tops of his shoes. Improvising can work wonders.

Repairing Gaiter Straps

The nylon straps or cords that come with some gaiters go under the shoes and boots and will wear out over time as the trails and rocks take their toll. Wrapping the straps with duct tape can help extend their life span. Then simply replace the tape when it wears through.

There are several methods to replace the worn-out straps. Mike Erickson uses swagged (pressed around the edges of the cable) 0.0625-inch stainless steel cable instead of nylon cord—he reports that these have held up for more than five years. Put a piece of duct tape over the swagged ends. Mike also reports using thin nylon everything nice and tight. The stretch cord is adjustable for length and is user replaceable. They are made out of durable Schoeller Dynamic stretch fabric that offers permanent stretch, durability, water and dirt repellency, and great breathability. Gore-Tex versions are also available. montbell.us

MOUNTAIN HARDWEAR GAITERS are offered in a variety of styles, high and low, strap and strapless. They are made with stretch nylon and fit easily over boots and trail shoes. mountainhardwear.com

OUTDOOR RESEARCH makes several gaiter styles appropriate for running and hiking. Gaiters are either step-in or open in the front with Velcro, have an eyelet on either side for a lace that goes under the shoe's arch, and a metal hook that fastens to a shoelace. outdoorresearch.com

RACING THE PLANET GAITERS are made from nylon and spandex and are above the ankle height. The **RAIDLIGHT** and **ROUGH COUNTRY** gaiters attach to the shoe's sole to provide sand protection. They suggest having a cobbler sew the Velcro onto the sole for strength. Also available is a Velcro strip and glue. racingtheplanet.com

REI makes several designs of gaiters. Its **TRAIL RUNNING GAITERS** are made from stretch-woven spandex/nylon fabric. The **TRAIL LIGHT GAITERS** are made with Cordura nylon. Each style has a side Velcro closure and an instep cord. Find them at local REI stores or at rei.com.

SIMBLISSITY LEVAGAITERS are ultralight and made from ultrabreathable Durastretch fabric. Uses a shoelace hook but no under-the-shoe cord or heel glue or Velcro. Offered in two sizes. simblissity.com

Custom-Made Gaiters

Cathy Tibbetts-Witkes and Lisa de Speville are two athletes who make their own gaiters. Both have made two sizes: ankle-length for the ordinary ultra and knee-length for sand dunes. They fit snugly over the shoe and attach to the outside with Velcro glued near the bottom on the sole of the shoe. Their gaiters are held up with elastic sewn into the top that is sized for the circumference of the leg either above the ankle or calf. "It took a few tries to work the bugs out," Cathy says, "but now I have totally sand-proof gaiters. Just keeping the fine dust out has cut down tremendously on blisters." Lisa calls her gaiters the most crucial piece of equipment she takes to a sand race. A critical component of gaiters worn in sand events is to have them attach to the sole of the shoes. The 4 Deserts Gaiters from Racing the Planet are made to attach to the shoe's sole to provide sand protection. With a little time and minimal expense, you can also make a set of gaiters. Lisa offers instructions on her website: adventurelisa .blogspot.com/2009/11/make-your-own-mini-gaiters.html.

cord doused with super glue and then wrapped with a couple layers of duct tape. Others use Kevlar shoelaces or picture-frame wire. Improvise to find other creative methods. A tough polyurethane strap that attaches to gaiters with adjustable fasteners can be found online at dgioutdoors.com.

TIP: A Simple Slit Saves the Strap

Some athletes use a serrated-edge file or a knife to make a slit in the sole into which the strap or cord fits. This can protect them from fraying or being worn through as quickly. If you choose to make this modification to your shoes, be careful not to cut too deeply and compromise the integrity of the sole.

Do-It-Yourself Strap Replacement

To replace the nylon strap itself, use the method recommended by ultrarunner Kirk Boisseree, using the following materials, which are usually found in fabric stores: 1-inch-wide nylon webbing, size 24 (0.625-inch) metal large snaps (four sets of male and female pieces), and a snap installation tool. The snap tool can usually be found in craft or sewing stores. Make the new straps as follows:

1. Using the old strap as a guide, cut two pieces of webbing the same length. Use a lighted match to slightly melt the ends of the straps to prevent fraying. Be careful to not touch the melted nylon until it cools.

2. At each end of the replacement straps, install a female snap. Use a center punch or a nail to make a hole in the center of the strap 0.75 inch from each end.

3. Push the snap through the hole and set the snap using the tool, following the instructions on the package.

4. Repeat for all four female snaps, making sure the snaps face the same way on each strap end.

5. Install the male snaps on the old straps about 0.5–0.75 inch from the gaiter. Using the center punch and installation tool, center the male snap in the hole, facing the outside of the shoe, and set the snap.

6. Remove the middle portion of the worn strap, cutting it down to about 0.5 inch from the new snaps.

7. Snap on the new straps and check for a proper fit.

Lacing Options

There are many options for lacing shoes or boots. The way you lace can accommodate many common foot problems or foot types: narrow or wide feet, high arches, localized foot pain, heel control, toenail and corn problems, and more. According to Australian mathematician Burkard Polster, there are 43,200 possible ways to tie a shoe with two rows of six eyelets. For those intrigued by shoelaces, Polster is the author of *The Shoelace Book: A Mathematical Guide to the Best (and Worst) Ways to Lace Your Shoes* (American Mathematical Society, 2006).

Tying laces too tightly can create pressure on the bony, thin-skinned tops of your feet. This can be worse if you have high arches or your shoes have thin tongues. Some athletes have problems with laces causing friction and pressure, occasionally resulting in blisters. After a long run or hike, some runners and hikers experience bruising over the instep where the laces tie. This sore, red spot is often called shoe-related neuritis because the laces irritate the nerves on the top of the foot. Occasionally, this can cause numbness of the toes. Laces can be adjusted to fine-tune the fit of the shoe or boot and to relieve pressure over the instep.

The lacing variations described on the following pages can make a shoe fit better and allow for needed spacing in the tongue area or provide for better heel control. The conventional method of lacing—crisscross to the top of the shoe—works best for the majority of people. But in some cases, other lacing patterns may alleviate trouble arising from the shape of a foot or the construction of the shoe. In the illustrations in this chapter, dotted lines show where laces are hidden from view.

Other than changing your lacing patterns, you might consider several lacing products that work well for running shoes, some boots, and many types of shoes. For instance, Easy Laces have been around for more than 25 years and are a favorite with many athletes. These products replace the normal shoelaces and end the problem of laces coming untied or breaking. Experiment with stretch laces to find the most comfortable degree of lace tightness that does not cause undue pressure on the instep and yet controls the heel. A tongue cushion can help with instep irritations.

Lacing Tips

To prevent laces from untying, don't double-knot at the top. Instead, gather the loops and lace ends and tuck them through one or two of the cross strands toward the toe of the shoe. This prevents laces from coming untied as effectively as double-knotting and is easier to untie. Also, when you're running through brush, it keeps the laces from getting snagged or picking up debris.

Physician's assistant and ultrarunner Rich Schick suggests another method for keeping laces tied. First, make your laces as short as possible so the loops are not too long. Then add a simple knot at the ends of each lace. When tying your shoes, instead of leaving extra lace, pull on each of the loops until each end knot is snug to the bow. Finally, tuck the loops under one or two of the lace crossings. Another method to keep your laces tied is after tying a regular knot, tie the bows into a second knot.

Ian's Shoelace Site (fieggen.com) describes and shows a variety of knots for tying shoes. Ian's Secure Shoelace Knot is the best for active athletes. His website is a wealth of information about shoelaces, knot-tying ideas, and lacing products.

If you will be in wet or cold weather, steer clear of loosely woven or cotton laces. Check your local outdoor store for laces made of polyester, nylon, or a blend of materials. Many athletes find their round laces come untied faster than any other design. Kevlar laces are very strong but may have to be double-knotted to stay tied.

Try flat instead of round laces, use one of the elastic laces below, or lace your shoes according to the issue you are experiencing (see the illustrations on the following pages).

Many shoes and boots are made with speed lacing hooks instead of eyelets. To keep laces secured with these hooks, wrap the lace over the hook, around it again, and then to the center for the knot.

For those wanting other options, Easy Laces, Lock-Laces, and the Yankz Sure Lace System feature elastic laces with a locking device. Each has a unique locking system.

Lacing Methods

Flat feet, high arches or not enough support in the arches, narrow or wide feet, and heel-control problems can be helped, to varying degrees, by lacing techniques. Several of the lacing techniques described on the following pages work best with shoes having alternating eyelets spaced in a zigzag pattern, rather than in a straight line.

Lacing pattern for narrow feet

For Narrow Feet

For narrow feet, use the eyelets farthest from the tongue of the shoe. This will bring up the sides of the shoe for a tighter fit across the top of the foot. This method works on shoes with variable-width eyelets.

For Wide Feet

For wide feet, use the eyelets closest to the tongue of the shoe. This gives the foot more space by leaving more width across the lace area. This method works best on shoes with variable-width eyelets. An alternative method is to pass back under the lace as it emerges from the second eyelet. This prevents the lace across the first eyelets from getting tighter as you run.

Lacing pattern for wide feet

Lacing pattern to prevent heel slippage

To Prevent Heel Slippage

For heel slippage, or heel problems, use every eyelet, making sure that the area closest to the heel is tied tightly and that the area nearer the toes has less tension. When you have reached the next to the last eyelet on each side, thread the lace through the top eyelet of the same side, leaving a small arch of lace between the eyelets. Then thread the opposite lace through each opposite arch before tying the laces together at the top. Wendy Holdaway found a solution by having a shoe repair shop put in a second set of eyelets from the top-most eyelet, around the heel at the top of shoe. She says, "It looks odd but gives me room in the toe box while holding the shoes to my very narrow heels."

For Instep or Top-of-the-Foot Pain

For instep or top-of-the-foot pain, use one of two lacing methods. The first is to lace using the instruction to prevent heel slippage above. The second is to leave a space in the lacing before the top eyelet. Depending on your shoes and the number and layout of eyelets, you might be able to skip at least one or even two sets of eyelets. It would be similar to the illustration for lacing over painful areas, but up higher.

For High Arches

For high arches, lace the shoes so the laces go straight across. After lacing the bottom two eyelets on the outer side to the inner two eyelets, lace up two eyelets on the same inner side and cross over to the outer side. Lace through these two eyelets and move up two eyelets on the same outer side. Continue this alternating method until one set of eyelets is left. Continue lacing up to the top eyelets on each side.

A high-arch lacing alternative is to string one lace through the first two bottom eyelets and then every other eyelet to the top. A second lace is threaded through the remaining eyelets. This allows tighter lacing at the ball of the foot and the ankle

Parallel lacing
for high arches

Double lacing
for high arches

while the midfoot is laced more loosely. With this method, quick adjustments are easily made for uphills and downhills.

For Narrow Heel and Wide Forefoot

For a narrow heel and wide forefoot, use two laces per shoe. Lace one through the bottom half of the eyelets tied loosely. Lace the other through the top half of the eyelets tied more tightly than the bottom lace. Another option is to lace the first few loops loosely, tie a knot, and then lace the rest of the way up the shoe. Doug Freese suggests skipping the first one or two bottom most eyelets rather than deal with two sets of laces.

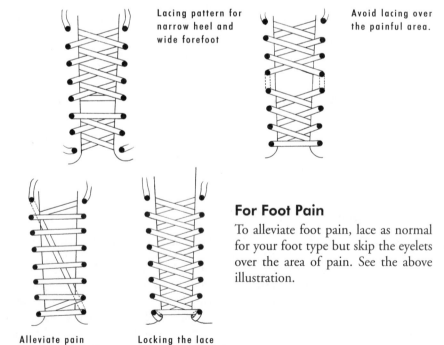

Lacing pattern for narrow heel and wide forefoot

Avoid lacing over the painful area.

For Foot Pain

To alleviate foot pain, lace as normal for your foot type but skip the eyelets over the area of pain. See the above illustration.

Alleviate pain caused by toenail trouble or corns

Locking the lace maintains constant pressure at the toes.

For Toenail Problems or Corns

For toenail problems or corns, lace down from the top eyelet opposite the problem toe to the bottom eyelet on the side of the problem toe, leaving enough end to tie the laces together. Then lace from the bottom up, side to side, until the top eyelet is reached. This method creates an upward tension on the bottom eyelet over the problem toe, relieving pressure. See the illustration on the bottom of the facing page.

For Constant Toe Pressure

To maintain constant pressure at the toes, lace the bottom eyelets as usual. Then lock the lace in place by looping the lace around and back through the same eyelet. Continue lacing as normal. Locking the lace at the second or third eyelet can modify this technique. This allows you to tie the laces as tight as you want above the lock while keeping the laces as loose as desired below the lock. See the illustration on the bottom of the facing page.

LACE PRODUCTS

EASY LACES are lockable shoelaces featuring a stretchy elastic cord with a lock where the usual bow is tied. You can slip your foot into the shoe or boot without releasing the lock, or you can release the lock to open the shoe farther. The laces are available in myriad colors. easy-lace.com

HAPAD TONGUE CUSHIONS prevent rubbing and alleviate other irritations at the instep. If you have narrow heels, they also hold the foot back into the heel of the shoe for a better fit. The coiled, springlike wool fibers provide firm and resilient support. The pad attaches to the underside of the tongue of the shoe. hapad.com

LACE LOCKS, sometimes called cord locks, are simple plastic cylinders with a button that locks or releases a lace run through a center hole. Two laces easily fit through the hole, which secures the laces at the desired tension. These are usually found in sporting goods stores.

LOCK LACES feature specially designed elastic laces combined with a spring-activated locking device. The high-tension springs are made from a metal alloy that won't rust or corrode. The locking device holds the laces (when knotted) in place so they stay secure and maintain the same constant tension on the foot. Available in a variety of colors and lengths. locklaces.com

SPEEDLACES come in two styles with two lace options. Choose either the regular **IBUNGEE** stretchy laces or the **RACE RUNNER** laces (stretchy or nonstretchy) consisting of six Zero-Friction eyelet fittings, laces, and cord locks. The fittings fasten into the lace holes and allow the laces to tighten evenly above the surface of the shoes. The cord locks and lace pulls allow self–adjusting equal tension of the laces. speedlaces.com

THE YANKZ SURE LACE SYSTEM includes expandable cord laces and locking devices with two points of adjustability, providing a custom fit. A toe-clip hook holds the extra loop of lace. Shoes can be changed without unlocking the laces. yankz.com

Self-Care for Your Feet

Skin Care

In order to keep our feet healthy, it is necessary to give them the attention they need. But then how many of us know what our feet really need?

It's relatively easy to tell how healthy someone's feet are—for me anyway. I just run my hands up and down their feet, and over and between their toes. That's about as up close and personal as you can get. The skin on healthy feet will feel soft and supple. The skin feels somewhat smooth and moist as opposed to feeling dry and flaky. Many people treasure their calluses and do everything to keep them, while others work hard to rid themselves of the rough skin. No corns, plantar warts, or athlete's foot will be seen or felt—just soft and supple skin. Notice how I come back to that again?

I'll also look closely at their toenails. These are a great indicator of the health of the feet. Are they properly trimmed and filed? Have the nails been picked at, which leads to ingrown toenails? Are the nails soft, flaky, thickened, and discolored? Is there nail fungus? Nice healthy nails are firm and strong and are trimmed well.

Because our feet have more than 250,000 sweat glands, the mixture of sweat and bacteria in our shoes and socks is what makes our feet smelly. Medically known as bromodosis, it is a common problem. Clean, dry feet and clean shoes and socks can lower the risk of foot odor and fungal infections. A tip for making sure your socks are really clean is to turn them inside out before washing. This way, all the dead flakes of skin have more chance of being washed off.

Take the time when showering to use soap and a washcloth on your feet. The rubbing exfoliates dry skin and helps do a thorough cleaning. Then dry your feet, taking extra care on the toes and between the toes. If you tend to forget washing your feet, get the FootMate System, a brush system that adheres to your shower floor and has two sets of scrubbing bristles to clean your feet (footmate.com).

A foot soak can help revitalize your feet, and Epsom salts are commonly used. Here's an alternative that Carey Lynn used at a multiday race and learned about from Claire Denise Johnson, a doctor friend. Carey soaked runners' feet for 15 minutes in a mixture of water, a quarter cup each of Listerine and baking soda, and a half cup of Epsom salts, pouring enough to cover the tops of their feet. She said the mixture seemed to revitalize, clean, and disinfect the runners' feet. Runners gave her high praise for the soaks. Try it after a long training run or if your feet are sore and tired.

Others use a foot soak with one part apple cider vinegar to two parts water. Soak for 15 minutes at a time. Adding one-quarter cup of baking soda is an option. This will help if you have smelly feet. Do not use this soak if you have scratches, open sores, wounds or cuts on your feet. If a rash, redness, or itching develops, discontinue the soaks.

In the summer when we are most active, our feet are often abused. They become hard, callused, or blistered by our multiday hikes, long training runs on back-to-back days, or cross-sport training, as well as by going barefoot or wearing sandals without socks. We repeatedly stress our feet without giving them time to recover and heal. In dry, cold weather our skin becomes dry, resulting in splits in the skin. Deep cracks are called fissures and are often accompanied by calluses. Dehydration can also cause these cracks and fissures.

Specialized tools are now available to reduce calluses. The Amope Pedi Perfect, Dr. Scholl's Express Pedi, and similar products make quick work of hard calluses. These are battery operated and use a wide roller head with micro-abrasive particles to remove excess hard skin. They excel at removing calluses on heels, bottoms, and sides of the foot. Refill roller heads are available for all models. All models are designed to stop when too much pressure is placed on the skin, preventing overexfoliating, which can damage the skin. The downside to these tools is the roller style has limited value on toe calluses.

The Heel Smoother Pro is the perfect tool for reducing calluses on toes. This two-speed, battery-operated pedicure appliance smooths calluses and removes dry skin anywhere on your feet. The shape of their DuraCrystal Power Tips is the perfect size to work on toes, but also works well on other areas of the foot. Even though this company has closed, you can find these by searching online.

Use creams or lotions that help improve the skin's texture and tone by exfoliating dry and dead skin and allowing newly rejuvenated skin to emerge. Some creams contain alpha hydroxy acids, which are all-natural substances found in fruits and sugar cane that generally speed up the exfoliation process.

The use of a deep-penetrating hydrating cream twice a day will help your feet stay soft and supple by restoring your feet's natural oils. Ultrarunner Roy Pirrung uses flaxseed oil products to keep his skin well conditioned. Pay close attention to your heels and the balls of your feet, two of the places where fissures and calluses typically form. To help the cream work its magic, at bedtime rub in the cream and place plastic wrap over your heels. The wrap seals in the cream to enhance the moisturizing effect. In the morning after showering, use the aforementioned callus-reducing tools, a pumice stone, or callus file to buff the skin and reduce calluses. After this buffing, rub in a small amount of cream to keep them soft during the day.

A good testimonial for soft feet comes from racewalker Dave Littlehales:

> I used to think that tough, callused feet were the way to go. But after the '97 Vermont 100, where I developed huge full-bottom-of-the-feet

blisters bilaterally, my podiatrist convinced me to go 100% in the other direction—soft and supple. Now I get a pedicure at least once a month, which smooths out all calluses and rough spots. I also put creams on my feet on a daily basis. When I hit the trails or roads, I use foot powder. Things have improved greatly.

Keeping Feet Fresh

It's very easy to keep your feet and shoes fresh by using a small amount of baking soda. Use it as a powder on your feet or sprinkle a bit into your shoes to control odor. A short spray of Lysol into each shoe is another option to help control odor.

Long-distance hiker Brick Robbins finds that after several months on the trail, he has a hard time with "stuff" growing on his feet. He has solved this common problem by soaking his feet for 20 minutes in a solution of about a gallon of water and 2–4 ounces of povidone-iodine every week or so. He says that it has kept his "feet from smelling too bad and seemed to kill the stuff that had started to grow under one of my big toes." Betadine can be used as an alternative to povidone-iodine.

If your shoes get stinky or have a mildew smell after getting soaked in rain, wash them with soap and water and let them dry naturally. After they have dried, give each shoe a couple shots of Lysol. Do not put your shoes in the dryer.

By the end of summer many athletes are suffering from dry and cracked feet—usually from going barefoot or wearing sandals. If you have not had success with your current choice of foot lotion or cream, try Vicks VapoRub. Larry E. Millikan, MD, a professor of dermatology at the Tulane University School of Medicine, says the petroleum in VapoRub holds in moisture, may have antifungal properties, and can reduce itching.

Occasionally check your feet and ankles for small areas of pigmented skin, moles that have changed in size or appearance, and any unexplained discoloration under a toenail. These could be early signs of melanoma and need to be checked by your doctor. Melanomas on the feet or ankles have a higher mortality than other melanomas because they are usually discovered at a later stage.

Pedicures

I asked Denise Jones, the Badwater Blister Queen, to write about pedicures. She shares her insights:

Why would an athlete or runner consider getting pedicures? Surely such a lavish bubbling foot treatment in a spa or salon might sound way too frilly and out of the ordinary for such a sport. Think about it this way: Your feet get you there in ultras. If your feet are in bad shape, they can greatly hinder your long-distance adventures.

Consider getting a pedicure for the health of your feet, not just for the aesthetics. You may think that the callus you've developed is your insurance and a means by which your foot protects those friction areas better. Quite the contrary; calluses are never normal. Rather, they are a sign of poor biomechanics or ill-fitting footgear.

Unless a callus is troublesome, most runners tend to ignore it. Once you have experienced a deep blister underneath a callus, you are more likely to rid your foot of it or at least minimize it. So consider getting pedicures. Also, warn your manicurist/pedicurist that you are a runner and you do not want your calluses shaved off, but rather you'd prefer having them gently removed a little at a time with a pumice stone or a buffing pad. Getting feet in better shape is a process, not instantaneous.

Additionally, problems can arise from poorly filed and trimmed toenails. Many runners have paid a high price for untrimmed nails, where an edge can catch on the sock and thus cause the entire toenail to lift after enough miles. Not only is this painful, but most of the time, it's also preventable. So get those toenails in good shape too with a pedicure. Then there is the foot massage. Ahhhh, it is therapeutic and just plain feels good! Until I get a good foot massage, I don't even realize how sore my feet are.

When you get a pedicure, your toenails are often cut and shaped before being soaked; however, some salons do this after soaking. Make sure, as a runner, that you get those toenails short enough and filed down smoothly. Then your feet will be soaked in a large basin of warm water. One foot at a time is removed from the water, a cuticle lotion is applied to the edge of the toenails, and your cuticles are trimmed and returned to soak. Then one at a time, each foot is removed from the water, and a pumice stone is used to remove calluses and dead skin from the base of the foot. Both feet are patted dry with a clean towel. Finally, toenails may be buffed or polish applied and lotion is massaged into each foot and leg.

If you are not sold on pedicures, listen to a few athletes. Karen shared her view:

I love my pedicures. I'm with the others in that regular upkeep of my nails makes them less prone to have issues. The biggest issue for me is nails that get too long banging against the end of my shoes. [The pedicurists] seem to be able to cut them short but not too short. Although I never let them touch the calluses on my toes, they do a great job of bringing down the ones on the backs of my heels, which get quite painful when I run. I also like that they make me stick to a moisturizing regimen on my feet, which generally keeps the calluses down to a dull roar.

Terri Schneider wrote:

I try and get regular pedicures for a few reasons: 1) I have very tough feet, which isn't necessarily a benefit for ultras, as I get thick calluses, then

SKIN PRODUCTS

A wide assortment of skin products that are useful for athletes is readily available at your local health-food store or drugstore.

AMOPE PEDI PERFECT ELECTRONIC FOOT FILE uses a roller to quickly reduce calluses. amope.com

AQUAPHOR HEALING OINTMENT can be used for dry, cracked, and blistered skin. aquaphorus.com

BURT'S BEES COCONUT FOOT CREAM and **PEPPERMINT FOOT LOTION** are made to revive and rejuvenate your feet. burtsbees.com

CORRECT TOES are a polymer material that separates toes into a natural alignment. correcttoes.com

DR. SCHOLL's makes the **EXPRESS PEDI FOOT SMOOTHER, ULTRA OVERNIGHT FOOT CREAM,** and **ROUGH SKIN REMOVING FOOT CREAM.** drscholls.com

FLAXSEED OIL products contain sources of essential fatty acids for proper skin conditioning.

FLEXITOL HEEL BALM has a combination of emollient ingredients that actively replenishes moisture deep below the surface of the skin. flexitol.net

FOOTHERAPY NATURAL MINERAL FOOT BATH for soaking and softening corns and calluses.

FOOTSMART carries a complete line of skin-care products made for the feet: **TOTAL FOOT RECOVERY CREAM, NIGHTTIME HEEL TREATMENT CREAM, CALLUS TREATMENT CREAM,** and **CALLEX CALLUS OINTMENT.** footsmart.com

GILDEN TREE makes products for feet: **NOURISHING FOOT CREAM, EXFOLIATING FOOT SCRUB, REVITALIZING FOOT SOAK,** and **95% SHEA BUTTER BALM.** gildentree.com

THE HEEL SMOOTHER PRO by Artemis Woman is an excellent tool made for callus control on toes. The DuraCrystal Power Tips do quick work on heel, toe, and other calluses. It comes with two tips for curved areas of the foot. Search for them on ebay.com.

JOHNSON'S NO MORE DIAPER RASH is a unique three-in-one formula that promotes effective healing; soothes red, irritated skin; and forms a protective barrier. It

blisters under them (very deep and painful) in 100-milers. The pedicure cuts away all thick areas and dead skin, nail pieces, and things that might dig in and cause blisters or problems. It keeps your skin a healthy and even thickness. 2) My feet look and feel much healthier when I get pedicures regularly. Dead skin is scraped away, allowing for a continual natural sloughing of skin. 3) It also keeps the shoe smell down dramatically!

Before getting a pedicure, ask how the spas are disinfected. Typically, the disinfectant takes 10 minutes to work.

contains zinc oxide and skin conditioners such as lanolin, petrolatum, and vitamins E and B5.

KATHY'S FAMILY FOOT BALM, FOOT SCRUB, and **FOOT BATH** is made with 100% natural and organic ingredients. kathysfamily.com

KERASAL ULTRA 20 EXTRA STRENGTH FOOT CREAM for dry heels softens even the driest feet. kerasal.com

KINESYS SPORT'S SOOTHING FOOT SPRAY has peppermint and menthol.

NEUTROGENA FOOT CREAM, a Norwegian formula, both moisturizes and softens dry skin. neutrogena.com

ON YOUR TOES works as odor control and an antibacterial foot powder. footodor.net

PRETTY FEET & HANDS ROUGH SKIN REMOVER is made to exfoliate rough skin away. prettyfeetandhands.com

SKINMD NATURAL, a shielding lotion that adds moisture while stopping the loss of your natural moisture to heal dry and damaged skin. skinmdnatural.com

SQUIRREL'S NUT BUTTER is an all-natural antichafe and restorative skin salve that is also useful as a lubricant. squirrelsnutbutter.com

TINEACIDE ANTIFUNGAL SHOE SPRAY for eliminating fungi and bacteria in footwear. drblaines.blainelabs.com

TRIPOD LABS' HYDROSTAT foot cream works on dry, rough skin on heels and feet.

UBALM offers three versions of their unique formulation with antioxidants, emollients, humectants, and lubricants for dry, cracked, and chapped skin. ubalm.com

XZUBER foot cream is an all-natural product that will eliminate the odor-causing bacteria on your feet. xzuber.com

VOGEL'S HOMEOPATHIC 7 HERB CREAM, a combination of herbs and oils in a natural base, is formulated to soften and smooth rough, dry, or cracked skin. avogelusa.com

ZIM'S CRACK CREAM moisturizes, soothes, and softens dry, cracked, and painful skin. There are two formulas: a nighttime liquid and a daytime cream. The creams are formulated with a unique herbal base of arnica and Myrcia oil. zimsusa.com

For several days after the pedicure, check your feet for infection. Don't get a pedicure if you have cuts or abrasions, even open blisters, on your feet. Women should not shave their legs, wax, or use hair removal creams within a day before getting a pedicure.

Foot Massage

Massage is great for the feet. It helps increase circulation to injured areas, and the increased blood supply helps speed recovery while reducing swelling. Sports massage focuses on releasing tight, contracted, or overworked muscles used in your sport or activity to restore them to their optimum condition.

Inflexibility associated with tightness can hinder efficient training and performance. When muscles are relaxed and receiving better circulation, they are stronger and tolerate higher levels of training with less pain and breakdown. Tight muscles can lead to strains and soft-tissue injury. Chronic tightness can cause muscle and connective tissue injury and inflammation, resulting in biomechanical imbalances, back pain, Achilles tendinitis, and plantar fasciitis. This is where massage and stretching can help.

Jillian Standish is a certified massage therapist whose typical clients are average athletes who need the benefits of massage to enhance their running. She devotes time during her massages to the feet since the lower leg muscles attach into the feet. As a prerace conditioner, the massage helps loosen the muscles, often lengthening the runner's stride. As a postrace conditioner, she massages knots out of tired and stressed muscles.

Healing from many injuries can be speeded with massage. Mild strains can be eliminated with a few sessions of deep-tissue muscle massage. When a serious strain involves torn muscle fibers, scar tissue develops, which can cause pain when the muscle contracts. Stretching and joint movement combined with deep longitudinal massage strokes can help break down this scar tissue. Chronic tendinitis associated with scar tissue and adhesions in tendons may be resolved with sessions of deep cross-fiber friction massage. Some practitioners use active release techniques (ART) for soft-tissue treatments. This treatment softens and stretches fibrous scar tissue, resulting in improved circulation, increased range of motion, and increased strength.

Robert F. Rusnak, DC, a certified chiropractic sports physician and ART practitioner, explains ART: "The ART technique consists of specific movements of the body to make layers of soft tissue slide over one another, while at the same time, specific pressure is applied to split and strip away the scar tissue that is sticking structures together like glue. The 'release' is accomplished by lengthening muscles, ligaments, and tendons or freeing a nerve along its path."

Look for a licensed massage therapist online, ask other athletes for referrals, or check your local sports stores for practitioners in your area. Likewise, physical therapists, sports-medicine chiropractors, and specialists in sports and orthopedic rehabilitation often incorporate massage into their practices.

Self-Massage

To do a self-massage of your feet, start by warming your feet in a bath or with warm, moist towels. Cross one leg over the other with the sole facing you. Use both thumbs to massage your feet in a deep, circular motion, working small areas at a time. Work from your toes toward your heel, and then to your ankle. Use various movements and pressure to find what feels best. All movement, and pressure, should be toward the heart—moving the old, stagnated blood back to your heart. The use of massage oil or creams can help with the kneading of the skin and can soften dry heels and calluses. Self foot massage is easier if you're limber, but even

MASSAGE PRODUCTS

DUE NORTH'S FOOT RUBZ MASSAGE BALL and **MASSAGE ROLLER** are made from hard rubber with stimulating nubs to massage. available through amazon.com

GAIAM RESTORE HOT/COLD FOOT MASSAGE ROLLER can be used cold or hot to roll out tightness. available through amazon.com

MOGI 360 FOOT MASSAGER has rotating massage spheres to relieve pain and tension. gomoji.com

NATURAL FOOT CARE: HERBAL TREATMENTS, MASSAGE, AND EXERCISES FOR HEALTHY FEET, by Stephanie Tourles, published by Storey Publishing in 1998. This book presents a holistic approach to caring for feet, introducing alternative and natural treatments for good foot health.

REJUVENATION REHAB makes a muscle massage kit with a nubbed ball and companion tension relief bar. rejuvenationrehab.com

RUMBLEROLLERS have firm but flexible bumps that work around bones to hit muscles and muscle attachments. rumbleroller.com

THE STICK is a massage tool that can be used on any major muscle groups through clothing or directly on the skin. It provides instant myofascial release, which promotes healthy and relaxed muscle fibers and good circulation. It comes in four sizes and can be used before and after exercise to aid strength, flexibility, and endurance. thestick.com

TRIGGERPOINT PERFORMANCE THERAPY has rollers in multiple styles that can be used to massage muscles and tissue, including the Nano Foot Roller and massage balls. tptherapy.com

if you're not, you can probably manage it. If possible, have a partner massage your feet. Another option is to use a product like TriggerPoint foam rollers, Rumble-Rollers, or a similar product to work the muscles and tissues of your feet. Other products are listed above.

Foot Massage Techniques

- **BOTTOMS OF THE FEET** Place your thumbs on the heel of one foot. Apply pressure to the underside of the foot, starting at the bottom and slowly moving toward the toes.

- **BALLS OF THE FEET** Make small circles using your thumbs. With fingers on top of the foot and thumb on the ball of the foot, push from toes toward the heels to roll the metatarsal heads.

- **ARCHES OF THE FEET** Massage the center of the arch with mild to moderate thumb pressure. The correct point is halfway between the heel and the ball of the foot and halfway between the inner and outer edges of the sides of the foot.

■ **HEELS** Massage the bottom and sides of the heel using thumbs or knuckles.

■ **TOES** Stroke between the toes upward toward the heart.

■ **TOPS OF THE FEET** Using your fingers, massage the top of the foot, focusing on soft points between the bones of the forefoot upward toward the ankle.

■ **STROKING THE FEET** Using both hands, place your fingers on the top of the foot and the thumbs underneath. One hand at a time, stroke upward (slide your hands toward the ankle).

■ **WALKING BAREFOOT** Especially if done outdoors on a variety of surfaces, walking barefoot stimulates the muscles, nerves, and joints of the feet.

Hydration, Dehydration, and Sodium

A subject often overlooked by athletes is the effect on the skin of dehydration and the loss of important electrolytes. Long periods of physical exercise cause stress to the extremities as fluid accumulates in the hands and feet. Fingers and toes often swell as they retain fluid because of low blood sodium (hyponatremia). This causes foot problems as the soft, waterlogged tissues become vulnerable to the rubbing and pounding as we continue to run and hike.

Make sure that you replace electrolytes, especially on long events. Drinking water or even sports drinks may not provide the proper replacement of sodium and other important electrolytes. The popular energy bars and gels may also be low in the electrolytes needed by the body.

Karl King, developer of the SUCCEED! Buffer/Electrolyte Caps, points out that the maintenance of proper electrolyte levels will reduce swelling of hands and feet even after many hours of exercise, and reduce hot spots and blisters on the feet. "When there is heat and humidity, the sweat rate is high and sodium is usually lost in significant amounts," he says. "The sodium comes from the blood stream, and when the plasma gets too low, the body reacts to maintain the minimal tolerable level by pushing water from the blood into extracellular spaces. Thus, hands and feet swell. When the tissue on the feet swells, the feet become soft and more susceptible to blisters and damaged toenails. The feet swell inside the running shoes, putting extra pressure on the tissues, and those tissues can be rubbed to the point of physical damage. We see blisters form as layers of skin separate, and we see toenails move more, damaging the weakened tissues that normally anchor them." Many times the water that creates blisters is underneath the skin, not on the surface.

As ultrarunner Jay Hodde notes, "The terms *proper hydration* and *well hydrated* should not be used interchangeably. Being well hydrated with fluids says nothing about the sodium content of the fluid; both are important." When you are well hydrated yet have low sodium, extra fluid accumulates in the tissues of the feet and the likelihood of blister formation increases. When you become fluid deficient, the skin loses its normal levels of water and in turn loses its turgor. Then it easily rubs or folds over on itself, which leads to blisters.

HYDRATION AND ELECTROLYTES

E-CAPS ENDUROLYTES are formulated to counteract the effects of electrolyte deple-tion and imbalances of hot weather. The caps can be taken as a supplement or mixed in any fluid replacement drink. The Endurolyte caps contain calcium, magnesium, potassium, sodium chloride, L-tyrosine, vitamin B6, and manga-nese. hammernutrition.com

S! CAPS replenish in the proper proportions electrolytes commonly found in blood plasma, supporting hours of exercise. They are designed for individuals engaging in physical activities where people sweat heavily. The caps contain a chemical buffering system of sodium chloride, sodium bicarbonate, sodium citrate, sodium phosphate, and potassium chloride, which neutralizes the acids formed during heavy exercise. This both reduces nausea associated with exercise, particularly in the heat, and reduces the swelling of hands and feet common after many hours of exercise. Using the caps often leads to a reduc-tion in hot spots and blisters. They should not be used when water is in short supply. succeedscaps.com

THERMOTABS are buffered salt tablets that can be taken to prevent muscle cramps or heat prostration due to excessive perspiration. The active ingredi-ents are sodium chloride and potassium chloride. Look for Thermotabs at your local drugstore or pharmacy.

Rod Dalitz comments, "I am now convinced that electrolyte balance may be a big factor in blisters. With too much or too little salt, the layer just under the skin swells, and your skin may separate from underlying tissue—*creating* a blister." Many athletes have found out the hard way that simply drinking a fluid replacement drink often will not provide the necessary electrolytes in the proper concentrations that the body needs. The use of a sodium replacement product in prolonged physical activity can help in the prevention of blisters.

Electrolytes and Black Toenails

Karl King emphasizes, "Black toenails are often a result of insufficient electrolyte management. Too little sodium makes hands *and* feet swell. You can see your hands, but you can't see it happening with your feet because they are in your shoes. When the tissues swell because they have excess water, the mechanical strength of the nail footing goes down. Then any movement will do tissue damage. Most of the damage is done in the second half of an ultra when electrolyte status is often thrown off if you don't take care of it. Not many people get black toenails from a 15-mile run. Before I figured out electrolytes, I had black toenails like all of my ultra friends. After improving the way I handled electrolytes, my toenails gradually healed and black toenails were a thing of the past."

Strengthening Your Feet

We've looked at skin care, pedicures, foot massage, and hydration, dehydration, and sodium. One more important area important to foot health is strengthening your feet. This can be done through exercises to build strength in your feet and ankles. Small movements and exercises like balancing on one foot, writing the alphabet with your toes, flexing and pointing your toes and feet, and even going barefoot at home—done consistently—can make a big difference in building foot strength. The more you strengthen your feet, the better they will perform and stay healthy. Check the "Strains and Sprains" section of chapter 21 for additional exercises for ankles.

Changing Your Shoes and Socks

Whether you are close to achieving an age-group win, reaching a personal best, simply finishing within the time limit, or reaching a specific trail destination, the 3–10 minutes necessary for foot care may seem like a lifetime. Only you can make the decision on taking the time to care for your feet. I have seen many runners take off their shoes and socks to reveal skin that falls off the bottoms—not small pieces but enough to cover half their foot! It cannot be emphasized enough—take the time necessary to manage your feet or they will manage you.

When possible, change shoes and socks before problems develop. You may opt to carry an extra pair of socks and a small foot-care kit in a fanny pack, allowing for road or trailside foot care as necessary. Dry skin is more resistant to blister formation than skin that has been softened by moisture. Depending on the event, you may choose to change at predetermined points or predetermined times. At these times, you should inspect your feet for problems and treat them appropriately. Reapply powder and/or lubricants when changing socks.

For long runs, determine in advance how often you will change your shoes and socks. Aid stations that are accessible to crew support or aid stations that have your drop bags are the best places to change shoes. On a 24-hour run having additional half- or full-size-larger shoes available may save your feet.

Changing shoes can help tired feet become refreshed. Because cushioning and support is different in each style of

The skin creases on this severely macerated foot, which resulted from not changing shoes and socks.

TIP: Horning In

Whenever you change shoes and/or socks, be sure to smooth your socks to avoid problem-producing wrinkles. Run your hand inside the shoe to smooth the shoe's seams and check for any irritating debris. When changing socks or shoes, too many athletes simply shove their feet into their shoes. This puts pressure on the heels and tender skin. Use a shoehorn when changing shoes to ease sore feet back into the shoe. The shoehorn will also help keep intact any taping you may have done to your feet. If you have an untaped blister on your heel, the pressure can tear the skin off the blister. Plan ahead and add an inexpensive shoehorn into each drop bag or aid station foot-care kit.

---

shoe, your feet may feel better in changed shoes. Each shoe's fit and dynamics has the potential to alter your gait and bring relief to your feet, ankles, knees, hips, and back—but a change can cause problems too. If you are changing shoes to get rid of a hot spot, be aware that sometimes relief new shoes bring to one area can result in other problems elsewhere. Simply pay close attention to your feet as you start out in your changed shoes. Sometimes it is necessary to go back to the old shoes.

Trail running and hiking often make for wet shoes and boots that become dirt caked. Change shoes and socks as soon as possible after getting wet. Even though shoes and socks do dry out after a stream crossing or in rain, continuing to run or hike may cause the skin on your feet to become overly soft and tender and more prone to blisters. Softening of the skin, called maceration, can cause skin over and around blisters to separate. Where the blister is already ruptured, the skin then opens up. When the skin has been wet for long periods of time, it is not uncommon, when removing socks, to find the skin as shriveled as a prune and the skin separating. The use of high-technology oversocks (see page 101 in the "Socks" chapter) to keep the feet dry can help reduce maceration and blisters.

Hikers need to carry a basic foot-care kit as part of a first aid kit. They should wash their dirty socks daily and dry them on the back of their packs. Some hikers will wisely choose to change socks several times a day. If possible, take a short 5–10 minute soak in a cold stream or lake to refresh your tired feet. Before putting socks that were washed in a stream back on your feet, turn them inside out and fluff up the fabric to restore some of their loft.

In extremely cold weather, it is important to keep feet dry and warm. Socks and footwear that are too tight can cause constriction and impede circulation. Changing from wet into dry socks helps keep the feet warm. The use of moisture-wicking socks also is helpful.

Keeping Your Shoes Fresh

We have all been around them at one time or another. Or maybe you are one too! You know, those who can't shake smelly feet. You can take steps to control your smelly shoes.

There are many products on the market to control odor, from baking soda balls to absorbent volcanic stone. Results are often so-so. For the absolute best treatment, try what many bowling alleys use on their often-worn shoes: Lysol disinfectant spray. To use, pull out your shoe insoles and spray the entire surface, giving a spritz inside the shoes too. Let all parts air out for a few hours before wearing.

The unique and innovative Fresh Force upside-down aerosol dispenser blasts odor in both the forward and rear part of the shoe, heel to toe. Simply insert Fresh Force into the shoe and press down, and the dual-action spray effectively controls odor on contact all day (kiwicare.com).

A more natural approach is taken by aromaweb.com. They give instructions to make a shoe deodorizer from natural ingredients. They suggest 4 tablespoons cornstarch, 4 tablespoons baking soda, 20 drops tea tree oil, 10 drops lemon oil, and 10 drops lavender oil. Sprinkle the deodorizer lightly into shoes in the evenings or at times when the shoes will not be worn for a few hours. You will not see a cure for smelly shoes the first time you use the deodorizer. The magic occurs after regular uses.

Stuffitts Shoe Savers are a cedar-filled fabric sleeve that is inserted into shoes to absorb moisture and odors and are available through online stores.

Extreme Conditions
and Multiday Events

Aching feet, cold and wet, maceration, trench foot and chilblains, frostbite, snow and ice, heat, sand, and jungle rot are conditions that adventure racers, ultrarunners, and travelers need to understand, especially during a multiday event. Many of these conditions can be experienced in the same event.

During the ELF Adventure Race, Steve Gurney's team had to deal with many foot-care issues: hot spots, blisters, grit, water, swelling, water, jungle rot, water—all common elements in a multiday adventure race. Some sports test and challenge us in different environments. These events will also challenge your foot-care skills. Because of the uniqueness of each event, there are tips that will work in one environment and not in another.

Jane Moorhead worked on participants' feet at the 2003 Primal Quest Adventure Race. Her experiences second Steve Gurney's points about planning for foot care under various conditions.

Never assume that you are blessed with such tough feet. Use the following tips based on the event's location, weather, terrain, and length, as well as how your feet have held up in past events. Read the whole section on multiday events, because extreme and multiday events are often related.

Aching Feet

Wayne "Smiley" Herrick calls it thru-hiker foot pain: "It's that aching pain that many (most) long-distance hikers get on the bottom of their feet from overuse. It feels as if someone has repeatedly taken a hammer to the bottom of your feet."

Others can also feel the ache and pain of too much time on their feet. Sudden increases in mileage put undue pressure on the bones, tendons, ligaments, and muscles of the feet. If you are typically walking 3 miles a day and then suddenly walk 10 miles, you can expect your feet to feel sore, hot, and painful. Increasing your

personal experience

"I'm convinced that one of the key factors in [our success] was conscientious foot care. We realized that with such a wet course, damaged feet would be the telling factor. We actually learned from the horse-riding stage—gee, if the horses are having problems with their feet, we will have it worse. It was exceptionally wet.

"Our simple strategy was to keep our feet as dry and undamaged as possible. Prevention is infinitely better than cure, but be efficient about it. At every rest or stop, we made sure that we immediately dropped to the ground and elevated our feet to reduce swelling. If the stop was a long one (more than 60 seconds), we took our shoes off and allowed our feet to dry. This was especially effective in the sun. The heat helped to dry and the UV killed some bugs.

"Cleanliness was important, and as I started to get jungle rot, I used copious quantities of that magic Betadine. We cleared grit out frequently but quickly. Several times our feet started to swell to the point that we could feel damage occurring, so we stopped to allow the swelling to go down. When we did move, we moved quickly and efficiently so as to reduce time on feet.

"I used insoles that molded to my feet and shoes, which also helped to reduce blisters, and they proved easy to modify with a knife to relieve hot spots. Several teammates used SealSkinz socks to keep the grit and infection out. We used a silicone lubricant to attempt to seal out moisture and to lubricate. I guess the ultimate key is to thoughtfully think about the conditions and plan smart."

—Steve Gurney, on winning the ELF Adventure Race

running miles from 10 kilometers (6.2 miles) to a half-marathon (13.1 miles) will result in similar complaints. The same goes for other distances. Ultrarunners can feel this after a 100-mile, 24-hour, 48-hour, or 72-hour race. Adventure racers can feel it after a 6- to 10-day expedition race. Typical causes are

- the day-after-day stresses of walking, running, or hiking long distances;
- trying to do many miles too fast;
- not properly conditioning your feet;
- pushing too hard in an event or race for which you are not fully trained;
- encountering conditions for which you are not prepared;

personal experience

"In the day I worked we saw almost 20 racers. Close to 75% of them had at least some degree of immersion foot, and they all had blisters in various stages. One racer told me that he had taken three pairs of socks and changed them religiously when his feet got wet. Another team cut the toes out of their $90 shoes in order to promote draining. Most of them had applied tape, moleskin, or some other type of dressing.

"So why were their feet in such bad condition? My husband worked the race as the support team leader for an Australian team. Out of the four people on his team, two had badly macerated tissue from broken blisters on the balls of their feet and two did not. Why? I wish I had an absolute answer, but I think there are many factors.

"Keeping feet dry is a must. One racer had such bad immersion foot that when he removed the tape from the bottom of his foot, he took a couple of layers of skin with it. We began turning people away from the tent until they had washed and dried their feet and let them bake in the sun awhile to dry the tissues out. The best taping in the world wasn't going to work on wet feet.

"*Know your feet!* Those who had used taping or moleskin going into the event fared better than those who didn't. If a racer knows that he or she tends to get pinch blisters on their little toes, they need to tape at the start of the race, not during.

"Racers should stop at the first sign of foot trouble to tape their feet. This was a demanding race, so even the most experienced racers may have underestimated the toll it would take on their feet. However, my impression was that many teams just wanted to keep moving and didn't take the necessary ten minutes to tape.

"And finally, sometimes you are just blessed with tough feet. Sorry, but it's true."

—Jane Moorhead, after working on feet at the
2003 Primal Quest Adventure Race

- wearing footwear—such as shoes, insoles, or socks—that is worn out;
or

- having preexisting foot conditions, such as flat feet or plantar fasciitis, which contribute to the overall demise of your feet.

The rule of thumb for runners has always been to increase weekly miles by no more than 10%. This is good advice for all of us.

What Smiley learned can help anyone who experiences this same ache or pain. Read what he describes has worked for him and other hikers and apply it to your situation. For some, the ache and pain in their feet may take months or longer to resolve itself. He shares his experiences with aching feet and foot pain:

> Do the bottoms of your feet still hurt or ache after changing shoes? This is a common, almost universal, complaint of long-distance hikers, and I was no exception. The daily high mileage and long hours of hiking invited problems. At the beginning of each part of my two-part A.T. hike, I endured intense foot pain of a variety I'd never experienced, even running marathons and ultras and being on multiweek climbing trips. I've since contacted a podiatrist and a sports trainer specializing in foot care. The only advice I got was, "Don't hike so much" and "Buy these $200 custom insoles."
>
> Some of the following is not scientific and only proven to work for me and other long-distance hikers. I was desperate and tried everything I heard and anything I could think of. First of all, reducing pack weight helps sore feet, and carrying a lighter pack to start with is a good preventive step. A solid training base is a strong preventive step. Changing to a new or different pair of shoes, especially a more supportive and/or cushioned model, could help. Taking a day off is an often overlooked, quite successful remedy. I've found that taking off my shoes and socks and elevating my feet and legs provides immediate, although somewhat temporary, relief. Elevating my feet and legs at night while sleeping was also helpful, as was getting a good night's sleep.
>
> A self foot massage and stretching the legs help by increasing blood circulation to the feet. The variety provided by occasionally walking around barefoot at camp and in town helps. Avoiding pavement and particularly avoiding concrete in towns is a good thing and becomes more important while standing still. If you pay careful attention, especially while running, the difference in hardness among various surfaces is perceptible.
>
> Maintaining a very high level of hydration also helped. I noticed several of my days of more extreme foot pain on the A.T. were at times when I was not as well hydrated. I'd try to drink 8–10 liters/quarts of water on a hot day. Soaking (numbing) my feet in a cold stream was very beneficial. While in a resupply town or after you get home, icing your feet is a good idea. I made use of snowfields along the Colorado Trail to ice my feet when they hurt.
>
> I've found that the surest cure for aching feet is time. Three weeks of breaking my feet in using the above tricks and treatments brings an end to the pain for me. I've talked to others who just learned to accept their foot pain as a permanent part of their thru-hike.

Cold and Wet

At one time or another, every one of us has trained or competed in an event in which our feet were cold and wet for long periods of time. In a short event, these conditions could persist for a couple of hours. In a one-day event, they could last 4–8 hours, and in a long event they may last 4–8 hours a day for continuous days. However long the period, this wet condition can have a negative effect on our feet.

Tips to Help Aching Feet

Constantly aching feet can be depressing and affect one's race, particularly in a 100-mile race or multiday event. Here are tips to help with this bothersome condition.

- Make sure you are well hydrated.
- Rest your feet whenever possible by removing your shoes and socks and elevating them above the level of your heart.
- Massage your feet (refer to chapter 14's section on foot massage).
- If you can, change into a fresh pair of socks.
- Take the weight off your feet by sitting whenever stopping.
- Use anti-inflammatories.
- Make sure you have a good training base of miles (duplicating race conditions, that is, pack on your back, same shoes, and so on).

Blisters may go from being minor inconveniences to major problems. Maceration can happen. In severe cases, chilblains or trench foot can become a real medical issue. When these conditions set in, you will be at the mercy of your hurting feet.

When treating blisters in cold and wet conditions, it is important to be careful in how blisters are lanced. Making too large a hole or too many holes in a blister allows moisture inside. This can lead to tissue swelling, making further patching hard to do. In wet conditions, use a waterproof dressing as described in the "Beyond Blisters" section of the "Blisters" chapter.

A macerated foot resulting from exposure to moisture

Wet, cold feet can lead to long-term or even permanent disability. Even at temperatures above freezing, the combination of cold and moisture can lead to serious injury. Chilblains and trench foot can occur even when temperatures are in the mid-60s in such activities as backpacking. Frostbite at lower temperatures can be debilitating. The care of your feet in cold weather is crucial in all sports. A study published in the *Journal of Athletic Training* found that an athlete who has sustained a previous cold injury has increased chances of subsequent cold injuries by a scale of two to four times in the same area again, given similar environmental conditions.[29]

Tips for Managing Cold and Moisture

Consider the following pointers when planning any training or competitive event in which cold and moisture will be an issue.

■ For high-intensity, fast-paced sports, lightweight, fast-drying shoes are best.

■ If you wear shoes with a Gore-Tex fabric, remember that your feet will sweat and create moisture inside the shoe—therefore moisture-wicking socks should always be worn. *Note:* Once a Gore-Tex fabric shoe has water inside from a stream crossing or other water source, it will stay wet inside for a long time.

■ Treat your shoes with a waterproof spray to protect the shoes from the elements and, in turn, keep your feet warmer.

■ If your shoes have a breathable upper, a layer of duct tape over the upper can keep the wind and moisture out.

■ Wearing shoes that do not have adequate draining capabilities will subject your feet to extended periods of moisture. Use a heated nail or a drill to make a few small holes where your upper attaches to the lower part of your shoe or boot. Make one on each side of the heel and one on each side of the forefoot. Some athletes prefer holes in the sole of the shoe for faster draining.

■ Wear socks that have moisture-wicking capabilities. Choose synthetic fabrics such as Drymax, CoolMax, Olefin, or a blend of materials. SmartWool, Icebreaker, or Darn Tough socks, made from merino wool, are good in wet conditions. Whatever socks you wear, change them frequently and dry the old socks.

■ Be careful not to wear thick socks or layer socks that are so tight that blood flow is restricted.

Rich Schick, an ultrarunner and physician's assistant, gives important advice about being cold:

The first thing to remember is that at any level of activity, you only have a limited total amount of heat produced by the body. The body is going to give priority to the vital organs and only send what is left over out to the hands and feet. This is why the first step to keeping the feet warm is to make sure that the torso and especially the head and neck are kept warm. Likewise, if the legs are bare or inadequately protected, a lot of heat will be lost before it ever reaches the feet. Next, you must understand the principle of how insulation works. Clothing traps air and allows the body to heat it. If insulation is compressed, it is no longer insulation. In the feet this translates to you can't have tight footgear and expect your feet to stay warm.

■ Consider wearing waterproof socks. You have many choices, including SealSkinz socks, Hanz oversocks, Dexshell Waterproof Socks, Showers Pass Crosspoint Waterproof Socks, Seirus Stormsocks, Rocky Gore-Tex oversocks, and eZeefit socks. Even with these socks, if your feet get wet from sweat, they will still suffer, albeit to a lesser degree. Refer to the "High-Technology Oversocks" section on page 101 for more information.

■ Some recommend using a plastic bag over your socks or between two pairs of socks. While this can keep your feet from getting soaked, your feet will get wet from sweat.

■ In hot conditions, sometimes aid stations offer wet sponges over your head to cool off. Be aware that this water can run down your body and into your shoes. Bend forward and keep the water off your body and especially from running down your legs.

■ In humid conditions, make a cuff out of a highly absorbent, microfiber towel (such as those sold in backpacking stores). A 3-inch-wide cuff around the top of your socks will catch much of the moisture running down your legs. Made with elastic or a Velcro fastener, it can easily be removed, wrung out, and reapplied.

■ Foot powders that absorb moisture can help keep your feet dry. Put small containers of powder into your drop bags and in your pack. Reapply powder when changing socks. Zeasorb or Odor-Eaters both make a good moisture-absorbing powder that does not cake up into clumps. Wipe off the old powder and grit before applying new powder.

■ When resting or sleeping, always take off your wet shoes and socks to allow your feet to breathe.

[A key problem is that] feet either get cold and wet from environmental conditions of rain or snow or as a result of wet snow or especially slush on the ground. Terrain factors of stream crossing and standing water also are sources of wet feet. Surprisingly, the most common cause of wet feet is the enemy within, perspiration. This combination of factors usually makes the reality of the situation a matter of how to deal with wet feet rather than how to keep your feet dry.

The choice of socks is crucial. The basic principle is that the thicker the sock, the more moisture it can hold and the longer it will take to dry. Furthermore, heavy socks are most often overkill and will lead to continuously wet feet from excess perspiration. For any activity of greater intensity than a leisurely walk, bulky socks are not necessary. For stop-and-go activities, carrying a pair for use when at rest is a good idea. I recommend a very light sock liner of a hydrophobic material such as Thermax or Capilene. Over this a lightweight sock of similar material, merino wool, or even nylon can be worn for additional warmth if needed. This combination won't pick up much weight and will dry quickly. Avoid wearing cotton socks in wet and cold conditions. Merino wool is a good choice.

Also remember what you may have learned as a child. When your head is cold, the rest of you will be cold. So warm your head with a hat or cap, knit cap, or some form of headgear. Keeping your head warm will help warm your feet.

Maceration

Maceration is an issue at many races and almost always common in multiday events. Maceration in the simplest description is pruned feet, similar to when one is in water too long and the fingers and toes look blanched and wrinkled.

Rich Schick, an ultrarunner and physician's assistant, continues his advice from the previous section on being cold and wet:

> So what happens when your feet are wet and cold and how can that affect your racing? As your skin becomes wet, it softens and becomes more susceptible to blisters. If a blister forms, it is more likely to rupture. The skin then separates further. Maceration happens when skin becomes soft and wet for long periods of time. When you take off your socks and find that your feet look like prunes, this is what has happened. The skin is tender and can fold over on itself, separating and creating problems. As layers of skin separate, blisters spread, the skin becomes whitish in color, and it can split open and bleed. It is very hard to patch feet when this has happened. Feet become so tender that every step is painful.

Again, Rich offers good advice: "You must protect the feet from maceration or skin breakdown. A beeswax and lanolin preparation such as Kiwi's Camp Dry can be effective. It is designed to waterproof footgear but has more durability than the Vaseline-type products. For those with especially sweaty feet, a quick spray with an antiperspirant prior to the application of the barrier ointment can be very helpful." Commonly used diaper rash treatments such as Desitin Maximum Strength Original Paste or Boudreaux's Butt Paste are inexpensive options to control moisture and can be found at drugstores and pharmacies. Zinc oxide and runner's products like Trail Toes and RunGoo work well too. Podiatrist Rob Conenello likes either Gordon Labs' Forma-Ray or Pedinol's Formaldehyde-10 Spray to dry the skin.

Many athletes with macerated feet feel as if the whole bottom of their foot is blistered. In fact, there are often no blisters. The skin is so soft and tender that every step is painful. Many times the skin has folded over on itself or has lifted to form deep creases, which can split open.

I have seen maceration go through several stages:

First, the skin begins to soften and becomes tender. Second, the pruning starts as the exposure continues. The skin wrinkles and softens even more. The third stage is when the skin can form creases and folds over onto itself. The creases may be shallow or deep but are painful. The fourth stage is the most severe. The folds split open and/or the skin may tear.

If there are blisters, they must be drained and covered with a waterproof dressing to help keep tissue swelling under control. Tissue swelling leads to cold and damp skin, swollen and difficult to patch. Refer to the "Beyond Blisters" section in the "Blisters" chapter for information on waterproof dressings.

The photo shows John DeDoncker's feet at the end of the 2015 Western States 100-Mile Endurance Run. His feet were at stage four maceration. Note the creases and folds, and torn skin in the upper arch. By mile 43, his arch was macerated, so medical staff applied 2nd Skin and wrapped the foot. By mile 65, the skin had lifted and torn from his heel. Medical staff cut away the heel flap, applied antibiotic cream and a nonstick pad, and

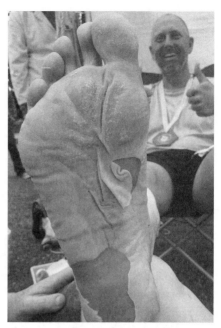

Severe stage four maceration—but a finisher's buckle

heavily wrapped the foot. He changed shoes and socks, but not until mile 78, after the damage had been done. The photo shows what we found at the finish line after cutting away the wrap. I applied a wound care dressing and wrapped the foot with Coban. A week later he was walking pretty normally and was reading a copy of *Fixing Your Feet!* I commend John for finishing and for his great attitude and smile at the end of a difficult race. I wish he had stopped at my aid station at mile 57. He recovered and ran another 100 three months later with a sub–20-hour finish and no blisters. He wrote, "With the aid of your book, I was much better prepared."

What would I have done had I seen him? I would not have put 2nd Skin on his foot because it is mostly water and contributed (in his case) to further maceration. I suspect this led to the skin on his heel tearing under his arch. I would have insisted on sock and shoe changes, dried his feet with powder while he sat for a bit, warmed and massaged the feet, and put an adhesive felt pad under the most severe parts of his foot, covering that with StrengthTape (a kinesiology tape). I would not have removed the flap on his heel. No matter how loose, it exposes new, raw skin, which is painful.

Preventing maceration is difficult, especially in events where there is prolonged water exposure. Shoes must drain well, even if you have to make holes with a heated nail where the upper meets the midsole. The use of high-quality moisture-wicking socks is mandatory. Use a product like Desitin Maximum Strength Original Paste, zinc oxide, Trail Toes, or RunGoo liberally on your feet before running.

And reapply it when you stop to rest. Wearing waterproof oversocks like SealSkinz or Hanz can he helpful.

Treating Macerated Feet

Macerated feet need to be dried as much as possible by removing them from the moisture source, applying drying powders, warming them, and exposing them to air. There is no quick fix for macerated feet.

At a race such as a 100-mile trail race, you have limited options. Most runners won't want to sit for an hour to try and dry their feet. The best you can do is to remove their shoes and socks, dry their feet, and apply powder. Massage their feet if you have time. If they have clean socks and a change of shoes, use them. If not, sprinkle powder into their wet shoes. If they have blisters or other foot issues, treat them as you normally would.

If you are at a multiday event, and it's a middle aid station, follow the above instructions. If it's the end of the day's stage, do the same but encourage them to get into their camp shoes and keep their feet powdered. Generally after a few hours or by morning, the skin is back to normal.

When runners have severe maceration and are continuing on, you have several options. The first is to liberally apply powder to their feet and inside their socks. The second is to apply a piece of adhesive felt to the worst area and use tape to

Tips to Avoid Maceration

Maceration of the skin can cause a great deal of pain and interfere with walking and running. These steps should be taken prior to exposure for the best effect. Also see "Tips for Managing Cold and Moisture" on pages 190–191.

■ Apply a beeswax and lanolin preparation such as Pro-Tech-Skin from Atsko or Kiwi's Camp Dry because of their moisture-repelling capabilities.

■ Use a moisture-controlling agent like Desitin Maximum Strength Ointment, zinc oxide, Trail Toes, or RunGoo liberally on your feet before running.

■ Some athletes have success with a moisture barrier product like Critic-Aid (available through amazon.com).

■ Try the above products in training runs and purposefully get your shoes and feet wet for long periods of time to see the difference in products to find one that works well for your feet.

■ Reapply the skin protectant at frequent intervals or when changing socks, making sure to clean the feet first.

■ Make sure your footwear drains moisture out of the inside of the shoe.

■ Warm your feet when stopping, resting, or sleeping.

■ When resting or sleeping, remove footwear, dry your feet, and allow them to air.

hold it in place. I have done this successfully on the ball of the foot using Hapla Fleecy Web (medco-athletics.com). When the skin has folds or ridges, try to stretch the skin as flat as possible when you apply the Fleecy Web. I prep the skin with benzoin and then put kinesiology tape over the Fleecy Web and onto the top of the foot to help hold it in place.

In many multiday events, the runners' feet are wet the majority of the time. When I worked the Jungle Marathon–Amazon, a seven-day stage race, most runners had some degree of maceration going on every day, and as the week progressed, it got worse. Events with rain or with stream and river crossings are just as bad. In reality, some runners in every race are simply predisposed to having issues, whether it's blisters or maceration. Other runners will come though the race fine or with minor problems.

Drying Your Shoes

Drying your footwear can help your feet. During a race, the sun may be your only drying agent. Use it. Remove the insoles, spread the laces, pull the tongue up and out, and put everything in the sun. Even if there is little or no sun, it can help to air your shoes and insoles. Sprinkle powder in your shoes too.

Drying products are made to cut the drying time of wet footwear, quickly absorbing moisture from your footwear, which improves your comfort, prolongs their life, and reduces the likelihood of mildew forming. Stuffitts Shoe Savers (available online) are filled with cedar chips and absorb 60% of the moisture from shoes in 1 hour and 80% in 6 hours. Stuffitts go inside your shoes and can be used anywhere to absorb moisture and eliminate odors. For home use, check out the Peet Dryer or the Go! Peet Dryer with adapters for home and car use (peetshoedryer.com).

Trench Foot and Chilblains

Chilblains and trench foot occur in similar environments, but chilblains is a more superficial injury and can develop in a shorter time than trench foot.[30]

The name *trench foot* originated during World War I when the troops stood in cold, wet trenches for days without relief. It is sometimes known as immersion foot. Trench foot is a serious nonfreezing cold injury that develops when the skin of the feet is exposed to a combination of moisture and cold for extended periods. It typically occurs with exposure to cold and wet conditions in temperatures ranging from 32°F to 65°F (0°C–18°C).[31] Tissue death can occur in feet exposed to moisture and cold in boots or shoes that constrict the feet for periods of 12 hours or longer. It can occur in temperatures as high as 65°F if the feet are constantly wet—in other words, it does not have to be in winter conditions.

Trench foot is caused by factors common to athletes participating in extreme sports: dehydration, wet shoes and socks, poor nutrition, inadequate and too-tight footwear, and cold. Many of the multiday ultramarathons and adventure races can create conditions right for trench foot. Under the right conditions, even a one-day event could jeopardize your feet. Similarly, hikers can find themselves in the same conditions. Footwear that does not breathe or drain can lead to moisture inside your shoes and socks, which can result in trench foot. Wearing any kind of vapor-barrier sock or shoe can lead to trouble. The continued wearing of wet socks and/or footwear is the most common mechanism for developing trench foot.

Due to the cold, wet, and constricting environment inside the shoe, vasoconstriction (blood vessels constricting) reduces circulation to prevent heat loss. With the resulting lack of oxygen and nutrients in the blood, toxins build up and skin tissue begins to die. Signs of trench foot include swelling, burning, itching and tin-

A bad case of trench foot

gling pain, loss of sensation, cyanotic or blotchy skin, pain or sensitivity, blisters, and skin fissures or maceration.[32] If trench foot is left untreated, ulcerations and gangrene may occur, and amputation may be required. It's a consequence of how damp and cool your feet are, no matter what you wear on your feet.

It can take 24–48 hours before the severity of the damage is fully apparent. If your feet are painful, swollen, and blistered, you need medical attention.

Chilblain, also known as pernio, is an injury due to 1–5 hours of extended exposure to cold and wet conditions. The higher the temperature (generally between 32°F and 60°F [0°C and 16°C]), the longer the exposure time required to develop chilblains. Common signs of chilblains are tenderness, itching, numbness, burning or tingling, skin necrosis, tissue swelling, an increased temperature, and red or cyanotic lesions.[33]

Tips for Managing Trench Foot and Chilblain

Trench foot and chilblain are caused by factors common to athletes participating in extreme sports: dehydration, wet shoes and socks, poor nutrition,
inadequate and too-tight footwear, and cold. There are specific ways to
reduce your chance of getting trench foot.

- Use a moisture-controlling agent like Desitin Maximum Strength Original
  Paste, zinc oxide, Trail Toes, or RunGoo liberally on your feet while running.

- Wash and dry your feet, patting them dry.

- Maintain, as much as possible, dry socks and footwear.

- Do not sleep in wet socks—sleep with dry, warm socks.

■ Avoid socks and shoes that are too tight.

■ Do not add socks if your feet are cold. This causes more constriction inside your shoes. Move up to a larger shoe.

■ Rewarm gently with warm packs or soaking in warm water (102°F–110°F [39°C–43°C]); do not use a strong heat source.

■ Do not rub the skin; instead, use passive skin-to-skin contact.

■ Elevate the feet above the level of the heart.

■ Start an anti-inflammatory drug program.

■ Consider the use of an antiperspirant with aluminum hydroxide to reduce sweating—use this on your feet for a week before anticipated exposure.

■ Do not pop blisters, apply lotions or creams, or walk on injured feet.

Frostbite

Frostbite occurs when tissue actually freezes. There are three phases. The frostnip phase occurs with superficial skin cooling below 50°F (10°C). The mild frostbite phase begins as skin drops below 28°F (-2°C). Phase three is severe frostbite, result-ing in microvascular collapse and leading to tissue death.[34]

Toes are particularly susceptible to this serious condition. Factors that contrib-ute to frostbite include exposure to wind, wet skin (even from sweat), and tight socks and shoes that constrict blood flow.

Early signs of frostbite include numbness, a waxy or pale discoloration of the skin, and pain in the area. The tissue may also become firm to the touch. As frostbite progresses, the skin gets paler and the pain ceases. Often frostbite will thaw on its own as the person keeps moving or gets into a warm environment and out of the wind, wet, and cold. As the tissue warms, there can be redness, itching, and swelling.

In severe cases of frostbite, the skin becomes immobile as it freezes with under-lying tissue. Blisters can form with clear or milky fluid. Blisters filled with blood indicate deeper damage. Leave all blisters intact. If they rupture, treat to prevent infection. While the skin may change color, or even darken, do not assume that you will lose the toes. It may take weeks or months to know if amputation is required. Check with your physician as soon as possible to determine what care is necessary.

Be aware of moisture inside your shoes and socks in extreme cold conditions. Sweat and outside moisture can change to ice inside your socks, leading to frostbite.

Snow and Ice

Hiking or running on snow and ice can be challenging. Traction is often severely compromised and unless one is careful, falls are common. Snow can cover a variety of rocks, roots, and other obstacles that can cause you to trip. Ice is a hard and unforgiving surface. The two most important factors in traveling over snow and ice are keeping your feet relatively warm and dry and obtaining traction.

Tips for Managing Frostbite

■ Use a moisture-controlling agent like Desitin Maximum Strength Ointment, zinc oxide, Trail Toes, or RunGoo liberally on your feet while running.

■ Do not rub your toes to warm them—that causes even more tissue damage.

■ Do not rub the frostbitten area.

■ Unless absolutely necessary, don't walk on frostbitten feet or toes.

■ Get into a warm environment as soon as possible.

■ Immerse the affected area in lukewarm—not hot—water, or warm the affected area with the body heat from another person. Thawing is complete when the tissue is soft and color and sensation have returned to normal. Water temperatures greater than 98°F–104°F (37°C–40°C) should be avoided.

■ Do not use a heating pad, heat lamp, or the heat of a stove, fireplace, or radiator for warming.

■ Do not rewarm or thaw frostbite unless you are sure that you can keep the area warm. It is important to remember that thawing the tissue and then allowing it to refreeze can be devastating. Get professional medical help if possible.

■ Dehydration will make you more susceptible to frostbite.

Moisture-wicking socks are a must. Merino wool is a good choice. Also consider wearing waterproof socks. You have several choices in waterproof socks: Seal-Skinz, Hanz, eZeefit, Rocky Gore-Tex, and Serius socks. These socks are described in the "Socks" chapter.

Cole Hanley runs with hex screws in the soles of his shoes during the winter and has been pleased with the traction they provide. He adds that no screws have ever fallen out and no screws have ever poked the bottom of his feet.

An alternative is to use one of the traction devices that fit over the soles of shoes. Dot Helm, from Alaska, has tried many of these traction devices. She comments:

I should note that the 200 meters between my home and neighborhood mailbox is one of the most treacherous stretches of ice around on a small

Tips for Managing Snow and Ice

■ Consider wearing one of the newer Gore-Tex fabric shoes to repel some of the moisture that will lead to wet and cold feet.

■ Use sheet-metal hex screws or one of the traction devices on page 200.

■ Use high gaiters to keep the snow out of your shoes or boots.

■ Wear the best moisture-wicking socks available. Drymax or wool blend socks are a good choice.

TIP: Hex Screws for Ice and Snow

Sheet-metal hex screws can be used in the soles of your shoes to get better traction. This is a cheap and easy way to modify your shoes or boots to be safe in snow and ice. Use 0.375-inch screws in the lugs of your shoes' soles. Put 10–18 of them around the edges of your shoes' soles with several at the toes and heels. Be careful if your shoes have an air or gel insert. Use a ratchet screwdriver or a drill with a 0.25-inch socket to make the job easier. Dipping the screws into epoxy before screwing them into the shoes will help them stay in place. For more detailed instructions, check out Matt Carpenter's (of Pike's Peak fame) screw shoe page at skyrunner.com/screwshoe.htm.

Ryan Wixom tried this with success: "It works great. I bought some small hex head screws and washers, and put about 13 into the bottom of an old pair of Montrail Vitesse. I used a couple of washers under each screw head to keep them from screwing in too deep." Doug Freese makes a good point when he adds, "Washers mean less screw in the shoe and are more likely to pull out so I would try to buy the right length." He also suggests using a hex head ratchet rather than a hand screwdriver. Doug even keeps an old pair of shoes with screws on hand for muddy races.

---

hill, maybe 15–20 feet high at a 10% slope. So traction devices get tested here. If the snow is soft enough for Yaktrax, I can usually snowshoe run. On the ice near me, the Yaktrax Pro doesn't have enough sharpness to provide traction on ice, like studded shoes do. They also keep my shoe off the ice, so I frequently have less traction than without them. I've also used ice joggers (studs like car tires) of one sort or another over the years to negotiate ice and they do fine, except when you have the rough ice and not enough of the studs contact ice.

Two cautions are necessary: If you use traction devices that fit around or over your shoes, be aware that they may fit differently on different shoes. Secondly, each traction device may work differently on different snow and ice surfaces.

Shoes are being made for the extreme conditions of snow and ice. Examples include Saucony Razor Ice +, Salomon's Snowcross, the Adidas Adizero XT Boost, and Merrell's All Out Terra Ice. Vibram's new Arctic Grip Compound (on the Saucony Razor Ice +), an advanced wet-gripping compound, will likely be found on other shoes soon.

Shoe companies are introducing shoes that incorporate some form of spikes for traction. Be on the lookout for these and similar shoes. The Icebug is a shoe and boot line from a Swedish footwear company. With their BUGrip technology, their shoes have 15–16 smart studs that work independently to grip surfaces. The carbide-tip steel studs are set in the hefty rubber lugs on the shoe's sole. Four varieties of shoes and boots are offered: racing, training, active, and winter. Icebug shoes can be seen at icebug.com.

WINTER TRACTION PRODUCTS

DUE NORTH EVERYDAY G-3 TRACTION AID is designed for people who walk, run, or hike and want greater stability on ice and snow. It fits over your shoes and has bidirectional tread and six tungsten carbide Ice Diamond spikes for maximum grip on ice and snow. It is made with a special compound rubber that retains elasticity in all temperatures. duenorthproducts.com

ICEBUG SHOES have 15 carbide-tip studs in their outsoles to grip snow and ice. The studs retract into the sole upon contact with rocks. They include a pull-on BUGweb that provides an additional six points of traction. icebug.com

ICESPIKE DELUXE is a package of 32 notched screws tested to 500 miles. These turn any pair of trail shoes into winter shoes (tool and instructions included). icespike.com

ICETREKKERS DIAMOND GRIPS are made from case hardened steel alloy, strung on steel aircraft cable, with their patented Diamond Beads with hundreds of biting edges to grip in all conditions. Other options include spikes and chains. icetrekkers.com

HILLSOUND has a line of crampons for ice: **TRAIL CRAMPON ULTRA, FREESTEPS6 CRAMPONS, TRAIL CRAMPON,** and the **TRAIL CRAMPON PRO.** They utilize stainless steel chains and spikes. hillsound.com

KAHTOOLA MICROSPIKES, a flexible traction system, is designed to be used with any common footwear, from trail-running shoes or hiking boots to snow boots. Kahtoola's 10-point gripping system is made from the strongest stainless steel. Straps and quick-release buckles make it easy to put the system on any shoe. They also offer **NANOSPIKES** and, for serious ice conditions, their **KTS CRAMPONS.** kahtoola.com

SNOWLINE CHAINSEN'S line of spikes includes **PRO, CITY,** and **LIGHT** versions. Distribution in North America is by Camp USA (camp-usa.com). kochalpin.at

STABILICER SPORTS are traction devices that have an aggressive cleat-and-tread combination held in place with their tension-fit binding. They are made with dual-density TPE elastomer construction with a traction tread outsole and replaceable cleats. They offer multiple versions for all types of footwear and conditions. 32north.com

VARGO POCKET CLEATS are made from titanium, weigh just 1.9 ounces each, and fold up for easy carrying. vargooutdoors.com

YAKTRAX PRO is a lightweight traction device made of rubber tubing covered with stainless steel coils that fits across the soles of your shoes. The coils are protected against rusting and hand-wound to give you 360 degrees of traction on ice and snow. A removable performance strap fits across the top of the shoe for stability. The newer **XTR** features heel and forefoot antisnowballing plates surrounded with steel spikes connected to a stretchy band that slips onto your shoe. Although Yaktrax makes a **WALKER** model, the Pro and XTR are best suited for athletes. yaktrax.com

Heat

Heat can affect your feet when running on roads, as at the Death Valley Badwater Ultramarathon or in the desert. We can learn from athletes who have been there. Cathy Tibbetts-Witkes, who has raced at Death Valley, the hottest place in America, describes running in the extreme heat:

> Unless you train [in the desert heat], your feet just aren't going to get used to pavement that you can cook fajitas on. With temperatures best measured with a meat thermometer, runners attempting Badwater have to figure out how to make their feet last 135 miles (bad enough as it is) in almost that much heat. Not only will your feet sweat, but also your crew will be spraying you with water to cool you down. As dry as the desert is, your feet will be wet at Badwater.

Denise Jones, the Badwater Blister Queen, tells of doing a heat-training clinic in Death Valley:

> I did a PowerPoint presentation on blister prevention and care and went over all the aspects. I did one demo the first night on a callus that had blistered and opened on its own on the ball of the foot. . . . Her feet were a mess—callus everywhere, black toenails, and nails too long. [This person] has done some amazing things in running, and yet it was clear to me that she wasn't practicing preventive measures at all. This is all the more reason for pedicures.

Five-time Marathon des Sables finisher and 2002 Badwater finisher Blaise Supler was surprised at how few blisters she got at Badwater compared to the Marathon des Sables held in the desert of Morocco: "The pounding at Badwater killed me, especially on the downhill. Plus the skin on my feet turned white and soft, with creases—I guess from the feet being so wet. It made the soles of my feet seem like they were on fire." This fire sensation is caused by maceration of the feet, which happens when feet are wet over long periods. Blaise admits that she "never changed my shoes or socks past mile 72. I was afraid to see my feet; they were so painful. But it turned out that they were hardly blistered." Maceration is preventable by using moisture-wicking socks, changing them frequently, and allowing the feet to dry and the skin to return to normal.

Clive Saffery ran the extreme Badwater Ultramarathon from Death Valley to Mount Whitney and came up with a creative method of protecting his feet from the heat. In the 1999 Badwater race, he added an extra precaution to his usual regimen of using lubricant and powder. To reduce heat on his feet, he duct-taped a cut-up space blanket on all the nonwhite parts of his shoe uppers and lined the underside of his shoe insoles in the same way, using small pieces of duct tape to hold the silver blanket on the shoe and insole. Aside from one small heel blister at 122 miles, he was trouble free the whole race in spite of the temperatures. The space blanket under his shoe insoles fared worse, however— when it was removed after the climb out of Death Valley, it had been reduced to a transparent piece of cling film! Some hot water heater blankets are thin enough to be used the same way.

Probably no one has had the opportunity to work in the heat as much as Denise Jones, the Badwater Blister Queen.

personal experience

"The heat of the desert has melted shoes. Imagine what it does to feet! Over the past ten years I have seen and worked on feet so unbelievably blistered from this event that it would make one think they have been boiled in oil. I have used a myriad of combinations to ensure that feet could handle the stresses of the Badwater Ultramarathon. Through this trial-and-error method, I have devised a system of foot taping that seems to work specifically for racing on pavement in temperatures exceeding 120°F. It has been my experience that if I can get a runner to pretape, it helps prevent a lot of wasted time as the race progresses. Blistering, if it does occur, is subsequently not as major and more treatable.

"Try this method in training first to see if it works for you. In the 2003 race Ben's feet did perfect. In the horrific heat, he had no blisters. I used a combo of my taping, the Injinji socks, and Hydropel, as well as powder, before placing his feet in the socks.

"I don't recommend duct tape. All tape should be breathable. This is very important in desert heat. We have found that duct tape doesn't breathe and causes the area that has been taped to become edematous, sometimes causing worse blisters underneath the tape."

—Denise Jones, the Badwater Blister Queen

Sand

It's all about the sand. Anyone who has traveled across sand knows how it gets into everything. Your goal is to keep it out of your shoes and socks. Take one race as an example: The Marathon des Sables (MdS) is a 150-mile race across the Sahara Desert of southern Morocco, which requires competitors to carry all their food and gear for the weeklong duration of the race.

Cathy Tibbetts-Witkes has done the MdS several times and has mastered the sand:

> With a little training, feet can get used to running long distances with a 15- to 20-pound pack. What your training at home can't replicate is the relentless sand, which commercially made gaiters don't sufficiently keep out. The trick to saving your feet at the MdS is to make your own

Denise Jones's Tips for Controlling Foot Heat

- Pretape any potential problem areas on your feet. In the desert, a breathable tape such as Kinesio Tex is essential.
- Make sure the shoes aren't black, as they absorb heat.
- Wear moisture-wicking socks.
- For those prone to toe blisters, Injinji toe socks help protect each toe.
- Orthotics or extra insoles provide extra insulation from the heated pavement.
- Take several pairs of shoes in larger sizes, so if your feet swell in the event, you can change to a larger size.
- You can also keep your shoes and socks cooler by placing them in zip-top bags in the coolers.
- It's also a good idea to keep the tape in a zip-top in your cooler too, because the adhesive melts in the desert heat, even in the foot box. When it melts, it won't adhere to the foot.
- Have some substantial scissors available, so if need be, you can cut your shoes in areas where friction has blistered you.
- Have a foot-care plan and the equipment to fix your feet.

gaiters, which completely cover your shoe and go up to your knee. I use 70- to 80-denier uncoated nylon and fasten them to my shoes with Velcro epoxied to the shoe.

Cathy's gaiters attach to the edge of the soles and end just below her knees. Check the "Gaiters" chapter for more information on using gaiters in the sand. Several types are there that are made for sand.

Whether or not you wear gaiters, try to use shoes that are not mesh (unless you use gaiters like those of Cathy Tibbetts-Witkes). The mesh allows sand to get inside your shoes, where it gets under your insoles, into your socks, and onto your feet. The sand, along with the movement of your feet inside the shoes, can tear up the shoes' inner material, causing even more irritations to your feet.

On the next page, Jim Benike tells of what he learned about this event and the effects of the sand on his feet.

If you use a lubricant on your feet, watch for sand buildup on your toes and feet. The sand will stick to the lubricant and rub between your toes and feet, creating a coarse friction. When changing socks, wipe off any old lubricant and clean your feet before applying any new lube.

You may have noticed a theme in the advice from all these sand veterans: sand can ruin your feet, and you need to do everything possible to keep it out of your shoes and socks.

personal experience

"The Marathon des Sables is unique in that it lasts seven days, so one has to run every day. One thinks in terms of sand, but there is so much grit and dust that is smaller than the sand. The grit will get into everything. Every crack and crevice—nothing escapes the grit. It will get into the mesh of any shoe. With that preface one can begin to discuss foot care.

"I used double-layer CoolMax socks, which I have been very satisfied with, but they are the wrong sock for this race. The grit and sand gets trapped between the two layers, so after a day or two the socks turn into sandpaper. Hand washing will not remove the sand and grit. Plan on three pairs, which I think is the right number—one pair for the first three days, one for the long day, and one for the balance of the race.

"I wore gaiters every day. Aside from gaiters one needs to cover the mesh of the shoe for the dune day and the long day. I saw several versions of a full shoe gaiter, but they didn't seem to hold up. I tried duct tape on the toe box, but it fell off one shoe. I could have used more duct tape. I think nylon over the toe box might work—the grit would still get into the shoe, but at least heat could escape. Some people just used a large sock over the toe box.

"I wear size 12 shoes but ran in 13s with an extra shoe insole. I took the extra insole out after the second day because my feet were swelling as expected. I had sandals for after the race. My feet were almost too big. I saw several people who couldn't get their feet into shoes or sandals and walked around with shoe insoles duct-taped to their feet.

"The race is about blister prevention, then blister management. It is just a question of how soon the blisters start. I used New Skin on my blisters and potential blister areas. It made the skin tougher and didn't attract grit or sand. I also used duct tape over the ball of my feet, which is where I normally blister. Pretaping might have helped, but I didn't do it. I know of others, veterans of this event, who did pretape. The needle-and-thread method of draining blisters worked for me. I didn't have any infections. The air is so dry that your feet dry out after each day's run. They never stay 'punky.'

"The French take the skin right off the top of the blister. In my opinion this is a bad idea because you still have to run the next day. A visit to the medical tent was a sure sign of someone in deep trouble."

— Jim Benike on the Marathon des Sables

Tips for Managing Sand

■ Avoid shoes with mesh materials.

■ Avoid double-layer socks.

■ Keep your feet as clean as possible.

■ Wipe off any old lubricant before applying a new coat.

■ Use gaiters that keep the sand out of your shoes and socks.

■ Stop and check your feet regularly.

Jungle Rot

Jungle rot is a skin disorder induced by a tropical climate. In long adventure races or ultramarathons, particularly in foreign countries, feet are often exposed to all sorts of organisms and nasty creatures. The ELF Adventure was one such race. It was held in the Philippines and Brazil, places where a racer can be exposed to unfriendly parasites.

It's easy to pick up a few bugs—protozoa or mites or who knows what—especially when going through streams, rivers, and damp caves. Many of these parasites enter the skin through open blisters, cracks between the toes, fissures on the skin, and scratches. Some may lead to a hemorrhagic appearance under the skin. They may ooze fluid, often yellow with pus, from infection. The feet may be painful and itch unrelentingly.

In most cases, a diagnosis will have to be made by a physician and oral antibiotics are prescribed. Some of these organisms will take weeks or months to be eliminated from your body. Many times the race organizations will be aware of the potential for this type of exposure and have medical recommendations for its control.

Tips for Controlling Jungle Rot

■ Do your utmost to keep your feet as dry as possible.

■ Air your feet during rest breaks or food stops. If you can, expose them to sunlight when resting.

■ Use a water-repelling ointment such as zinc oxide, Desitin Maximum Strength Ointment, Trail Toes, or RunGoo to keep moisture at bay.

■ Change into dry, clean socks as often as possible.

■ When changing socks and shoes, check your feet for open skin and treat those areas with Betadine and an antiseptic ointment. Some lubricants are made with antibacterial properties. The "Compounds for the Feet" chapter lists several of these lubricants (page 128).

■ If you suspect a parasite, get medically checked as soon as possible.

personal experience

"Having experienced the worst foot problems I can imagine at the ELF, I can share what happened. What is it that allowed some teams to totally avoid foot problems while others had to quit? Should some of us spank our parents for bad genes or will enrolling in an Anthony Robbins fire walking course do the trick? My team took no special precautions and might be a good control group to help generate some ideas to prevent these problems for racers in similar environments in the future.

"Although the race's website listed only three official withdrawals for sore feet, it's likely that feet played some part in many withdrawals. You could see many competitors hobbling. At one point my feet were swollen to twice their normal size with distention where there should have been arches. They had taken on a mottled white, blue, and pink coloring, and I'm told that I probably had a fever due to the infections raging within.

"The doctors have told us that we experienced a combination of fungus and hookworms on top of the general blistering and swelling we had expected. The race conditions were very wet, and so were competitors' feet, from a combination of creek crossings and rain. Wet feet and fine grit led to blisters, which in turn allowed penetration by the fungus under the skin, moving us from athlete's foot to Stay Puft marshmallow feet. Subcutaneous fungal infections were the largest cause of pain and severe swelling. The doctor said hookworms are generally acquired in sandy soil that enters shoes and carries the organisms, allowing them to burrow in. One teammate wore SealSkinz socks that kept the sand out and she didn't get hookworms. Those of us without SealSkinz were infected with the hookworms. I counted around 30 in my feet!

"Here is what little I learned. Betadine rocks. One of the French doctors suggested mixing Betadine with petroleum jelly, coating the feet, and wearing socks (and the obvious and ever so useless, 'Keep zee feet dry'). This really helped kill the external fungal infection as the stuff kills everything. Hookworms are easily treated by a single dosage of a prescription medicine that for me worked almost overnight.

"Hiking poles are a must for races this length, especially if there is any chance you may become foot impaired. I put 40% of my weight onto my Leki hiking poles for a good portion of the hiking sections and wouldn't have been capable of finishing without them."

—David Schmitt, who has raced in the ELF Adventure

Foot Care in Multiday Events

Multiday events are a challenge to even the experienced athlete. There may be changing weather conditions: water from rain, wind and cold, and heat and humidity. No two multiday events will be the same. You must be prepared for whatever is thrown at you. Proper pre-event planning with your shoes, socks, and foot-care kit, along with your other gear, is crucial. Whether you are doing a 100-mile trail run that takes 40 hours, a six-day road race, a three-day adventure race, or a two-week backpack, you must take care of your feet from the start. Some suggestions are appropriate for road races but not for trail races or events that are a mix of road and trail. Modify the suggestions to fit your event.

Rob Byrne has participated in the Marathon des Sables in Morocco, the Gobi March in China, and the Sahara Race in Egypt, each a seven-day stage race about 150 miles in length. He uses petroleum jelly on his feet, and then a polypro liner sock and a cotton sock on top. Each day he gets a new pair of liner socks and replaces the cotton socks every other day. I cringe at his use of petroleum jelly and cotton socks, but they work for him. He had no blisters even with all the river crossings in the Gobi event. He does wear gaiters.

I love the last line of this quote from the Marathon des Sables website: "As to your feet, there is nothing better than training before the race to ensure the good condition of your feet during the race. They will carry you throughout the race if you take good care of them. During the race they will be subject to constant friction, and blister treatment at night is the daily routine of the medical team. Shoes two sizes larger and with a wider fitting at toe level will be more comfortable when your feet swell due to the heat . . . or plasters! All too few competitors go to the chiropodist to prepare their feet, a mistake that many regret afterward."

Terri Schneider, an ultrarunner and adventure racer, talks about managing her feet in the seven-day Sahara Race in Egypt: "In a stage race, as long as you are draining blisters and airing your feet out each day after running, the blisters will start to heal by week's end (as long as you don't get more). I would take all tape off when I was done running each day, clean the feet (as much as possible without having showers), drain them, and let them dry out as much as possible. Using benzoin each day to keep the tape on was a problem, as over days it dried my skin out too much and they became irritated. I must say that the heat and pack weight didn't help our feet at all. Elevating my feet as much as possible postrunning helped, and I slept each night with my feet on my pack as well. By week's end my blisters started to heal—though I did lose a few toenails."

Adventure racer Ian Adamson gives three prerace tips for multiday events:

First, choose shoes that breathe and drain well. Water and moisture always get in, but you want to make sure they get out, and fast. Waterproof shoes have their place, but rarely on the feet of an ultra-endurance athlete because they have the propensity to turn your nicely conditioned feet to mush faster than you can say "hop, skip, and jump."

Second, look for adequate midsole cushioning. Racing flats are nice and light, but over a few days it will feel as if you are walking with bare feet over the rocks. Too much cushioning is also bad because it elevates your feet, sacrificing lateral stability.

Third, some form of stone bruise protection is essential. The Salomon adventure racing shoes all have superior stone protection in the form of an outsole Kevlar or plastic plate. Carrying extra weight in uneven, off-trail terrain can wreak havoc on the soft tissues of your feet with inadequate defense.

More Tips from Ian Adamson for Healthy Feet

Try a silicone-based lubricant, which helps drive moisture away from your skin and reduces friction between your feet and shoes. Sportslick, Trail Toes, and ChafeX are all good products.

Empty your socks of rocks and junk. The debris that accumulates as you thrash around in the forest can cause blisters, sores, abrasions, and cuts, all highly contraindicated for happy feet. Best of all, use a light gaiter to keep things out to start with.

Walk through very cold water whenever you can. Cold water is extremely useful to reduce swelling and has some lovely, if painful, therapeutic and preventive effects while racing on your dogs. Don't worry about the moisture; if you have fast-draining shoes and use a silicone lubricant, you will be fine. Otherwise, soak your feet in whatever cold water is available.

Dan Brannen, an experienced multiday ultrarunner, has several ideas for the problem of swollen feet in multiday races:

In the latter stages of multidays on tracks or road loops, my enlarging feet felt best with no socks and open-toe running shoes. The biggest cause of serious swelling during a multiday is, ironically, being off your feet. The best way to avoid really troublesome foot swelling is to stay on the track as much as possible. Any rest breaks longer than a few hours are just going to make your feet bigger. Forget icing, elevation, and rest during the race. Their effect will be inconsequential.

Dan also recommends wearing socks and sandals when traveling home after the event (especially when flying). Or wear your shoes loose and untied—even when walking through the airport.

Peter Bakwin, a veteran multiday trail runner, observed a multiday race and offered the following: "I noticed a lot of the multiday runners had the toes cut out of their shoes. We camped next to one runner, and she had several pairs like that and her shoes were probably two sizes bigger than you would normally use. She changed her shoes and socks frequently, rotating socks to get dry ones. I also noticed that a lot of the six-day guys were using very thin nylon stockings under

As odd as it may look, cutting the toes off shoes helps prevent common foot problems.

their regular socks." Trauma shears make short work of cutting shoes and should be available at any race that has medical support.

Sharon and Chuck Chelin share a good suggestion for staying on top of foot-care issues. Their suggestion can be used by anyone, from hikers to adventure racers:

> Except for urgent daytime events, evening is when feet are inspected and maintained. This includes cleaning, as best we can under the circumstances; inspection and repair of any blisters; sandpapering of any dry, rough, or cracked areas; trimming and smoothing of nails; and application of a favorite conditioner, such as lotion, salve, alcohol, powder, and so on. This is also the time shoes are inspected. Out come the insoles and inserts, so the dirt can be removed and an inspection can be made for nasty little sharp burrs and stickers that like to work their way through the fabric, padding, and linings.

Off with the Toes

If you choose to cut the toes out of your shoes, use EMT scissors or utility shears, not a knife. Plan ahead and have a pair in your medical kit. Using a knife can lead to injury when trying to cut through tough shoe uppers. Here are a few tips.

- Cut from just below the bottom pair of eyelets or the trim piece of fabric that the eyelets go through.

- Cut down to where the upper joins the sole, from one side around to the other side.

Tips for Multiday Events

- Train your feet for the rigors of carrying a pack by training while wearing your pack with approximately the same weight.
- Use rest periods and food breaks to air your feet. This is crucial to let the skin dry and heal.
- Cut the toes out of your shoes (if the location and terrain allow). If necessary, cover the opening with duct tape or glue a piece of spandex or other stretch material to keep out trail debris.
- Frequently ice your feet or immerse them in ice water during occasional break periods.
- Elevate your feet when resting.
- Rotate your socks to keep your feet as dry as possible.
- Have extra shoes that are a size or two larger than normal, with interchangeable insoles.
- If you cannot change into larger shoes, start with shoes larger than normal and add a flat insole to help them fit from the start. Remove the insole as your foot swells.
- Use different thicknesses of socks.
- Use anti-inflammatory medications.
- Change shoes and socks frequently.
- Have a pair of lightweight sandals, flip-flops, or Crocs to wear around camp at the end of each stage.
- Use Super Salve, Bag Balm, Brave Soldier Antiseptic Healing Ointment, or a similar ointment to keep your feet as healthy as possible.

- Trim as much as necessary to clear the toes.
- If trimming the heels, keep the top part of the heel counter. Trim under this down to where the upper joins the sole.
- Use duct tape or an ENGO patch to cover any rough edges.

Ray Zirblis writes from the experience of 24-hour and multiday stage races. He knows firsthand that foot swelling can trouble racers: "After the Orlander Park 24-Hour, my feet are typically quite swollen for four or five days. Air and auto travel home is always excruciating. Once home, I keep a bucket of ice water by my bed and every couple of hours, when those 'dogs begin to bark,' I get up and soak them."

When I did a 72-hour road race, I learned that a quick 20-minute nap every 6 hours helped me stay sharp. From 12 hours on, I took these quick catnaps for the remaining 60 hours, and during each nap I slightly elevated my feet—with my shoes off.

Going into a multiday event without knowing the best way to care for your feet and how to fix blisters or a turned ankle can spell disaster. Practice before your event, and if you have a team or crew, or are on a team or crew, learn everything you can about how to take care of and fix your feet.

Saving Your Feet

In a multiday event, you'll have time at the end of each day where you'll be walking around your camp. Here's where you'll want to have lightweight sandals, flip-flops, or Crocs to wear. These will save your feet by allowing them to air and dry out. If you have had work done on your feet and they are patched or taped, try and keep dirt, sand, and moisture away from the treated area. Nothing will destroy a good patch job faster than sand and water. Pick your camp footwear based on the setting of the event. A good choice for sandy conditions is Crocs without holes in the toe area (crocs.com). Otherwise sandals like Xero Shoes' Z-Trek and Z-Trail (xeroshoes.com), Bedrock Sandals (bedrocksandals .com), Luna Sandals (lunasandals.com), or Oofos sandals (oofos.com) are good. Inexpensive flip-flops would be my last choice. I have seen athletes using homemade flip-flops made from cardboard or old insoles with duct tape straps and even dry bags to try and protect their feet.

Teamwork
and Crew Support

There may be times when you are involved in a team sport or a sport that utilizes a crew. Adventure racing is typically done as a team. Backpacking and hiking, while not team sports per se, may be done as a group. Crew support is found in ultramarathon events, adventure racing, and team sports: football, soccer, and so on. Before your race or activity, develop a plan, draw up a list of supplies, and clarify all the responsibilities of each team or crew member. And be sure to discuss your group's notion of teamwork.

Teamwork

Any time you are with a group, teamwork is vital. You are only as strong as your weakest member and as fast as your slowest member. If you have a crew supporting you and you need foot care, can any crew member manage your feet—or only one? Do team members know how to care for each other's feet as well as their own?

For adventure racing, this is of particular importance. As you train and race, your team will learn from each other's strengths and build on each other's weaknesses. It may sound easy, but this aspect is rated as one of the most complex and difficult of all adventure-racing components. Each team member must have some degree of skill at all of the disciplines—including foot care. The same can be said for all members of a backpack or hike. The story of one team's experience during an adventure race will illustrate this point.

Patty Hintz, a member of Team R.E.A.R., participated in a two-day adventure race in the Shasta-Trinity Alps. She describes the race:

> The mileage for the running section was about 35 miles and one of my teammates had a problem with blisters. Being an experienced ultrarunner I brought along extra Spenco 2nd Skin. When she said blisters, I had no idea we were talking both heels, both forefeet, and multiple toes on each foot!

We had three different types of tape to put over the 2nd Skin. I first tried moleskin—but a few miles later it was off. Next was cloth tape, but it did not hold either. Finally, I remembered the duct tape in our team's mandatory gear. I don't know how she managed, but she said her feet felt 100% better. She was able to continue the race and the duct tape never came off.

This story is important in that Patty had anticipated foot problems and was prepared. She knew the value of 2nd Skin and knew how to tape the feet. She also knew how to improvise. If she had been on a team where no one knew how to properly drain blisters and tape over them, they may not have finished the two-day event. Patty describes some problems they encountered:

> Later we talked about what caused the blisters. [My teammate] had great running-type socks to reduce friction. Her shoes had plenty of break-in time and fit her feet properly. I personally think that it was not enough experience with time on her feet. I honestly feel that if your shoes fit properly and are the right type of shoe for the way you run, you wear appropriate socks, and you spend time breaking in a new pair of shoes before you race in them, blisters are still going to come until your feet have enough distance and time to toughen up. Until then, I'm a firm believer in duct tape and 2nd Skin. As far as my teammate's feet, I'm happy to say they healed very quickly—in about a week.

Planning for Foot Care

People participating in the same activity or on the same team would be wise to sit down before an event, particularly if it is your first or second event together as a team, or your first multiday event, and talk about foot care. Who has the most foot-care experience? What is the best way to prepare your feet—pre-event taping, toughening your skin, better socks, and/or better-fitting shoes? As Patty asks, "Does each member have enough time on their feet to toughen them for the distance?" What is the best method to use when fixing blisters? What about really big blisters? What is the minimum amount of foot-care knowledge expected of each person? What foot-care gear will you carry and how much of each item? Foot-care kits are useless if only one

All team members need to be able to work on each other's feet. Here, a teammate wraps Coban over 2nd Skin on a toe blister.

person knows how to use the materials in them. Who then will fix that person's feet if problems develop? And who will manage the team's feet if that person is injured or has to be pulled from the race?

Planning should also include preparing a foot-care kit. The chapter "Foot-Care Kits" includes a list of what to include in your kit.

Team Responsibilities

You need to know how to use each item in your foot-care kit. Each member of the team should know how to tape their feet to prevent and fix blisters. Each team member should work at finding what is best for his or her feet—lubricants or powders, two pairs or one pair of socks, double-layer or single-layer socks, the best way to lace shoes for specific foot problems, and the best-fitting shoes for his or her feet. It is the responsibility of the whole team to be sure each member is adequately trained in proper foot care. It can mean the difference between a good race and just finishing—or even not finishing.

Crew Support

If you will be participating in an event where you have crew support to help you at aid stations, be sure to discuss foot-care issues with them before the event. Let them know if you are planning shoe or sock changes at particular aid stations, and if so, what specific shoes or socks you will want. Let them know all of the following:

Denise Jones tapes feet at the Western States 100-Mile Endurance Run.

- how to take your shoes and socks off to avoid making any foot problems worse,

- how to put new shoes and socks back on,

- what powders and/or lubricants you use and where on your feet you use them,

- how tight you like your shoes tied and whether you use single or double knots, and

- how you want to deal with hot spots, blisters, toenails, or other unique problems.

Practice this with your crew at home, well in advance of the run. By trial and error find what works and what doesn't work. It is important to know the amount of time these activities will take.

When arriving in the aid station, let them know what you need for your feet. Advise them of any hot spots or blisters. Never let them pull shoes off your feet without proper unlacing. This action, however unintentional, can rupture a blister or cause increased pain to already hurting feet. A shoehorn can be a lifesaver—use it to easily slide the heel out of and into the back of the shoe without too much pressure on sore and tender heels.

18

Providing Foot Care
for Athletes

Providing foot care for athletes is a huge responsibility. Their feet are what keep them going, and if you are known for providing foot care, the athletes will be appreciative of whatever you can do. If you are simply helping one runner, you might be a bit more casual. But if you will be part of a foot-care team, you need to be prepared.

In 2015 race directors of several multiday ultramarathons in Europe were overwhelmed by the sheer volume of runners seeking medical attention for blisters. They said it took upwards of 30 minutes per foot to treat most of the runners, which caused a significant drain on the medical team's ability to look after more serious problems. In 2016 these races began introducing a triage system for medical care. Patients are assessed prior to treatment, with the neediest being treated first, regardless of how long others have been waiting. If the assessment indicates "minor" blisters, advice is provided and runners are expected to treat their own feet. All runners must have their own blister treatment kit as part of their mandatory gear kit. Event staff candidly state that foot care is easily divided into several phases—what they call the six Ps (Proper Preparation Prevents Piss-Poor Performance)—and provide a thorough list of preparation, prevention, assessment, and treatment suggestions. *Proper Preparation* means in the months before the event, *Prevents* means during the race, and *Piss-Poor Performance* is what happens if you fail to follow the first three Ps.

Rebecca Rushton, an Australian podiatrist and owner of blisterprevention .com.au, and I agree that foot care at multiday events is vital. I consider a 100-mile ultramarathon a multiday event. The problem is that many runners have become dependent and expect that events will have medical personnel providing even the most basic foot care. Participants have come to treat foot-care services at events as a perk of the event. While it's nice to have, it's not practical and sustainable long term. Race directors need volunteers with the time and expertise in foot-care techniques, as well as the budget for supplies and equipment. The larger and longer the event, the more volunteers are needed and the more costly it becomes.

I wrote in a blog post, "At some events participants will move along the trail from aid station to aid station and, at each one, require some degree of foot care. What was patched at an earlier aid station didn't work or didn't hold up, and they want someone at the next aid station to redo their feet. That's a lot of work and supplies." Rebecca wrote something similar: that many athletes fail to take care of their feet and fail to plan, and in many cases fail to take common sense action (reduce calluses, trim toenails, perform self-care, and so on) that could have prevented or reduced the problem. Rebecca and I support what we call assisted self-management. In the aid station, provide a table, a few chairs, and basic foot-care supplies. Medical personnel will be available to give advice and tend to more serious treatment. It could even be that runners are shown how to patch the first blister and then manage the rest themselves. It's a workable model and builds on today's popular do-it-yourself (DIY) method of learning new skills.

This leads to a new mind-set among many medical professionals who manage medical direction at races and multiday events that is worth considering. An article in the April 2014 *Sports Medicine* summarized it well. "Although participants in ultra-endurance events should be educated and prepared to prevent and treat their own blisters and chafing, blister care will likely be the most frequent use of medical resources during ultra-endurance foot races."[35] The mind-set is that participants need to shoulder some of the responsibility for managing their feet. Medical staff at aid stations can quickly become overwhelmed even to the point of running out of supplies. We can help promote and support this new mind-set in several ways:

- Give participants tips to prepare their feet in advance of the event. (Refer to "Foot Care in Multiday Events" in chapter 16.)

- Give participants tips on the best footwear selections for the event (types of shoes, gaiters, oversocks, camp shoes, and so on).

- Give participants a list of foot-care gear they must carry. A section on mandatory foot-care gear can be found at the end of this chapter. Even runners in a 100-mile race can carry a small zip-top bag pinned to their bib number or in their hydration pack.

- Advise participants whether foot-care services will be provided and, if so, to what degree: no foot care nor supplies, limited self-management, or full service.

- Provide a self-service table of supplies for runners to use in DIY patching of their feet. This can speed up their in-and-out times at aid stations.

- Stress the importance of knowing how to work on one's feet (by reading this book or through other sources, or workshops).

- Stress the importance of runners having crews knowledgeable in foot-care work and prepared with a well-stocked foot-care kit.

How you implement the principles of self-management or whether you decide to provide full-service foot-care services depends on several factors: the number of participants, the difficulty, the remoteness, the number of medical volunteers, the availability of supplies (and ability to absorb the cost), and the number of aid stations and how far apart they are. It should be a well-thought-out and joint decision of the race director and the event's medical director.

I have taught many people how to patch feet. Some of these, in turn, have taught others. Ordinary folks can patch feet as well as medical professionals can. Over the years, I have taught podiatrists, doctors, nurses, paramedics, emergency medical technicians, athletic trainers, and many other people who simply want to learn what to do. The skills to get an athlete back on the trail or road whose feet are badly blistered are not typically taught to medical professionals.

My goal when patching feet during an event is to get the athletes back in the race. That goal is the same regardless of the length of the race—a marathon, 50-mile, or multiday race. I need to be as prepared as possible to do whatever it takes to patch them up. That should be your goal too.

While you are working on runners' feet, educate them about what you are doing and why. Tell them what you see on their feet (calluses, untrimmed or thick toenails, toenail fungus, and so on) and what they can do about it, what you are doing to their feet and why (cleaning, draining blisters, patching, and so on), and what they can do to be better prepared (better socks, gaiters, and so on). We need to do as much as we can to educate runners so they can manage their own feet.

Some medical directors advise their team to patch the first blister, while talking the athlete through the process, so the athlete can patch the next one. If this is the plan, work with the race director to convey this to participants ahead of the race starting. Taking this approach will require careful preplanning to have enough supplies, or making sure the athletes do.

Being Part of a Foot-Care Team

Whether working as a crew member or as part of a medical team doing foot care, it is imperative to have a solid understanding of all aspects of foot care. Blisters will be a large part of your routine, so knowing their types and how to drain, patch, and tape them is vital. Whether pretaping over potential problem areas for an athlete before a run, over a patched blister during a run, or redoing a blister patch during a multiday event, taping skills are a huge part of providing high-quality foot care. Knowing how to drain a blister under a toenail is a good skill to learn. You need to learn what causes blisters, how to trim toenails, the problem with calluses, treating maceration, and more.

Make sure you study the following chapters in this book: "Taping for Blisters"; "Extreme Conditions and Multiday Events"; "Blisters"; "Strains and Sprains, Fractures and Dislocations"; "Tendon and Ligament Injuries"; "Heel Problems"; "Toe Problems"; "Forefoot Problems"; "Skin Disorders"; and "Cold and Heat Therapy."

In addition to having the practical skills, and just as important, one needs the ability to talk to the athletes you are treating and to listen to their concerns. When

I am patching feet, I run my hands over the feet and ask what's going on. I always try to examine the whole foot, and both feet when possible. As I patch blisters, I try to educate the athlete about blisters, calluses, or whatever the issue is, and explain what I am doing and why. I believe strongly in helping athletes understand the ins and outs of foot care. While I'm patching their feet is a good time because they are a captive and interested audience.

If you are working with others who are also helping with foot care, be conscious of the degree of their skills. They may not know as much as you and will welcome you sharing your expertise.

This is no time for shortcuts. Not using compound tincture of benzoin will result in tape coming off and bunching up in the socks. Using the wrong tape, white athletic tape as an example, will result in the tape peeling off and causing further problems. Using a needle and not enlarging the hole will result in the hole sealing up and the blister refilling. Slapping on tape with folds and creases in the skin can cause discomfort to the athlete. You owe it to yourself and the athletes to do the best possible job.

Setting Up Your Station

A great tool to use for foot care is a chaise folding recliner. These adjustable chairs are perfect for patching feet because they provide full body support while the athlete reclines. The feet are lifted up for easy viewing. A low stool or chair for you to sit in while working will save your back. A massage table works well too. It is nice to have a table on which to spread out your materials. Plan ahead for events where you will be working at night. A good headlamp is vital. Even with indoor lighting, a headlamp can help you see blisters more clearly. Remember to have a container for trash and take care of your sharps.

Tips on Managing Blisters

Over the years I have worked aid stations at single-day and multiday events. I have patched thousands of feet of professional athletes, weekend athletes, and walkers who are not athletes. The one thing all these people had in common was their propensity to get blisters—often really bad blisters. Here are my tips on managing blisters.

PREPARATION

- Any blister should be drained. If the blister is causing discomfort to the athlete, drain it before it presents bigger problems.

- Use an alcohol wipe to clean the skin surrounding the blister.

- Cold and/or damp skin makes for difficult taping—try to dry and warm it.

- If the feet are macerated, apply powder generously. Try and warm the feet at the same time. In a multiday race, doing this for several hours can help restore the skin's integrity.

DRAINING BLISTERS

■ If using needles for draining blisters, move the needle side to side to enlarge the hole so it won't close up on itself.

■ A #11 scalpel or pointed scissors can make a small cut, which will promote continued draining.

■ Plan several drain cuts/holes in places where gravity and ongoing foot pressure will aid with continued draining.

BLOOD BLISTERS

■ If draining a blood blister, warn the athlete about signs of infection.

■ Usually it is better to drain and patch a blood blister in a controlled environment than to have it rupture out on the course.

■ Add a dab of antibiotic ointment in or over the blister before patching.

MULTIDAY BLISTER TIPS

■ If the feet and conditions are wet, at the end of the day or of a stage, remove any tape or dressings to allow the skin to breathe and dry out.

■ Patch and tape feet after feet have been cleaned or washed. If athletes have downtime during an event, encourage them to let their feet air out in order to dry the blisters.

■ Use a syringe to inject a dab of zinc oxide in a blister to help the new skin dry and harden faster.

■ Expect to redo blister patching and taping during the event.

PATCHING BLISTERS

■ Spenco 2nd Skin patches are sufficient for short events but will lead to cold and damp skin on longer events, making further patching difficult.

■ Use a waterproof hydrocolloid dressing if the race conditions are wet.

■ Blisters under toenails, if visible at the tip of the nail, can be drained there; otherwise, drilling the nail will be required.

■ Tape can be applied directly over a blister as long as a dab of zinc oxide, antibiotic ointment, or blister patch prevents the tape from sticking to the roof of the blister.

TAPING

■ Compound tincture of benzoin will help the tape stick better. Avoid getting it into open skin as it will sting.

■ Round all corners of tape.

■ Avoid folds and creases in the tape.

■ If using kinesiology tape, remember to rub the tape for about 20–30 seconds to warm and activate the adhesive for better bonding.

■ Avoid tape that does not mold or shape to the contours of the foot.

Working a multiday event will teach you more about foot care, often in an intense setting. You'll see runners day after day, and get to see what works and doesn't work on their feet. For instance, using powder to reduce macerated feet, modifying footwear, using dental floss to stitch damaged shoes, and more.

Carey Lynn worked a multiday race and learned about a foot soak from Claire Denise Johnson, a doctor friend. Carey got the runners to come in as soon as they felt a hot spot. She soaked their feet for 15 minutes in a mixture of water, a quarter cup each of Listerine and baking soda, and a half cup of Epsom salts, pouring enough to cover the tops of their feet. After the soak, she dried and wrapped or taped the area. She said the mixture seemed to revitalize, clean, and disinfect the runners' feet. You can use cold water for runs in hot conditions and warm water in cold conditions. She mixed it up for each runner and preferred this to mixing a larger batch up ahead of time—saying it seemed to work better as a fresh mix each time. Runners gave her high praise for the soaks. In shorter races, whenever possible and runners were willing to take the time, she washed their feet with soap and water. If time was short, she just used alcohol as a wash.

Modifying Footwear

There are times when shoe modification is called for. Runners will complain of a sore area under a certain part of their shoe. Most often it's when toe boxes are too short or too low and the athlete's toes are hurting. In road races, it's common to cut away the toe box or a portion over the affected toes. Cut from just below the bottom pair of eyelets or the trim piece of fabric that the eyelets go through, down to where the upper joins the sole, from one side around to the other side. Trim as much as necessary to clear the toes.

If cutting around the heels, keep the top part of the heel counter. Trim under this down to where the upper joins the sole. The back of the heel counter can be cut out for those with heel bumps or Haglund's deformity.

Try to keep the cut edges as smooth as possible. Use duct tape or ENGO patches to cover any rough areas.

The only tools you will need are a good pair of utility or EMT shears, a container of dental floss, and several large sewing needles. Use the dental floss to sew any tears or cuts in the shoe's upper. The tough nylon thread can also be used to repair a shoe's sole that has separated from the upper.

Any kind of shoe modification made to runners' shoes in a trail race can be problematic because of dirt, small pebbles, and rocks getting into the shoe. In those cases, you could try and cover the cutout area with strips of duct tape.

Advising about Postevent Care

After spending time patching a blister, or several blisters, you want your patch job to hold. The best way to assure this is to advise athletes to be careful as they put on and take off their socks. Tell them to bunch their socks up, top to toe, and then roll them onto or off the foot. This simple instruction can save your patch job and avoid having the tape come loose.

It is important for athletes to know how to manage their feet after the race or event. The most common issue is typically blisters, but sprained ankles and black toenails are two other common problems.

For blisters, advise athletes to expose the skin to air as much as possible by wearing sandals. Soaking feet several times a day in warm to hot water with a cup of Epsom salts helps dry out the blister. They should trim away any rough skin edges around the blister as they form. If there was blood in a blister, tell them to watch for signs of infection: redness and warmth at the blister site, red streaks going toward the heart, pus, tenderness, and/or pain.

Sprained ankles should be iced, wrapped with a compression wrap, and elevated above the heart. The ankle can be weight bearing as much as the athlete can tolerate.

Black toenails will benefit from Epsom salt soaks as well. Usually, black toenails will take months to resolve before the old nail falls off. If the nail is loose, wrapping a Band-Aid around the toe and nail will help keep it in place.

Epsom salts also help with muscle relief and recovery, either as a foot soak or a lower- or whole-body soak. A quart-size box or bag is very inexpensive and a good investment to have in your postrace kit. If you travel to a race, pack several zip-top bags with the salts for a postrace soak in your hotel room. Try for several soaks a day if possible.

The previously mentioned Dr. Johnson's foot soak can help your feet recover postrace. Pack the ingredients if traveling and soak your feet in a sink or bathtub. Just as with Epsom salts, several times a day won't hurt.

Your Tools

The final chapter in the book, "Foot-Care Kits" on page 341, lists items that should be in a basic event foot-care kit. When building a kit, add or subtract items based on your experience level. The quantity of supplies depends on the mileage, length of the event, the number of athletes you will be working with, and the number of days you'll be working. My kit fits in a yellow toolbox.

At the 2010 Gore-Tex TransRockies Run, a six-day stage race in Colorado, I used two rolls of Kinesio Tex 1-inch tape, three rolls of 2-inch tape, and one roll of 3-inch tape. I also used several yards of HypaFix 2-inch tape and 60–70 compound tincture of benzoin swabs. Miscellaneous supplies included latex gloves, eight #11 scalpels, a tube each of zinc oxide and antibiotic ointment, several hundred alcohol wipes, a large pack of 4-by-4-inch gauze, a container of hydrogen peroxide, a 10cc syringe and several 18-gauge needles, a bunch of ENGO patches in different sizes, several scissors, tweezers, a 1-watt headlamp, and several small bottles of hand sanitizer. There were 40 runners doing the three-day event and 220 doing the six-day event. In addition to me, two to three athletic trainers, who used supplies from their own trailer, were providing foot care daily.

Mandatory Foot-Care Gear

In the first part of this chapter, I mention the benefits of requiring event participants to carry mandatory foot-care gear. While this may not be feasible for a short
race, or even a 100-mile race, it is important in a multiday event. It doesn't hurt
to stress the importance of knowing how to patch one's feet with the supplies. You
don't want to burden runners down with a large kit, but the following list can
easily fit in a medium zip-top bag. Customize the list for your event—its length
and conditions.

- 10 feet of tape (like Hypafix, kinesiology tape, or Leukotape)
- Several needles
- A small pointed scissors
- 20 alcohol wipes
- 8 compound tincture of benzoin ampoules or 8 Skin-Prep Protective Wipes
- 10 3-by-3-inch or 4-by-4-inch gauze pads
- A small tube of antibiotic ointment
- A small container of lubricant
- A small tube or container of Desitin Maximum Strength Original Paste,
  zinc oxide, Trail Toes, or RunGoo for moisture control
- A small plastic bag with several each of small and large ovals, and rect-
  angle ENGO Blister Prevention Patches
- A pair of camp sandals or Crocs (if a multiday event)

Part Four

Treatments

Treating Your Feet

The Fourth Law of Running Injuries:
Virtually all running injuries are curable. Only a minute fraction of true
running injuries are not entirely curable by quite simple techniques.
—Tim Noakes, MD, Lore of Running[36]

No matter how hard we try to prevent problems with our feet, there may come a time when they need repairing. Then you become reactive. Many athletes are forced to be reactive in treating problems because they fail to take the time to find what their feet need and how they respond to the conditions they subject them to.

The following chapters explain how to fix typical foot problems. It is always best to know how to fix problems before they develop. Beginning a long trail run or a multiday hike without preparing for the possibility of blisters, a sprained ankle, or other potential injury is foolhardy. One or two unexpected blisters at the wrong time can spell the end to a long-anticipated event.

I believe that every runner, hiker, adventure racer, walker—any athlete—should know how to do their own foot repairs. Bil Vandergraff, a 25-year veteran as a Search and Rescue (SAR) Ranger in the Grand Canyon National Park, made an honest comment, "I don't take care of blisters. I refuse to. If you can't take care of your own blisters, then you don't belong in the canyon."[37] I love that statement. Apply it to whatever activity you are doing. You shouldn't count on a crew or aid station volunteers, or even medical staff, to take care of your foot-care needs.

A similar perspective was taken by the race directors of a European multiday race when they described foot care as having several phases—the six Ps: Proper Preparation Prevents Piss-Poor Performance. The medical staff had been overwhelmed at several races with excessive foot-care demands, and they wanted to convey to participants the importance of knowing how to care for your own feet.

In 2000 I conducted a survey of runners, ultrarunners, triathletes, hikers, and adventure racers. While not a formal scientific survey, the 214 responses showed some interesting results:

■ Athlete's foot is more common in males.

■ Black toenails affect 71%.

■ Calluses affect 49%.

■ Ingrown toenails have affected 32%.

■ Morton's foot affects 30%.

■ Sprained ankles affect 11% now and have affected 36% in the past. Many participants have experienced this more than 15 times—the highest was 30 times!

■ Missing toenails have affected 57%.

■ Achilles tendinitis affects 11% now and has affected 25% in the past.

■ Plantar fasciitis affects 17% now and has affected 30% in the past.

■ Orthotics are worn by 36%.

As you can see from the results, most of us are not immune to injuries or problems with our feet. Of particular interest was that many of those surveyed had two or more problems with their feet at the same time. What the survey told me was that athletes need to know how to treat common foot ailments—not just what they now have, but what they might experience as a result of their activity. I have no doubt that the numbers would be similar were I to repeat the survey 15 years later.

David Hannaford, DPM, who wrote the foreword for the second edition of this book, sums up the complications of injuries. "Every foot is different and it is rare to find a foot that doesn't have some inherent flaw in one of these tissues [of the foot] that can leave a person susceptible to injury. These structural risk factors can exist within a foot for many years and then all of a sudden appear as an injury when enough forces occur at one time that exceed the strength of that particular tissue. Increased mileage, fatigue, shoe faults, weight gain, muscle atrophy, poor daily-wear shoes such as flat sandals, unfamiliar activities such as climbing ladders, age-related arch loss, and many others, may combine. Scientists have also noted chemical changes in the actual connective tissue with aging. If it sounds complicated, it's because it is." (*Ultrarunning*, 2008).

The Marathon des Sables, an extreme six-day, self-supported race in the Moroccan desert, treats runners to 150 miles of sand, sand, and more sand; 200-foot sand dunes; rocky roads with small odd-shaped stones; heat that sucks the moisture out of skin; and winds and sandstorms that torment every inch of your being. Robert Nagle, a highly experienced Eco Challenge adventure racer, ran the race in 1997 and had only one blister. He commented, "Many of the participants have neither the experience nor knowledge of foot care for ultras—so they suffer mightily." The name of the game is to plan ahead to finish well and with healthy feet. If you don't, you are at a disadvantage right from the start.

In 1996 Dave Covey, an experienced ultrarunner, participated in a competitive and challenging 25-day, 600-kilometer wilderness trek across Western Australia that stressed his feet beyond his wildest imagination. While working in a walking and backpacking shoe store, he studied the different types of boots and selected a nylon-and-leather boot with a Gore-Tex fabric interior. The combination of high temperatures, long pants, and wearing heavy-duty nylon gaiters to protect his legs from the spiny vegetation made his legs sweat constantly. With his feet always wet, and the terrain very uneven and rocky, his feet were subject to extreme punishment. Changing into dry wicking-style socks every 2 hours helped for the first two days. By the third day blisters had developed on the bottoms of his toes. Moleskin simply would not adhere to the wet skin. By the end of the eighth day he rested his feet for a few days to try to dry out the blisters. He then used Betadine and duct tape on the toes. By the 18th day, the skin finally began to callous over, and during the last six days of the trek, he did not have to use any tape. Dave gave his boots high marks for comfort, realizing the blisters were caused by other factors.

In the preceding two cases, Robert and Dave had done their homework. They knew what their feet needed to complete their extreme event. They planned and were prepared. Whether we are doing something similar or something much, much easier, we too need to have a basic understanding of treatments to fix our feet.

Some things are very basic. When your feet are tired, you have several ways to help them feel better. When changing socks, stopping for lunch, or whenever possible, take a few minutes and massage your feet and check for any hot spots. A short soak in an icy stream or in a bucket of cold water can revitalize tired feet. When you sit down to change socks or shoes after being on your feet for any great length of time, elevating your feet above the level of your heart will help reduce swelling of the feet. While hiking or on adventure races, try to wash your feet with soap and water at least once per day, preferably in the evening.

Other things are more detailed and complex and are included in the chapters that follow. The information includes descriptions of problems, ways to treat them, products that can help relieve or solve them, and, in some cases, exercises to strengthen the affected areas. Read the chapters that pertain to your injury history, and try the treatments and products to find those that will resolve your problems.

20

Blisters

An article in the August 2004 *Journal of Emergency Medicine*, "Event Medicine: Injury and Illness During an Expedition-Length Adventure Race," reported: "blisters on the feet [represent] the single most common injury at 32.8% of all reported and treated cases." The article was written by David Townes, MD, an ER doctor who led the medical teams at the Primal Quest Adventure Races, and three other MDs.[38]

A newer 2014 article in *Sports Medicine* provides even more statistics, "Blisters are the most commonly encountered medical problem in ultra-endurance foot races, representing 17%–40% of injuries at continuous ultramarathons and 33%–74% of injuries during multistage ultramarathons. Although typically minor in nature, they can have serious adverse affects on race performance."[39]

Before we go any further, I suggest reading the new chapter 9, "Blister Prevention: The New Paradigm." This important chapter spotlights how blisters form, introduces the new concept of shear, and talks about how shear relates to heat, moisture, and friction, which were always thought to be the culprits that caused blisters. Understanding that information will help you to better understand how to treat blisters.

Most athletes hold a common misconception about blisters—that blisters are simply a fact of life that one must learn to live with. Most athletes try tips that they have learned from others. If those don't work, they move on to another idea. Most try for a while, then give up and spend the rest of their lives fixing their inevitable blisters. The fact is that there are many ways to prevent blisters.

Blisters start out as hot spots. If caught in time and treated, hot spots can be controlled. Left to their own, they will develop into an irritating blister that can stop you in your tracks, end your athletic event, and sideline you for weeks. Blisters can be painful but can also cause you to change your gait to avoid putting pressure on the spot, thereby changing your stride, which can lead to injuries. Hot spots are simple to prevent and treat. Blisters are different. Many athletes think that there is one way to patch blisters. This chapter will show you many different ways to manage pesky blisters. Some are simple and quick. Others are complex and take more time—because they are meant to last during an ultramarathon or adventure race.

Part of caring for blisters is to also identify and eliminate the problem that caused them in the first place. One runner reported having developed the first blisters he had ever gotten while running, though he didn't notice them until afterward. After a 50-mile trail run he had two identical blisters, one on the tip of each little toe. Here is where detective work can get tricky. The blisters could have been caused by the seam welt over the little toes on the inside of the sock (a very common problem in a very common spot). It could have been the fit of the shoes—perhaps the shoes and/or the toe box were too short. The toenails could have been the culprits if they were too long, catching on the socks and making the socks bunch up at that point. Or the downhills could have been the culprit. Then too, the runner could have had a problem with his little toes—perhaps they were longer than normal or angled in such a way as to be more prone to friction. This is a perfect example of all the factors that go into the fit of your shoes and socks and how everything on and around your feet works as a unit. Simply patching a blister and continuing on is fixing only part of the problem.

Athletes talk about repeatedly getting blisters in the same place over and over and of getting blisters where they never had them before. Blisters can occur anywhere and at any time. When someone asks me about their specific blister problem, I always ask them, "What changed?" For more on this, read the section "What Changed?" on page 13.

Treating blisters takes time and practice. Denise Jones tells of a runner at the Death Valley Badwater Ultramarathon:

> He had a combination of the wrong socks (all cotton), shoes that became too small once his feet swelled after 115 miles, and virtually no adequate tape with which to repair his throbbing feet. After nearly an hour and a half, I was able to drain and dress his blisters and cut the toes out of his shoes so that the swollen nubs—his toes—could become less crowded. I was pleased to learn that after that session of repair, he was able to complete the distance and finish the race. He thanked me over and over for helping him.

Hot Spots

Most runners experience hot spots in the areas where they are susceptible to blisters forming. The area will become sore and red—thus the name *hot spot*. You may also experience a stinging or burning sensation. Around the reddened area will be a paler area that enlarges inward to where the skin is being rubbed.[40] The area becomes elevated because the surface skin is lifted as it fills with fluid. The hot spot has then become a blister. On feet, hot spots are an indicator of problems under the skin. Rubbing has not caused the blister, only the redness on the skin. Most likely, pressure and shear have combined to start the formation of a blister.

When you feel a hot spot develop, check your socks to be sure that they have not bunched up, retie your laces, and check inside your shoe to be sure that there is no debris that could be an irritant.

Treating Hot Spots

You must deal with these hot spots before they become blisters. By the time the hot spot has developed enough to be felt, protection is necessary. Take the time to deal with hot spots as you feel them develop. Continuing to run or hike on them will only make them worse. Untreated hot spots usually turn into blisters, which are harder to treat. Use your choice of one of the tapes or blister-care products described in this book to protect the area. If you have used lubricants or powders on your feet, clean the affected area with an alcohol wipe before applying tape, adhesive felt, or moleskin. In a pinch, when you are out in the middle of nowhere and develop a hot spot, use a dab of lip balm on the hot spot or put an energy gel wrapper or other slick paper over the hot spot between your sock and shoe.

Patty Gray, of the Muir Trail Ranch in the California High Sierra, learned of Dr. Scholl's lamb's wool years ago from a ballet dancer. Dancers use it in their toe shoes. She sees on average 1,000 backpackers through the ranch each year. Patty says, "I've suggested its use at the first sign of a hot spot, especially on/in the toe area to be wrapped around the digit. It stays in place nicely by itself and is also useful too in protection of the toes/toenails should they be bumping the end of the boot." The lamb's wool is a staple in their foot-care box.

It's important to find the cause of the hot spot and eliminate it. Hot spots typically develop from pressure caused by your footwear or socks. Examine your shoes or boots to determine whether you can modify them to remove the pressure point causing the problem. You may have to make a slit or cut out a small section in the side or toe of the shoe. Start with a small cut or hole and enlarge it as necessary. Be sure that your socks are not bunched up and creating pressure points. Run your hands inside the socks to remove any loose lint balls. After putting on your socks, use your hands to smooth the material around the shape of each foot. Consider applying an ENGO patch to your shoe or insole underneath the location of the hot spot.

Blisters

Basically, blisters are an injury. And as we all know, blisters can be painful. One blister in a sensitive place on the foot can easily ruin an otherwise good day. Blisters have often destroyed months of training and hundreds of dollars spent on a major event. Several blisters can drain your energy and reduce a runner to a walker or a hiker to a plodder, which in turn tends to create more blisters, which then slows forward motion even more. Too many athletes fail to educate themselves about blister prevention and how to do adequate blister care. Many runners and hikers think blisters are unavoidable and simply a part of the running or hiking process. Sometimes I think we should offer an award to the folks with the biggest blisters! Yet, somehow, when I remove a runner's shoe at the aid station and the skin falls off half of each foot, I realize that the runner should not get an award but an education on good foot care.

An Experiment of One

Ultrarunner Mark Williams has learned that the blister issue is an individual one: "What works for one may not work for the other. You must experiment, experiment, and experiment. If something doesn't work, don't try to make it work. I've had some nasty blister issues. I tried taping, Bag Balm, Runner's Lube, Vaseline, wider shoes, and longer shoes. I think the blister issue is an individual one." Consider the following experiences of a few runners:

- "These Band-Aids on my toes will work fine."

- "I get a lot of blisters on my right foot and very few on the left."

- "I constantly get blisters when I run any longer distances of 25-plus miles and only on the side of the two toes next to the big toe on my left foot."

- "Wearing orthotics, I am prone to continual blisters on the inside of my right heel where the foot hits the orthotic."

- "The only blisters that I get are on my little or big toes, and then only during races."

- "I never had a blister until today."

Some athletes claim to have feet with skin as soft as a baby's bottom while others take pride in having thick calluses on the bottoms of their feet. Both may claim to never blister and yet on another day, in a different race or activity with different conditions and variables, both may blister. Over time, our feet change. Other blister-causing factors also change from race to race—weather conditions, a lack of foot conditioning through training, the body's hydration level, the length of the race, choices in socks and footwear, and running biomechanics as the runner reacts to a sore hamstring or tight quads, for example. All contribute to potential problems.

Blisters come in a variety of sizes. They start small, from a hot spot, and can continue to grow until they are treated. One blister may not seem like much, but suddenly you have two, and then, maybe three. Multiply the pain of one well-placed blister times three or four, like some people get, and you can imagine how severe a seemingly minor problem can become.

Ron Jansen consistently got big, silver-dollar-size blisters under the balls of his feet and in the middle of the foot. He shared, "I suspect that I have metatarsalgia because that same area goes numb and eventually gets very painful right in the same spot where the blisters form. Sometimes the blisters are the standard variety and sometimes they're blood blisters. I've found that if I use Hapad metatarsal pads (or even just a cotton ball duct-taped to the underside of my insole), that's enough to support the metatarsals and keep my toes from going numb, and they also seem to help prevent the blisters. I still get them but not nearly as bad."

Keeping Stuff Out of Your Shoes

If you have ever walked or run a trail, or hiked with a backpack, you have probably had stuff get in your shoes. You know the stuff—small rocks, sand, grit, leaves, twigs, thistles and stickers, cattails—that kind of stuff. The problem is, this stuff often leads to blisters forming.

What usually happens is that you feel the offending stuff—and make a choice. Stop and remove it or continue. Sometimes we stand on one foot and kick the shoe against a rock to try and move the rock around inside the shoe. Other times we stop and take off the shoe and remove the offending piece. The sooner we remove the bad stuff, the better the chance that there will be no negative consequences.

It's when we ignore the stuff that we get into trouble. Small rocks, sand, and grit can cause a hot spot, which can develop into a blister. Other stuff can cause skin irritations and require an antibiotic ointment.

There is an easy way to keep junk out of your shoes. Gaiters. These can be homemade or store bought. In short, gaiters go around the top of your shoe and lower leg. They may zip, secure with Velcro, or pull on over your feet. They fit snugly at the top and keep stuff from getting inside your shoe. Styles fasten to the shoes differently. Some have a strap that goes under the shoe's arch while others fasten to the front and back of the shoe. Read more about gaiters beginning on page 162.

When ultrarunner A. J. Howie did the 1992 Trans-America, he described his blisters as "pepperoni pizza blisters," large enough to make the *Guinness Book of World Records*. Blisters can also become major nightmares. John Supler, participating in the Marathon des Sables, reported, "When I came in, my feet were shredded like noodles. And when I woke up, my foot was stuck to my silk sheet, with a pool of yellow pus underneath it, leaking out."

The time and conditions required for blisters to develop will vary from individual to individual. Runners and hikers tend to get either downhill blisters on the toes and forefoot caused by friction while going downhill, or uphill blisters on the heels and over the Achilles tendons caused by friction while going uphill. Blisters on the heel can also mean the heel cup is too wide. Blisters on the top or front of the toes or the outsides of the outer toes can indicate problems in the toe box. The chapter "The Best of 20 Years of Foot Care" includes a section on the little toe triangle where many athletes blister.

Kevin O'Neall has done dozens of marathons and ultras. He shares his attempts at preventing blisters:

> I have never done a long race without getting blisters. I've tried it all: lubricants; double-layer socks; size D, E, 2E, and 4E New Balance shoes; sandals; and military boots. I use a Dremel drill to sand calluses once or twice weekly, and a hacksaw and grinder to trim the insoles near blister

zones. I cut into my shoes for extra toe room, and then patch the hole with tape to keep dirt out. I've experimented with every kind of tape there is and used seven different brands of duct tape. Nothing works perfectly.

So what's the miracle? While surfing the Badwater website, I saw a mention of an ingenious toe product used by dancers. Bunheads (capezio. com) makes flexible fabric toe socks with a gel lining. Sounds dumb, but I ordered some. The box has a photo of a dainty dancer's leg standing on its toes. So far I've got about 40 miles on one tube with no breakdown. The box says they're washable, but I've run without washing them to see how they'd stand up to sweat and grime.

Kevin attempted the Leadville 100 in 2002 and got hot spots on his right big toe even though I'd applied tape. He rolled a piece of Bunheads Big Tips over the tape and was able to continue until a fall strained a calf muscle and forced him to walk. He eventually missed a cutoff and was out of the run, but the Bunheads kept him in the race up to that point.

The bottom line is that finding what prevents blisters on your feet can take much time and experimentation. It may involve one or more of the prevention measures in the previous chapters. It may also involve using one of the treatments in this chapter.

Blisters 101

A basic understanding of how blisters are formed is necessary to successfully treat them. In short, blisters are formed by shear and the five contributing factors: skin resilience, bone movement, pressure, friction, and moisture. Studies have shown that the foot inside the shoe or boot is exposed to shear at many sites as it experiences motion from side to side, front to back, and up and down. These shear sites also change during the activity as the exercise intensity, movement of the sock, and flexibility of the shoe or boot changes.[41] The complete explanation of blister formation is explained in chapter 9, "Blister Formation: The New Paradigm." Rather than retell it here, please refer to that chapter.

The friction against whatever is touching the skin causes the shear between the layers of skin. In order to prevent blisters, shear must be reduced. Friction can be reduced in many ways, all explained in chapter 9, referred to earlier. Some athletes unknowingly clench their toes. This curling downward of the toes can lead to toe blisters or toenail trauma during the transition through the foot strike from midfoot to push off with the toes.

Normal skin   Blister forming   Large blister

personal experience

"I had hoped that 15 years as a long-distance runner and back-packer had eliminated the element of surprise in regard to foot problems and their treatment. I was wrong.

"The first day of my 17-day hike required an additional 11-mile climb to the trailhead atop Mt. Whitney's 14,500-foot summit. On the way up, both heels started to blister. A little early in the trip I thought, but not unexpected. I immediately applied my favorite remedy, 2nd Skin. This was to become a daily ritual. The 2nd Skin would ease the soreness and keep the wounds reasonably clean, but the Adhesive Knit that held it in place could not withstand the rigors of such a brutal, rocky trail, and the blisters worsened to more than an inch in diameter. Every step was painful, distracting me from the trail's beautiful surroundings. Soon, I ran out of Adhesive Knit and resorted to that trusty standby, duct tape. This kept the dressings in place longer, but after clambering up and over yet another 12,000-foot pass, it too would slip. Then I got a rash from the tape's adhesive and smaller blisters from the tape's edges.

"At my resupply point, nine days into the trip, I stocked up on 2nd Skin and duct tape and padded the heel cups of my two-year-old broken-in boots with moleskin and more duct tape. This stopped any future heel blistering but pushed my toes forward in the boots just enough to cause a whole new set of foot problems for the final leg of my trip. Some days it just isn't worth getting out of bed!"

—Tony Burke recalling the way he approached his 1996 backpack of the 211-mile John Muir Trail in California's Sierra Nevada

---

Because your footwear causes blisters, the healing process truly begins when these are removed. If you have the option of a day's layover in camp without shoes and socks, this can speed the healing process and get you back on your feet faster and feeling better. Wearing sandals without socks exposes the blister to the air, which aids in healing.

Try to avoid getting blisters on top of existing blisters. When your skin is healing, protect or cushion the tender area.

Blisters Yesterday, Today, and Tomorrow

Most of us face it at one time or another: What worked for us in the past is no longer working. Ultrarunner Marv Skagerberg candidly warns, *"Caveat pedis,* or let the toes beware. I have completely solved the blister problem 12 times by perfecting various methods that allow me to run for 24 hours and up, blister free. However, the next time out with the exact same method, I have plenty of blisters." He has found that a combination of compound tincture of benzoin and silicone cream is by far the best for his feet (see page 153 for his method). Yesterday's method may have worked for years. Today's method may work for years. But then again, as Marv warns, it may not.

The late ultrarunner Dick Collins used to have problems with blisters. After trying recommendations from others, including tape, he formed his own conclusion. Dick learned, "Anything other than socks on my feet will over time become an irritant." He used only petroleum jelly on his feet and wore synthetic socks. Having completed 1,037 races, including 238 ultras, he found what worked for him and stuck to it. Like Dick, we each need to learn what works for us and be open to trying new ideas and products that could help keep our feet healthy.

We have no guarantee that what works one day will work another day. Ultrarunner Damon Lease experienced this frustration. By mile 20 of a 50-mile race he was feeling hot spots on his toes. By mile 38 he was reduced to a painful walking state. At the 42.2-mile aid station he made the difficult decision to stop. Damon noted, "I did nothing differently in this race than any other ultra." He had used the same shoe and sock combination in other ultras, but this course was steeper, with "more loose rocks and rough footing than the others." It happens. The trick is to play with all the variables in training to find what works best for your feet. Then be prepared with additional options in your gear bag.

Types of Blisters

There are many types of blisters. In my experience, toe and heel blisters are the most common, followed by ball of the foot and callus blisters. Sometimes though, the certain types of blisters will be common to a specific type of activity. Road races often lead to ball of the foot blisters, while trail runs lead to heel and toe blisters.

Toe Blisters

Shoes with a toe box that is too short in length and/or height often cause toe blisters. The toes rub against the toe box and blisters result because the moving toe bones stress the inner tissues of the toes. Improperly trimmed toenails are also a common cause. Socks will catch on the toenails and push them back into the cuticles, causing blisters or fluid under the nails. Blisters between the toes are commonly caused by pressure from skin on skin. Blisters on the bottom of the toes can be caused by pressure and friction from the insoles. Oftentimes the pinky toe curls under the neighboring toe, leading to blisters. Shoes with a good toe box and properly trimmed toenails are important to prevent toe blisters. Injinji toe socks can help those prone to toe blisters.

Ball of the Foot Blisters

Blisters on the ball of the foot are generally caused by friction and pressure on this weight-bearing area of the foot. Through the foot strike, the metatarsal bones slide back and forth, stretching the tissues in a shearing motion. This may be from the surface of the insole or from socks. Often a lubricant or powder will help prevent these. Trying another pair of insoles can also help because your insole coverings may be rough. An ENGO patch placed on your insole can effectively reduce friction.

Heel Blisters

One of the more common blisters found on athletes' feet is on the heels. Is there a reason for this? Why do so many athletes blister there? The best answer is that heels move around a lot inside shoes, both up and down

An ENGO patch applied to an insole can reduce friction.

and side to side—creating shear between the inner layers of tissue. Some shoes have plastic in the heel counters—a piece of plastic that is curved around the back of the shoe's heel counter. This plastic piece can sometimes be an irritant and rub on your foot, causing a hot spot that turns into a blister. Another irritant is the edge of the insole where it meets the inside of the shoe. Run your fingers around the inside of your shoe. Feel for seams or the hard plastic heel counter that can cause blisters. Feel the edge of the insole. Some insoles have a thick edge, while others are thinner. Another insole may fit better and not have the problem edge.

Bottom of the heel blisters can be caused by a rough surface of your insole or socks that are worn through or with a weave that has irritated the skin.

Steep downhills can lead to large blisters covering the entire bottom of the heel. These can be treated with an ENGO patch on the insole under the heel and by draining the blister. Injecting zinc oxide into the blister will help dry the new skin and, when taped, allows for walking or running.

Calluses and Blisters

An adventure racer told me, "My teammates who had calluses as protection from blisters had the worst blisters." I have seen this time and time again. Calluses can offer a bit of protection against blisters, but the trade-off is that when you do get blisters under calluses, the blisters are bad. Oftentimes they are larger and deeper because they are underneath the callused skin. And more important, these blisters are next to impossible to drain because the depth and exact location of the fluid pocket under the hardened skin is hard to determine. You are better off reducing your calluses and getting to soft skin.

Blister Look-Alike

Sometimes you find a blister on one of your toes—but it's not a blister. A mucocutaneous cyst is a small nodular single mass that forms on the top of toes. These frequently form at the joint just behind the toenail. Caused by a weakening of the joint capsule, they are firm and rubbery and filled with a clear fluid. A silicone toe cap can help when it rubs. Treatments range from doing nothing to surgical excision.

Gently push out the serous fluid.

Use a sterilized needle to make several small holes on the outside edges of the blister.

Draining Blisters

It's generally best to lance and drain a blister before it enlarges and ruptures, especially if you will be continuing to run or hike. Dr. Bergeron recommends draining the blister prior to applying a dressing when it is in a weight-bearing area and larger than 0.8 inch in diameter.[42] Blisters are usually drained with a needle. My recommendation is to drain any blisters that are in a pressure area (toes, arch, ball of the foot, and so on) or that are causing pain or discomfort. In my experience, it is easier to drain and manage them when they are small and before they become large and the roof tears off.

To drain a blister using the needle method, do the following:

1. Use an alcohol wipe to clean the skin around the blister.

2. Sterilize a pin or needle with a flame by heating with a match (avoid soot on the tip). Use it to lance two to four puncture holes. Move the needle side to side to make the opening larger so it will not seal up. Making a single large hole increases the possibility of the blister roof shearing off as you continue running or hiking.

3. Make the puncture holes on the sides of the top and bottom of the blister where ongoing foot pressure and gravity will push out additional fluid, generally to the back of the foot and toward the outside. Make at least two holes.

4. Use pressure from your fingers to push out the fluid and blot it away with a tissue.

5. Clean and dry the skin before doing further blister care. The outer layer of dead skin should not be removed.

It is important that the blister not be allowed to refill with fluid. Use one of the blister-care products in the next section to protect the blister. Occasionally recheck the blister and drain it if it has refilled with fluid.

If you are prone to getting hot spots and blisters, try dabbing on a bit of Anbesol or Cankaid before patching. These products, sold in drugstores, are numbing medicines for your gums but will also work to numb the painful spots on your feet.

Other methods for draining blisters include using standard nail clippers or small pointed scissors to clip a hole at the edges, or use a pointed scalpel. These can make a small V notch, rather than a simple hole. Podiatrist Dan Simpson reports, "I have never had a complication from this method and the clippers are easier to manipulate than scissors due to the shorter distance from your hand to the business end. The clipper also functions as a built-in depth gauge, preventing too deep an incision." Scalpels are great at making a clean cut.

Remember that the larger the puncture hole or holes made with a needle, or incision made with a scissors or scalpel, the more chance of getting sand or grit inside the blister. This is important when one will go through sand, streams, and rivers. If this happens, refer to the next section on degloving and irrigating blisters. Making too large a hole or too many holes in a blister allows moisture inside. This can lead to tissue swelling, making further patching hard to do. In wet conditions, use a waterproof dressing.

If you use a needle or scalpel to lance and drain the blister, make sure you properly dispose of them. Put them in a plastic container and save them until you can dispose of them according to your community guidelines. Many hospitals, fire stations, and hazardous waste sites will accept them.

However you lance blisters, the goal is to drain fluid so healing can start. This means making several holes where gravity and pressure, along with capillary action and muscular movement, fully empty the blister.

Picture a 1-inch blister on the side of a heel. I would make three holes—two on the bottom just inside each side edge and one on the top, also just inside the forward top edge.

Another method helps blisters drain better when further hiking or running is required. Ray Zirblis picked up this tip while running the six-day Marathon des Sables in Morocco, and it would be appropriate for stage races or multidays where a runner needs to keep running. At the end of the day's run or other effort, if you find

Thread through a side of a heel blister

A heel blister filled with blood

blisters, drain them and add another step: Sterilize a needle and a few inches of thread with alcohol. Then thread the needle and run it and the thread through one side of the blister and out the other, leaving the thread in place with a 1-inch tail hanging on either end. The thread acts as a wick to further drain any moisture in the blister while one is running or sleeping. Ray reports, "I found that my blisters dried more thoroughly overnight than normal for me, and the inside was much less raw and less sensitive than usual." Be alert for any signs of infection when using this method.

In some cases, you should not attempt to drain blisters. *Do not drain a blister when it is blood filled.* Doing so creates the risk of a serious infection, as bacteria is easily introduced into the dermis layer of skin and into the blood system. Pad around the blister with moleskin or adhesive felt. As the blister heals, the blood will turn from bright red to a reddish-brown.

Do not drain the blister if the fluid inside appears to be either cloudy or hazy. Normal blister fluid is clear and the change indicates that an infection has set in. If clear, the fluid can be drained, an antibiotic ointment applied, and a protective covering applied. Recheck the blister three times a day for signs of infection. Each time you check, apply a new coating of antibiotic ointment and change the dressing. Early treatment can keep the infection from becoming more serious.

If the blister has ruptured, the degree of repair depends on the condition of the blister's outer covering. Clean around the blister with an alcohol wipe and apply one of the blister-care methods described in the next sections. You can treat a ruptured blister—if the skin is generally intact.

If the outer layer of skin is torn off or only a flap of skin is left, carefully cut off the loose skin, clean the area, and cover the new skin with one of the blister-care methods described in the next sections. As the blister heals, trim off any rough edges.

Degloving and Irrigating Blisters

There are times when a blister's roof has torn and dirt or sand has gotten inside. You must get the irritant out, otherwise it will rub on the inner raw skin. Use a syringe and needle to irrigate the inside of the blister with water (sterile if available) to force the dirt or sand out. If you cannot get it out, use a scalpel or scissors to cut away (deglove) the blister's torn roof. Once the skin is removed, irrigation should be easier and successful. Because the blister's roof is gone, you'll need to cover the raw, exposed skin with a dressing. Use one of the dressings from the "Advanced Blister Patching" section or the "Beyond Blisters" section to cover the raw skin. When possible, use a waterproof dressing to avoid tissue swelling from the moisture.

Preventing Infection

Whether you get a blister or several blisters, whether you drain them or not, you need to watch them for signs of infection. If you pop a blister or you have a blister with its roof torn off, once you have the chance, apply an antibiotic ointment.

In 2005 news sources disclosed that actress Hilary Swank was nearly KO'd from the filming of *Million Dollar Baby* due to a foot infection—from a blister. It appears that she popped the blister on her own and continued with her workouts.

When the pain increased, she found streaks going up her foot. Going to the doctor, she learned that the blister had become infected. There is a lesson here that we all need to learn. Just as Swank thought a blister was a simple thing, as they usually are, they can also become serious health issues. Blisters are an injury and must be watched for signs of infection. I'd wager that 99.9999% of all blisters heal just fine. But if that 0.0001% is on your foot, or on the foot of someone you know or love, you'd be more careful.

For open blisters, using soap and water and an antibiotic ointment or Betadine is important for avoiding infection. Though you may not use these on an open blister during a run or in the middle of the day while backpacking, at the end of the event or day, take the necessary time to properly treat the open skin. Applying an antibacterial topical ointment will help the open blister heal up to 40% faster. Check your local drugstore for a broad-spectrum antibiotic ointment such as Neosporin, Bacitracin, or Polysporin that provides protection against both gram-positive and gram-negative pathogens. Green Goo and Brave Soldier Antiseptic Healing Ointment are excellent all-purpose salves to have on hand for blister care.

Recheck blisters daily for signs of infection. An infected blister may be both seen and felt. An infection will be indicated by any of the following: redness, swelling, red streaks up the limb, pain, fever, or pus. Treat the blister as a wound. Clean it frequently and apply an antibiotic ointment. Frequent warm water or Epsom salt soaks can also help the healing process. Stay off the foot as much as possible and elevate it above the level of your heart. If the infection does not seem to subside over 24–48 hours, see a doctor.

General Blister Care

From the perspective of runners and hikers, the goal of blister treatments is to make the foot comfortable because often running or hiking must continue. Bryan P. Bergeron, MD, identifies four therapeutic goals of blister management.[43]

He recommends that all blister treatments be considered with these four goals in mind:

- avoiding infection,

- minimizing pain and discomfort,

- stopping further blister enlargement, and

- maximizing recovery.

Ultrarunner Gillian Robinson of zombierunner.com has learned to "pay a lot of attention to healing, so I don't run on wounded feet. Even the worst blisters heal in about five days if you use Neosporin, cover it during the day, and leave it uncovered to breathe at night (if it's not too gross). My feet seem to toughen up after blister trauma, so I trim off the dead skin and keep going."

For years, normal blister care was gauze, moleskin, and petroleum jelly. Anyone can slap on a piece of moleskin, slather on some petroleum jelly, and hope for the

Moleskin with center hole cut out
for blister

Gauze taped over moleskin to
protect blister

best. But to really fix a blister so you can continue running or hiking is an art. Observing the podiatrists at the finish line of a marathon or ultra, one finds most blister-care practices incorporate these three materials.

The time-honored method of blister care uses moleskin to protect the blister. If the blister is intact, cut a piece of moleskin about 0.5–0.75 inch larger around than the blister with a hole slightly larger than the blister in the center. Press it on the skin around the blister and put an antibiotic ointment, Bag Balm, or medicated petroleum jelly in the hole over the blister. The final step is to place a piece of tape over the moleskin. Do not use gauze because it is too rough and can irritate the skin.

Personally, I am not a fan of moleskin. It does not stick well, even with a tape adherent; it is too thick; and it does not conform to the curves of the foot.

Alternatives to moleskin are Hapla Fleecy Web, ReSkin, or one of the tapes identified in the "Taping" chapter. You can also use one of the tapes or Spenco Skin Knit in place of the gauze. When using tape or moleskin over a blister, apply it as smoothly as possible. Use finger pressure to smooth it evenly across the blister, and then repeat the smoothing process several more times after the initial application. Remember to cut the tape or moleskin large enough to extend well beyond the edges of the blister. The most common failure in using tape or moleskin is not allowing enough necessary for good adherence. The larger the blister, the more the tape or moleskin should extend past its edges.

Advanced Blister Patching

There are as many ways to patch blisters as there are products that can be used to patch them. Learn advanced techniques before a race. Experiment with different products and different taping techniques. Find what works for your feet and then perfect the method. Practice on your good feet so you will know how to make the patch or tape stick when your feet go bad. Learn how to patch intact blisters, drained blisters, and blisters with the skin torn off. The more you practice taping and patching blisters, the better you will become. Trial and error is a good way to learn.

BASIC BLISTER-CARE PRODUCTS

ADHESIVE FELT is available in rolls in 0.125-inch and 0.25-inch thicknesses. This pink felt is extra thick and, compared to moleskin, provides extra cushioning and a stronger adhesive base. Check with your local drugstore, medical supply store, or podiatrist for availability.

BRAVE SOLDIER ANTISEPTIC HEALING OINTMENT was formulated for athletes and is popular among cyclists. Developed by a dermatologist to keep abrasion wounds moist and protected, Brave Soldier helps heal blisters, road rash, minor cuts, and burns. It's made with tea tree oil as a natural antiseptic, aloe gel for its natural healing properties, jojoba oil as a natural moisturizer, vitamin E to rebuild collagen and skin tissue, shark liver oil to reduce scarring, and comfrey to stimulate skin cell growth and wound resurfacing. bravesoldier.com

GREEN GOO is one of those salves that are good for everything. It's 100% natural with antibacterial and antiseptic herbs to help heal and repair wounds and chafing. sierrasageorganics.com

HAPLA FLEECY WEB is an extremely soft self-adhesive padding with a felt surface and two-way stretch. medco-athletics.com

MOLESKIN is a soft, cotton padding that protects skin surfaces against friction and has an adhesive backing that adheres to the skin. Dr. Scholl's makes **MOLESKIN PLUS** from thin cotton-flannel padding and **MOLESKIN FOAM** from soft latex foam. Moleskin is available in a variety of sizes in most drugstores, and it can be cut to the size needed. Moleskin should not be applied directly over a blister because it can tear any loose skin when removed.

RESKIN is a soft reusable bandage made with a perforated Lycra weave over a soft silicone gel adhesive. Its two-way stretch allows it to fit to the curves of your foot. It is easily removed and can be washed and used again. reskin.ca

Even though the time-honored general blister-care products are still used by many, there are more efficient products to both prevent blisters and promote healing. The chapter "Taping for Blisters" contains information that can be used as treatments for blisters. By following the methods described, you can apply tape over a blister whether the blister roof is intact or not. Tape wherever necessary based on experience and circumstances. You can also apply tape over Spenco 2nd Skin or other blister-care products mentioned above. In fact, often the tape will help hold the patch in place, especially in an ultramarathon or multiday event.

My method of patching blisters has changed over the years. The care I administer depends on the type of event. In all instances, I drain the blister and apply a small dab of zinc oxide to the top of the blister, as a drying agent and to control moisture, and to keep the tape from sticking to the blister's roof. Then I simply cover the blister with kinesiology or HypaFix tape. In some cases, I will use one of the blister patches on pages 248–251. Kinesiology tape is my tape of choice. And I always keep a supply of ENGO patches on hand to apply to the athlete's footwear. If the shoes are wet, as a last resort, you can apply an ENGO patch over the top of the blister patch.

Compound tincture of benzoin (or any tape adherent) applied around a blister helps protective layers to adhere.

Once the protective coating covers the blister, apply a light coating of powder to exposed benzoin.

For years the main product for patching blisters has been Spenco 2nd Skin. We have all seen the familiar blue squares of gel, either having them on our feet or applied to someone else's feet. The gel has helped many athletes make it to the finish line or get to the end of a hike or walk. The 2nd Skin cushions and protects the blister. Spenco 2nd Skin has two downsides, though. It requires a tape or dressing to hold it in place, and over long periods of time, the gel softens the skin—leading to a maceration appearance.

Several other products—Band-Aid Advanced Healing Cushions, Blist-O-Ban Adhesive Bandages, ENGO patches, GlacierGel dressings, LiquiCell Blister Bands, Skin-on-Skin, and Spenco Blister Pads—are designed to provide advanced blister care, and their information can be found in the advanced blister patching product list on pages 248–249. Band-Aid, GlacierGel, LiquiCell, Compeed, and Spenco Blister Pads are all similar in that they have a pad inside with an adhesive strip around the outside. Functioning as a second layer of skin, these pads cushion the area, virtually eliminating blister pain, while protecting it from further damage caused by friction.

Applying 2nd Skin to blister

These style pads are easy to apply and provide a waterproof barrier to the skin, which is important in events with prolonged water exposure. For larger blisters, put two pieces side by side. Their hydrocolloid dressings absorb moisture to form a gel. In medical terms, the moisture or fluid is called exudate. The dressing turns into a spongelike mass that cushions the blister. Whatever leaks from the blister is absorbed in the dressing and stays there. The hydrocolloid construction creates optimum conditions for rapid healing, while embedded cellulose particles absorb excess fluid and perspiration from the wound surfaces. Additionally, bacteria are sealed out, reducing the risk of infection. If left on long enough, the blister or wound dries out and the skin heals. These pads can be left on until they come off on their own.

Even though a blister has been lanced, it will continue to "weep" as part of the healing process. The fluid may work its way to the edges of the dressing, at which point the dressing should be changed. Once fluid has started to ooze out, bacteria can find its way inside and cause infection.

Compound tincture of benzoin applied to the area around a hot spot or blister will help blister products or tapes stick to the skin more effectively. Avoid getting tincture into a ruptured blister or other broken skin. After the tincture has dried and become tacky, apply one of the blister-care products from the following pages. Be sure to apply a light coating of powder to counteract the still exposed benzoin to prevent socks or contaminants from sticking to the skin. Be forewarned that forgetting this step when using benzoin on the toes may result in blisters resulting from two toes being stuck together.

Be sure to carefully roll your socks on and off. This keeps the patch from catching on the socks and pulling off or bunching up. The use of a shoehorn will save patches applied to your heels.

In a long race where athletes will rest or at the end of the day in a multiday stage race, remove any tape or dressings so the skin can breathe and dry out. Moisture and water can be held inside the blister site even as shoes and socks dry out. This can lead to tissue swelling and maceration under the patch.

There is another type of dressing that can be used for patching blisters. Xeroform is a yellowish petrolatum gauze dressing that can be cut and placed over a blister and then taped over. Also a small piece of 2nd Skin can be cut to fill an open blister and then covered with tape over the top. This allows a runner to continue with little pain. It's the fluid in the blister that causes the pain. Most blister patches require tape over the top to hold them in place.

To patch a torn or deroofed blister, trim off any loose edges of the blister's roof skin. You then have two choices. Apply one of the waterproof adhesive dressings from the "Beyond Blisters" section or cut a piece of DuoDerm or 2nd Skin in the shape and size of the open blister. Warm it in your gloved hands for a few minutes to make it soft. Peel off the backing and place it inside the blister cavity. This forms an airtight dressing, soothes the wound, and fills the empty space inside the blister. A DuoDerm or 2nd Skin patch will require tape over the patch. If the blister is infected with pus, remove the roof of the blister and clean the blister cavity.

If you have toe hot spots or blisters, you can use a gel toe cap to protect the whole toe. The caps are either solid gel or a fabric with gel inside. Bunga Toe Caps,

Bunheads Jelly Toes, Hapad's Pedifix Visco-Gel Toe Caps, and Pro-Tec Toe Caps are examples of these caps. With care these caps can be washed and reused.

TIP: Integrity Check

When using any of the products listed on the following pages on your blisters, be sure to occasionally check them. They may peel off, shift their position, or ball up under the stresses of hiking and running. When doing hills, the constant uphill and downhill movements of the feet combined with the pressures of the running body or the weight of a backpack may compromise their integrity. If you sense a change in how they feel, stop and check it out.

Instead of putting something on your feet, you can put ENGO patches inside your shoe or on your insoles. These thin fabric-film composite patches can greatly reduce friction in targeted locations within your footwear by giving a slick, slippery surface to the area of your footwear or insole where friction is a problem. They can also be used to patch over a worn spot inside the heel of the shoe. Scientific and field tests show that ENGO's slippery blue surface significantly reduces the shearing effect of friction and rubbing, providing immediate relief. The ultrathin patches leave footwear volume virtually unaltered, a strong plus.

Removing tape and blister patches can be tricky. If you pull the tape too quickly, you'll pull the skin too and risk pulling the top skin off the blister. Nik Weber has found that rubbing alcohol removes tape the best, but it will sting until it evaporates when applied to open wounds. But it still hurts less than lifting the blister skin up with the tape. He says, "I use a long cotton swab with a wood stick, soak the tape, then use the soaked cotton swab to peel the edges of the tape loose. You sort of push at the tape–skin interface with the cotton swab until the tape releases."

Extreme Blister Patching

Some athletes may choose to use extreme methods to treat their blisters in order to continue in a competitive event. These are aggressive methods. A competitive 100-mile, 24-hour, 48-hour, or six-day run may motivate a runner to want to try any means to keep running. Likewise, hikers may need to deal aggressively with blisters when in the middle of a multiday hike. The team participation rule in an adventure-racing event may force a team member to consider treating blisters in an extreme method.

Sealing Blisters

There are two extreme methods of blister prevention and care. Review the following methods to determine whether one may be useful for you in your running and hiking adventures.

One extreme method uses one of several products to glue the blister's roof to the skin underneath. Dr. Trolan has participated in several Raid Gaulloises and served as a medical consultant to adventure-racing teams in the Eco Challenge as well as to Naval Special Warfare. He describes two extreme ways of treating blisters, warning that they are "not for the faint of heart."[44] These methods have helped many adventure racers finish their events. The methods should not be used if the blister is infected. Likewise, the following technique with compound tincture of benzoin can lead to infections and should only be used if you accept the possible consequences.

At the 2010 six-day TransRockies race, many of the runners came to the medical station with huge blisters on the bottoms of their heels. We felt that the cause was the repetitive daily running on the course's steep downhills, probably with moisture on the feet. These blisters spread across the whole bottom of the heel, and oftentimes the skin tore. I found that the best treatment was to inject zinc oxide directly into the blister cavity once it had been drained. I gently massaged the zinc oxide to fill the whole blister. Then I taped over the blister as described in the "Taping for Blisters" chapter. The zinc oxide dries the inside of the blister, and the tape anchors the skin against the foot. This method is described below and is my favorite. I used 18-gauge needles because that was what I had on hand. A blunt needle is safer and can be used if the skin is torn. If the blister's roof is intact, you will need to use a pointed needle. A 16- or 18-gauge needle is recommended because of the thickness of the zinc oxide.

After you have opened the blister and drained it thoroughly, and the feet are dry, use one of the following methods to seal down the blister roof.

■ Use a syringe and a large-bore 18-gauge needle to inject zinc oxide into the blister. Because the zinc oxide is rather thick, warm it in the sun or roll the syringe between your hands. This changes the viscosity to make it easier to inject. Inject enough to fill the blister evenly, using your fingers to spread the zinc throughout the inside of the blister. The zinc dries the skin and makes it possible to walk and run when the blister is taped. It does not adhere the blister's roof to the inner skin as do the following two methods, but there is no pain and the possibility of infection is low.

■ Use a syringe, without a needle, to inject compound tincture of benzoin directly into the blister. Immediately apply pressure across the entire top of the blister to evenly seal down the blister's outer layer to the underlying skin. This also pushes out any extra benzoin. Be forewarned that injecting the benzoin is momentarily painful. Dr. Trolan rates it as an 8 on a 1–10 pain scale. New-Skin Liquid Bandage can be used instead of the benzoin.

In the Amazon Jungle Marathon the medical team injected benzoin into as many as eight blisters on one runner's feet. The blisters were first drained and then the benzoin injected, with immediate pressure applied to bond the two surfaces. I watched as he screamed as each blister was injected. Several of the blisters refilled, and he was back the next day. The lesson learned was the importance of injecting enough benzoin to completely fill the blister's cavity.

(continued on page 250)

ADVANCED BLISTER PATCHING PRODUCTS

BAND-AID ADVANCED HEALING BLISTER CUSHIONS are made with an elastic polyurethane film over a moisture-absorbing and adhering layer, or gel, both covered with protective silicone papers that are removed for use. They are not meant to be cut and can be worn for several days. There are large ovals and smaller cushions designed for toes and fingers. Look for Band-Aid products at drugstores and running and sports stores. bandaid.com

BLIST-O-BAN ADHESIVE BANDAGES from Sawyer use a patented dome, which externally reproduces the function of the body's internal bursa sacs. When force is applied to the area, the patch provides a gliding surface, reducing friction and shear forces. Blist-O-Ban Bandages consist of breathable plastic film layers bonded together, except for an area in the center, creating a dome-type area, allowing the plastic sheets to glide freely against each other—taking the pressure off the skin underneath. The patches are only 0.006 inch thick. The oval bandages have a medical-grade adhesive and are breathable and latex-free. sawyer.com

BUNGA TOE PADS AND TOE CAPS are made from a medical-grade polymer material to reduce pain, pressure, and rubbing. bungapads.com

BUNHEADS GEL PRODUCTS are made of a nonsilicone polymer, formulated with medical-grade mineral oils to cushion and protect those areas of the foot prone to friction trauma. They are washable, supple, hypoallergenic, nontoxic, dermatologist tested, and cost effective. The Jelly Tips, Jelly Toes, Big Tip, and Pinky Pads are designed specifically for toes. bunheads.com

COBAN is a self-adherent wrap that can be used around feet, ankles, and heels to hold blister products in place. Its elasticity and flexibility allows movement of the joints. Because it adheres to itself, it contains no adhesive. Because it is elastic, be careful not to apply it too tightly and cause constriction. Pharmacy or medical supply stores typically carry Coban or similar self-adherent wraps. Most are available in 2-, 3-, and 4-inch widths.

COMPEED BLISTER RELIEF PLASTERS absorb moisture and cushion blisters. The hydrocolloid action works well in blister healing. Made with a very aggressive adhesive, they come in medium, small, and toe sizes. compeedusa.com, compeed.co.uk, and amazon.com

DR. SCHOLL'S BLISTER TREATMENT sterile pads prevent blisters and help protect existing sores from pressure and abrasion. Cushlin pads adhere directly to skin, forming a tight seal around blisters. Available at most drugstores.

DUODERM CGF FLEXIBLE STERILE DRESSING is a polymer wound dressing used in hospitals. Packaged in a 4-by-4-inch size, it can be cut to fill the space inside an open blister. Buy the borderless dressings. Available in medical supply stores.

ENGO PATCHES are low-friction patches uniquely applied to blister-prone areas of footwear, insoles, socks, and athletic equipment—not skin—for easier, longer-lasting, blister-free protection. Ultrathin patches leave footwear volume virtually unaltered. Strong, latex-free adhesive prevents migration and movement, even through moisture and sweat. Scientific and field tests show ENGO's slippery surface significantly reduces friction and rubbing, providing immediate relief. Several sizes are available: small ovals for toes; large ovals for the ball of foot, arch, and heel areas; and rectangles for custom trimming. goengo.com

GLACIERGEL BLISTER AND BURN DRESSINGS contain 50% hydrogel to cushion, cool, and provide pain relief. They come in a kit with three large oval and three rectangle dressings and alcohol wipes. They are made to stay in place for three to four days, and they have an adhesive edge for easy application. adventuremedicalkits.com

HAPLA FLEECY WEB is an extremely soft self-adhesive padding with a felt surface and 2-way stretch. medco-athletics.com

The "Beyond Blisters" section of this chapter lists **HYDROCOLLOID DRESSINGS** that can be used to patch open blisters.

LIQUICELL BLISTER BANDS use an advanced liquid technology to place liquid in a cell, which circulates and moves in all directions against friction and pressure. They come in small and large sizes, with an adhesive backing, and are sold in packs of eight. pro-tecathletics.com

NEW-SKIN LIQUID BANDAGE is useful as a skin protectant or toughening agent. It comes in a spray or liquid, dries rapidly to form a tough protective cover that is antiseptic, flexible, and waterproof, and lets the skin breathe. Available at most drugstores.

Hapad offers **VISCO-GEL TOE CAPS** that can be used over toe blisters. hapad.com

PRO-TEC'S TOE CAPS, made from custom-grade silicone, are soft and stretchable to fit all toes. Locate a reseller through their website. pro-tecathletics.com

SKIN-ON-SKIN from Medi-Dyne is a product similar to 2nd Skin. It comes in 1-inch squares and 3-inch circles and is made with water, hydrogel, and vitamin E with a flexible adhesive knit that secures the hydrogel in place. medi-dyne.com

SPENCO ADHESIVE KNIT can be used to cover 2nd Skin pads or as a skin protector to prevent blisters. Spenco Adhesive Knit is a highly breathable woven fiber with the ability to stretch and conform, and it does not come off from sweat or bathing. It cuts to size and fits easily around toes and hard-to-tape areas. Adhesive Knit comes in 3-by-5-inch rectangles. spenco.com

SPENCO 2ND SKIN BLISTER PADS should be applied directly over blisters. Made with the 2nd Skin hydrocolloid pad bordered with a thin adhesive film, the pads keep blisters from drying out; absorb moisture and perspiration; and promote a scab-free, naturally healed blister. The small is great for toes, while the large works well for heel blisters. spenco.com

(continued on page 250)

ADVANCED BLISTER PATCHING PRODUCTS *(continued)*

SPENCO 2ND SKIN DRESSINGS are unique skinlike hydrogel pads that can be applied directly over closed or open blisters. The pads help reduce friction and the discomfort of blisters. They can also be used over abrasions, cuts, or similar wounds. Use one or more pads to cover the blister area. Remove the cellophane layer on one side of the pad, apply that gel side to the blister, and then remove the cellophane from the other side. The pads do not stick to the skin and require tape to hold them onto the skin. They should be kept moist and changed daily. Cover the 2nd Skin pads with either Spenco Adhesive Knit, one of the tapes mentioned, or a self-adhering wrap. These pads are available in a variety of sizes: 1-inch squares, 3-inch circles, and 2-by-3-inch rectangles. Be sure to keep your packet of pads moist or they will dry out. spenco.com

XEROFORM PETROLATUM GAUZE DRESSING is a sterile, nonadherent fine-mesh gauze wound dressing. This product can be used over blisters. Xeroform is packaged in a 1-by-8-inch strip, a 5-by-9-inch rectangle, or a 4-by-108-inch roll (for medical crews). It can be found in medical supply stores.

(continued from page 247)

Others have expanded on these injection methods with other products. Any method of gluing blisters should be used at your discretion and with a watchful eye toward later infection.

Lisa Bliss, MD, found, "Instant Krazy Glue works great, but I always seem to get into a battle with the bottle and end up gluing my fingertips together. I prefer to treat my own blisters, and I really don't want to have to put gloves on to do so, so I use either benzoin or Orajel (Orajel Maximum Strength Toothache Pain Relief Gel). In my opinion, benzoin works a bit better, smells better, and, yes, burns like hell for a few seconds. Orajel, on the other hand, is great for sticking down the roof of a blister after draining, and it has the added benefit of 20% benzocaine that helps soothe the burning. I've used Orajel both during and after runs to treat blisters. It's sticky enough to hold down the roof of a blister (just squirt a drop in the hole you've cut to drain), but I have always dressed the blister afterward because I'm not sure if it will hold if I have to continue to run. It's not as adhesive as benzoin and certainly not as much as Krazy Glue. It does help the sting somewhat, at least enough to get you running again. No problems with it. It doesn't glue fingers together, which is good for me!"

Instant Krazy Glue is now offered in All Purpose, Gel, and Maximum Bond formulas. It is best used on small- to medium-size blisters. When you want to apply Krazy Glue to blisters, here are some tips.

■ Make sure that the skin is dry and free of oils or powders.

- Use small, sharp scissors to trim the edges of skin to be as even as possible.

- Decide if you will inject the glue or just use it on the surface skin. Injecting it will produce a better and longer-lasting hold.

- If injecting, squeeze the glue in and immediately hold pressure on the blister's roof to help it bond to the inner layer. As much as possible, hold the edges of the blister's skin together.

- If applying to the surface only, apply light layers over the blister, allowing 20–30 seconds between layers.

- Cover the blister with your favorite tape, with a dab of zinc oxide over the blister's roof.

There are several alternatives to Instant Krazy Glue. Super Glue (supergluecorp .com), which has been around for years, and the newer Gorilla Super Glue (gorilla tough.com) are also good choices for sealing blisters.

Never underestimate the creative search for blister preventing ideas. Some athletes have found that Sno-Seal Original Beeswax Waterproofing is effective when applied over compound tincture of benzoin. Atsko's Pro-Tech-Skin is similar and is made for use on skin. Remember that any of these products needs to be reapplied when changing socks or every 4–6 hours when on your feet.

The choice is yours. These types of blister sealing work to seal the blister's roof to the inner skin so running and hiking can continue. But there is definitely pain and always the risk of infection, and other treatments are available.

After sealing the blister, Dr. Trolan suggests several options. Apply a coating of benzoin to help the tape better adhere to the skin. Or apply Instant Krazy Glue over the blister. This layer provides an extra layer of protection and helps your tape covering better adhere to the skin.

For severe cases, Dr. Trolan has used the tincture of benzoin injection, followed by a coating of tincture of benzoin on top of the blister, followed by a coating of New-Skin Liquid Bandage, followed by a layer of Krazy Glue, and finally followed by tape. He recommends using an emery board or fine nail file to smooth any rough spots on the blister coating before applying tape or moleskin.

Ultrarunner and Pacific Crest Trail record holder and former Appalachian Trail record holder David Horton recommends using the combination of an antibiotic and drying-agent zinc oxide on blisters when you have an overnight stop or a rest period for the zinc oxide to do its magic. He remembers using the zinc oxide method on blisters when running the Trans-America (across the United States). He advises that you "take a needle and drain the blister. Then using the same hole, inject zinc oxide back into the blister until it is full of zinc. Put a Band-Aid over that. Many times we would do that in the Trans-Am, and the next day the blister would be nearly dried up. It is still the best thing I have seen to do to a blister." David made this blister fix one time on ultrarunner Dusan Marjele, the eventual Trans-Am winner, and he came back several more times because it was so effective. For multiday events, this is a great method.

Using Syringes and Needles

You may see medical aid station people using syringes with needles to draw out the blister fluid and then to inject the tincture. Syringes with needles must be sterile in order to prevent infection. There is no safe way to dispose of the syringes and needles, or sharps, as they are called in the medical profession, except in a sharps container. If you use syringes and needles outside of a medical station, store the sharps in a hard-shelled container until they can be safely disposed of.

In this time of hepatitis, HIV, and AIDS, we need to practice universal precautions—in this case, hand washing and switching to new gloves before treating each person. An open blister must be treated as an open wound, and the blister's fluid must be treated as a bodily fluid. Additionally, there is a danger that using a syringe, you might inject more tincture than is necessary to get a good seal or not enough to cover all inner surfaces. By making several small puncture holes in the blister, excess tincture can be pushed out when pressure is applied to the roof of the blister. A good seal is then ensured.

Pushing a sharp needle into a drained blister must be done with care. The sharp point can easily penetrate the new, raw skin, which will be painful. Because needles have a beveled point, insert the needle with the tip toward the roof of the blister. An alternative is to use a blunt-end needle or a teat cannula, which is used on cow udders and can be found online.

Needles used to drain blisters can be any size. Needles are known by their gauge size. The larger the needle gauge number, the smaller the needle. A 25-gauge needle is very small and can be used for normal draining; however, a larger gauge 20- or 22-gauge needle will make a bigger hole and make draining easier. Needles used to inject zinc oxide should be either 18- or 16-gauge because of the viscosity of the zinc. Compound tincture of benzoin can be injected through a 20- or 22-gauge needle.

Deep Blisters

Deep blisters are blisters under a callus, which means they can be many layers of skin deep. Usually the only way to treat deep blisters is to use a syringe and needle to drain the fluid. The athlete knows that a blister is there—but it is almost impossible to drain because the fluid is impossible to see and finding the exact depth is hard.

Under extreme conditions, entire feet can blister and whole skin layers can separate. It's best to do all you can to prevent such dire circumstances.

personal experience

"Leukotape rocks! This was the best tape. Unfortunately, [at the Primal Quest Race] we had only one roll and went through it quickly. The adhesive was far superior to any other we had available and the tape shaped well to toes and feet.

"For blisters that were open with macerated or infected tissue, we used Xeroform gauze. This is the petrolatum- and antiseptic-impregnated bandage that is often used for sucking chest wounds. It worked particularly well for blisters in between the toes. We cut the gauze pads to size and wrapped them around the toes and then taped over them. Unfortunately, we could not talk to the racers at the end to see how well this worked, but it seemed like a good idea.

"We used syringe needles (mostly 18-gauge) to drain the blisters. The larger-size needle allowed the fluid to drain easily through the needle, without risk of it closing back up. Some also used the bevel edge to cut a slightly larger opening. We drained any blisters, large or small, that had palpable fluid. To clip or not to clip a blister was on a case-by-case basis. We never clipped intact blisters, but open or torn skin was often removed to prevent further tearing.

"If the area was tender, we taped it. Any reddened or sore area was either taped or covered with moleskin. If the racers had done this earlier, I think we would have seen fewer patients.

"A podiatrist showed us a trick to keep tape from curling at the edges. She takes a normal votive candle and, after taping, rubs it over the edges of the tape. The small amount of wax reduces friction and helps prevent curling. This is less messy than using Bag Balm or petroleum jelly.

"Two people had infected cuticles due to ingrown toenails. The doctor had to lift the cuticle and drain the pus. Obviously, these racers didn't read John's book on trimming your toenails!"

—*adventure racer and paramedic Jane Moorhead, relating how her medical crew managed feet in the 2003 Subaru Primal Quest Adventure Race*

Pressing on the callus to try to expel the fluid by hand is too painful. Using a pin or scalpel won't work. The blister is so deep that nothing else can get in that deep. Only in the biggest races with a full medical staff will there likely be a doctor who has the Zylocaine and equipment to properly care for these blisters. If I am treating an athlete with deep blisters, I will only use a needle or scalpel with their consent after I explain the problem.

Read the section on calluses on page 328 to understand how to soften these problem areas. It is true that many athletes value their toughened feet and calluses. For some, they help. For others, they mask hidden deep blisters.

personal experience

"Deep blisters are next to impossible to treat. I can think of one instance in which a runner used a combination of compound tincture of benzoin and Hydropel in combination to do a Badwater double. He got through the one way to the top of Mount Whitney, but his feet were a mess by the time he was ready to do the return trip. You see, he didn't want to bother with pretaping. I don't blame him; it's a time-consuming effort to do it. But he developed blisters so deep on his heels and the balls of his feet that he could not move forward. They became blood blisters. My husband, Ben Jones, who is a medical doctor, injected him with Zylocaine, so that the blisters could be drained and treated. Under normal race circumstances it's impossible to get an injection to drain blisters. Usually there isn't that resource in a race.

"That is why I recommend filing calluses down so that if one develops a blister on that area, it can be drained and treated. Otherwise, [the blister] just grows and it becomes impossible to move forward. Once the fluid is drained, the blister is treated with antibiotic ointment and 2nd Skin and taped. It's then possible to keep on moving quite comfortably."

—Denise Jones, the Blister Queen of Badwater

Beyond Blisters

There may be times when blisters develop and even with treatment, due to continued running or hiking, additional care is needed. Several things may happen. The skin may slough off and ball up in the sock, leaving raw exposed skin. The skin may stay in place but fall off when the sock is removed. The raw skin may bleed. When blisters have developed to this point, you have to make a choice. Continuing to run or hike may lead to infection and further damaged tissue. Ideally, stay off the feet as much as possible. If you must continue, treat the problem and recheck frequently.

Sterile wound-dressing products will help the healing process. Medical personnel should have several of these products in their kits to manage extreme blisters and cases where the skin has separated from the foot. These dressings are typically available only through medical supply stores and online.

■ AmeriGel's Hydrogel Formula Wound Dressing and Hydrogel Saturated Gauze Dressings

- Cramer's Nova Derm Sterile Wound Dressing
- DuoDerm CGF Flexible Sterile Dressing
- Ferris's PolyMem Wound Care Dressing
- Spenco's 2nd Skin Moist Burn Pads
- Postoperative dressing like Smith & Nephew's Primapore and Opsite FlexGrid

The above products, with two exceptions, are made with an adhesive edge around a center dressing and most are waterproof, making them excellent choices for wet conditions. They should be your first choice. Second, DuoDerm and 2nd Skin can be cut to the shape of an open blister and used to take the place of the blister's roof or applied over the blister and surrounding skin. DuoDerm's downside is that it adds a bit of thickness, and in the case of 2nd Skin, moisture. Leave the dressings on as the healing process begins from the inside. When the skin on the bottom of a foot has sloughed off or torn, the dressing can get an athlete back on his feet. Hypafix or Cover-Roll tapes are great for covering any of these dressings and adding another layer of protection. Nonadhesive dressings require a tape covering or self-adhering wrap to hold them in place. One of these carried on a multiday hike could easily save your feet.

Fixing Blisters, Their Way or Yours

You may find yourself entering in an event in which you do not have control over the blister treatments and how they are applied. Participate in a 100-mile trail event or an adventure race, and you will find medical aid stations manned by podiatrists, podiatry students, nurses, emergency medical technicians, and an assortment of individuals with various medical skills. These individuals will treat your blisters according to what they know and what materials they have available to them. How they treat your blisters may not be how you would like them treated. Most aid stations are stocked with moleskin, petroleum jelly, and gauze. They may or may not have 2nd Skin and compound tincture of benzoin. If you want your feet treated with a specific product, you will have to carry a few in your fanny pack. If you want a specific powder or lubricant, you will need to carry these in a small container. I am always happy to see athletes who are able themselves, or with their crews, to manage their own feet. It can be very taxing on a small medical staff and on their supplies to manage everyone's feet and special needs.

For example, the Marathon des Sables is unlike any other marathon or ultramarathon. The six-day, self-supported race in the Moroccan desert has 150 miles of sand, sand, and more sand. Cathy Tibbetts-Witkes, a many-time Marathon des Sables finisher, calls it a blisterfest: "Even people who never get blisters get them." While the medical care is adequate and very good, it is not everyone's first choice of blister care. Cathy reports the usual procedure is to lance the blisters, cut the skin off, apply benzoin, and then apply a blister patch. While this is not my first choice of treatment, it does work. Runners report a low incidence of infection despite the high level of open blisters. Remember: A lack of preparedness on your part means that you will be treated as the medical team has been taught.

Dr. Trolan stresses the importance of understanding how your feet change when you add things to them. Adding a bunch of moleskin and gauze to your foot can change the way your foot fits inside your shoe or boot. The extra thickness of the blister patch changes pressures and angles of the foot inside the shoe. This in turn changes the shoe from its usually broken-in fit to that of a mismatch. New pressure points develop, turning first into new hot spots and then into blisters. The biomechanics of the foot, ankle, and leg are altered and the gait changes. Additional problems are likely to develop. Dr. Trolan recommends using as little and as thin a blister patch as possible. This has become my teaching too.

Do not hesitate to give medical personnel at these aid stations instruction on how you would like your feet patched. I remember the bulky gauze patch put on the bottom of my right foot in 1986 during the final stages of my first Western States 100-Mile Endurance Run. While it was a good patch job, it simply did not fit right and turned me from a runner into a walker. Be aware of how medical staff are treating your feet. If you prefer a specific method of blister patching, you need to tell them, and be prepared to describe it to them—or better yet, be prepared to do it yourself.

Postevent Blister Care

I have worked the finish line of many events. Runner after runner line up to have their blisters lanced and patched. Most times, their feet are dirty and sweaty. My rule is that I don't patch anyone at a finish line unless they have washed their feet, and preferably after they have showered. I don't want to apply dressing only to have them get it wet.

Wrap Coban around the toe and then around the tip.

Many times, their blisters are small and not worth lancing. I recommend that at home or in their motel room, they soak their feet in hot water with Epsom or Pepsom salts several times a day, if possible. The salts help dry out the skin, and often the fluid will be reabsorbed into the tissues. Epsom salts are very cheap and I would encourage you to add a zip-top bag filled with the salts for your postrace supplies. Pepsom Salt and Pepsom Sports are a new class of Epsom salt products formulated for their first aid benefits (pepsom.com).

A foot soak can help revitalize your feet. This soak is one Carey Lynn used at a multiday race and learned about from Claire Denise Johnson, a doctor friend. Carey soaked runners' feet for 15 minutes in a mixture of water, a quarter cup each of Listerine and baking soda, and a half-cup of Epsom salts, pouring enough to cover the tops of their feet. She said the mixture seemed to revitalize, clean, and disinfect the runners' feet.

I never put tape on a foot at a finish line. I use only Coban or a similar self-adhering wrap. Rolls of the wrap in 1-, 2-, or 3-inch widths can be found in most drugstores. A tube of antibiotic ointment should also be packed for open blisters, scratches, and cuts.

As your blisters dry, if the skin has torn, it will harden. Keep this trimmed so it won't catch on socks. A nail file can be used to sand down any rough edges.

A simple postevent foot-care kit can be carried in a large zip-top bag. Being prepared with Epsom or Pepsom salts, antibiotic ointment, a roll or two of Coban, small scissors, and a nail file is always a good idea.

Strains and Sprains, Fractures and Dislocations

Ankle sprains and strains are common occurrences—some even with resulting fractures. Bones can break as a result of falls or twisting motions, and stress fractures can occur if athletes push themselves too fast and too soon, an unfortunately common tendency. A sudden fall with its resulting wrong landing can result in a dislocated ankle or toe. The cause may be rocks or tree roots hidden in leaves or grasses, unsteady footing while trail running at night, or twisting motions coming off a curb. Athletes need to be prepared to deal with these injuries quickly and appropriately, as late or inadequate treatment can worsen the injury, sidelining you longer and possibly setting you up for future injuries.

Strains and Sprains

A strain is the overstretching of a muscle or tendon—but without the significant tearing common to a sprain. There may be bleeding into the muscle area that can cause swelling, pain, stiffness, and muscle spasm followed by a bruise. Strains can come from overuse, repetitive movements, excessive muscle contractions, or prolonged positions.

A sprain is a stretching or tearing injury to the ligaments that stabilize bones together at a joint. Sprains are usually associated with traumas such as falling or twisting, and ankles are frequently the sprained or strained joint. During a fall or sudden twist, you may experience sudden pain or hear a pop. If you cannot walk after a few minutes of rest or if you heard the infamous pop, you can be fairly certain you have a sprain. After a sprain occurs, the fibrous joint capsule swells and becomes inflamed, discolored, and painful. An X-ray is in order. Delaying treatment for sprains or strains increases the risk of swelling and further injury.

One ankle sprain will make you more susceptible to repeated sprains, as the ligaments are left weakened, lengthened, and less flexible. Without proper care, you could get sprain after sprain and develop chronic ankle problems.

It is important to properly treat your sprained ankle. Swiss researchers analyzed health histories of 268 people and noted that 18% of those with osteoarthritis have suffered previous ankle injuries. David Weinstein, MD, head of the US medical staff at the 2004 Olympics, states that when ankle ligaments are stretched, the ankle bones slide against each other and wear down the joint surface. This may, over time, increase your risk of osteoarthritis fivefold.

Ultrarunner Sue Norwood calls herself the "queen of ankle sprains." She shares this advice: "I have learned from my 22 years of experience as a patient with recurring ankle problems from trail running. My ankle sprains got progressively worse until I ruptured two peroneal tendons in one ankle and had to have surgery to reattach them. It's better to learn effective preventive techniques than to let yourself get this injured!"

The most common ankle sprain is an inversion sprain, in which the foot rolls to the outside and the ankle turns out. The injured area is the lateral ligament just below the ankle joint on the outside of the foot. An eversion sprain, in which the ankle is turned inward and the medial ligament injured, is less common. In a serious sprain, both the lateral and medial ligaments can be injured. An X-ray will reveal whether there is a bone fracture that would require immobilization of the joint.

There are three degrees of an ankle sprain. A grade I sprain has minimal swelling, and the athlete can still put weight on the leg with the twisted ankle. The ankle's ligaments have been stretched and some are torn. A grade II sprain has moderate swelling and moderate pain when weight is put on the injured ankle. There is a partial tear of the ligament. A grade III sprain has a large amount of swelling, and weight placed on the ankle cannot be tolerated. Grades I and II will heal in about 4–6 weeks with full recovery in 10–12 weeks.

A grade III sprain requires medical attention. With a severe sprain there is the possibility of a related fracture. If there is a great deal of pain and swelling, and you are unable to bear weight on the foot, an emergency room visit and an X-ray are in order.

There are ways to minimize ankle sprains. Obvious but often forgotten, specific strengthening exercises can go a long way toward preventing strains and sprains (see "Strengthening Exercises," page 264). In addition, always be aware of how your feet land. If you sense your foot starting to roll over, quickly transfer your weight to your other foot. When on the trail, be attentive to changes in the terrain, especially on downhills and in the late afternoon and evenings, when shadows merge into darkness. On the road, be aware of curbs, manholes, and grates, as well as the slanted, concave surface roadway. On grassy areas, watch for hidden holes and roots. Any of these can trip you up and throw you off balance. Additionally, you are more susceptible to making wrong moves and being slower to respond to sudden terrain changes when you are tired.

Treating a Strain or Sprain

The initial treatment for a strain or sprain includes the classic RICE treatment:

■ **R** = rest　　■ **I** = ice　　■ **C** = compression　　■ **E** = elevation

Ice your injury within 30 minutes if possible. The first 24 hours are the most critical for beginning treatment. The typical sprained ankle takes four to six weeks to fully heal. Severe ankle sprains can require a cast for complete immobilization. Rob Conenello, past president of the American Academy of Podiatric Sports Medicine, says that for acute injuries, ice, when used correctly, is the gold standard for decreasing inflammation.

Early treatment within the first 24 hours decreases swelling and lessens the risk of additional injury. Initial rest of the foot is also important. A lightly applied Ace wrap will provide compression to help keep swelling down while providing support. Apply the Ace wrap from the forefoot toward the ankle. Do not wear the Ace wrap to bed at night. Apply ice for 20 minutes at a time at least four times daily. Six to eight times a day for the first few days is even better. The chapter "Cold and Heat Therapy" gives more information on making the most of icing techniques.

Elevate the injured area above the level of the heart as much as possible during the first 48 hours. This keeps blood away from the injured area and reduces pain and swelling. In bed at night, elevate the foot on a pillow. The treatment goal is to return the ankle to normal motion and to be weight bearing as soon as possible. The combination of rest, icing, compression, and elevation, especially in the first few days, will help the healing process and decrease the pain and swelling.

Heat increases blood flow to an injured area, which makes swelling worse. For this reason, the use of heat is not recommended for at least a week after an injury. Moist heat can be applied by using a moist heating pad, a warm towel, or a warm bath. Dry heat can be applied by using a heating pad for 20 minutes at a time.

The use of anti-inflammatory medications is usually warranted. Nonsteroidal anti-inflammatory drugs, commonly called NSAIDs, are used to control pain and swelling after an injury. The most common NSAIDs are aspirin, ibuprofen, and naproxen sodium (Aleve). These pain relievers should be taken according to their instructions and usually with food. Be careful if you continue training, because the NSAIDs block pain signals that would warn you of further injury. Overuse has also been linked to gastritis, kidney problems, and bleeding ulcers. For that reason, many medical directors of races have stopped giving NSAIDs to runners.

Fairly new to the market are several NSAIDs that are applied topically to the pain site. Three of these are Voltaren, a gel; Flector, a patch; and Pennsaid, a liquid. These have more reduced exposure than do the oral NSAIDs. Your doctor can help you decide if you would benefit from a topical NSAID.

Natural science can also help. Traumeel is a natural pain reliever that works with your body to promote healing while reducing recovery time (unitedremedies. com). Homeopathic treatments use minute doses of natural substances to stimulate the body's self-healing response. For sprains and strains there are three recommended remedies: *Arnica montana, Bryonia alba,* and *Rhus toxicodendron.*

Depending on the severity of the injury, you might be able to walk on it. With minimal pain and swelling, self-treatment at home can often be sufficient. If the pain is severe with a large degree of swelling and there is discoloration of the injured area, prompt medical attention is mandatory.

Bryan Whitesides, a board-certified orthopedic clinical specialist, suggests the following two tips to help athletes more quickly and completely recover from an ankle sprain. "First, the use of crutches for even a few days can dramatically improve recovery time," he says. "Encourage walking using the crutches to reduce weight on the ankle instead of keeping the foot off the ground. Second, a compression wrap with the addition of a horseshoe-shaped felt pad greatly reduces the effects of swelling." To wrap an ankle sprain, Bryan cuts 0.25 inch of thick felt into a horseshoe shape and places it so the U cradles the malleolus (ankle bone). Then he uses an elastic wrap to firmly compress the entire horseshoe against the ankle. He adds, "The horseshoe and wrap should be used until the swelling is nearly gone." Bryan maintains the website injuredrunner.com, which offers a DVD about stretching, strengthening, and balance training—vital for athletes.

Wrapping an Ankle

Bryan Whitesides offers the following tips for wrapping an ankle. This technique provides compression and support following an ankle sprain. Two-inch-wide elastic wrap works best, and the tension should be firm but still allow normal circulation.

1. Start the wrap 3–4 inches above the outer side of your ankle. Pull the wrap straight down under your heel and around to the arch.

2. From your arch proceed around to the front of your ankle and then around to the back of your heel/Achilles.

3. From the Achilles, continue diagonally along the inner side of your heel; then wrap under your arch to the outer side of your ankle and up to the front of your foot.

4. Proceed around the inside of your ankle and pull the wrap behind your heel/Achilles. Continue around the outer ankle diagonally, coming under the foot again and around to the front of your ankle. This pattern can be repeated for additional support/compression.

5. With any additional wrap, spiral up the lower leg.

There are two schools of thought on how soon to start running, exercising, or bearing weight on an injured ankle. One says to get out on it as soon as possible and let pain be your guide. If the ankle is stiff and sore when you first start, keep going and see if it loosens up. If the pain increases, you should call it a day, go home, and ice. If it doesn't get worse or feels better, you are probably OK. The other says to work through the healing process at the ankle's speed. You must choose your course based on available information. Even if you can't bear weight on the injured ankle, starting range-of-motion exercises or using a Thera-Band resistance band can help jump-start the rehabilitation process (thera-band.com).

Certified athletic trainer Jay Hodde, MS, ATC/L, points out the following dangers of running too soon on an injured ankle:

Running with a severe sprain can cause more problems than just reinjuring it. Several things may happen. First, your gait will change as you guard

When Your Ankle Still Hurts

Lisa Bliss, MD, shares some solid wisdom: "Soft tissue injuries should heal up within eight weeks with appropriate diagnosis and rehabilitation. If there is recurrent pain or swelling eight months after the original injury, there is either a missed diagnosis, insufficient rehabilitation, or recurrent injury.

"After my sprain at Western States, I rested the ankle and did the usual rehabilitation protocol consisting of range of motion, proprioception, strengthening, and plyometrics. I returned to running pretty quickly with the ASO brace, but the ankle never fully recovered. There was continued pain deep in the joint, especially with downhill running (when the joint is least stable and relies on ligaments for added stability). I never had real pain (such as when I had my toenails permanently removed!), only a vague discomfort, and only when running. After several attempts at running longer distances without pain failed, I finally got an MRI. It showed that I had completely ruptured the lateral ligaments in my ankle—the anterior talofibular ligament (ATFL) and the calcaneofibular ligament (CFL), and by exam and stress X-rays, the ankle was very unstable (grade III ankle sprain). No wonder all the rehabilitation in the world couldn't get me back to pain-free running.

"I elected to have surgical repair of the ligaments and am now three weeks post-op. Prognosis (my own) is a full recovery and return to running in a few months.

"The point I want to emphasize is that you should not take your ankles for granted! They should be in tip-top shape for the trails—no less. They should not be painful or swollen after a 'short' 50K. An ankle that's not 100% after eight months means that something is wrong. It may be as simple as weak peroneal muscles or as traumatic as a bruised bone or a cartilage fracture, but even a weak muscle can be a problem for an ultrarunner.

"I always recommend against surgery if there are other treatment options available. As most of us know, proprioception is key to nonsurgical rehab, but many of us fail to strengthen the peroneal muscles on the outside of the leg (those whose ankles evert). If the lateral ligaments are stretched out, then the muscles must be very strong to help stabilize against recurrent sprains. The other thing that is very important is protecting the ankle from reinjury. Wearing a brace will not make the ankle weak; not doing the strengthening and proprioception exercises leaves the ankle weak. The brace may prevent a severe injury."

the injury. Because your body is not used to these changes, overuse injuries may occur in other areas of the body. Second, the severity of the sprain may increase, prolonging recovery. Third, the ankle joint may develop the tendency to partially dislocate (subluxation). This is more common if the sprain is severe. Usually, there is some minor slipping of bone surfaces that can cause problems if the joint mechanics are thrown off by the sprain. Bruising of the bone surfaces can occur and can lead to complications later in life, such as an increased risk of arthritis.

When you can start to put weight on the ankle, begin with easy walking and slowly build back to the routine you had before the injury. Wear an ankle support if you cannot bear your full weight on the ankle. Walking even a little bit a few times a day will aid on the road to recovery. After each exercise period, ice as necessary. Following a few of the strengthening exercises described on page 264 will also help you gain back ankle strength and normal motion.

Ankle supports are an important part of treating an ankle sprain or strain. The support will allow you to be up and about faster and will provide comfort as the ankle continues healing. There are many types to choose from. The section "Ankle-Support Products" (on page 268) describes an assortment of available supports. But rather than becoming dependent on ankle supports, work on strengthening your ankles and sense of balance.

You can strengthen your ankles by focusing on proprioception, the neurological signals from your body to your brain that tell it where your body is relative to the space around it. It's a sixth sense that helps you feel secure in where you are putting your feet—without stumbling and often without looking. When you step on a loose rock, proprioception receptors in the muscles and tendons around your ankle register the sudden sideways movement of your foot and immediately notify your brain of the change in position. Your brain sends a message to your other foot to step sideways in order not to fall and to use your arms to gain balance.

Several exercises on the following pages focus on this aspect of ankle strengthening, which improves your ability to balance. Many athletes swear by proprioceptive reconditioning after an ankle injury. When you are able to make a midstride adjustment as your foot hits the ground, senses an uneven surface, and sends a signal to the brain, you are more likely to avoid a sprained ankle. The more we practice this on varying terrain, the quicker and stronger this process becomes. Proprioception can be enhanced by walking and running on soft and uneven ground at every opportunity. Practice proprioception at home or at the office when doing simple tasks by balancing on one foot. The use of a wobble or rocker board is also helpful. Because injuries often occur when we are fatigued, doing these exercises at the end of a workout when our muscles are already tired can be helpful. Proprioceptive exercises will help strengthen your knees too.

Josh Gilbert, a chiropractor, thinks a wobble or rocker board is a good tool. He suggests the following: "First, I would do a very simple activity. Stand on the injured ankle and balance for as long as you can. If you can do this for 30 seconds or longer, start doing the same exercise with your eyes closed. This helps to get your brain neurologically connected again with your ankle and the injured tissue and receptors. Only do this exercise if the ankle can bear your weight without pain (or not too much). Each joint in your body has receptors that tell your brain where it is. You don't have to look at your leg to know that it is turned in, out, pointed

Proprioception

Steve Gurney, an adventure racer (gurneygears.com), gives a good explanation of this important term. "Proprioception is the feedback between sensory tissue, our brain, and muscle. By sensing the angles and forces in each movement of our feet, the brain can fire the appropriate muscles for stability and then movement. The more we practice this on varying terrain, the quicker and stronger this process becomes. Proprioception can be enhanced by running on soft and uneven ground at every opportunity. Try making a rule to stay off sealed surfaces. Run on grass verge, in creeks and riverbeds, in parks, beside rail tracks, and in subdivisions. If you have to run on roads, then run up and down the gutters playing coordination games (for example, three steps in the gutter, two steps up on the curb).

"Balance practice is excellent, using such things as a wobble board or tightrope-style balance on gate chains, parking lot walls, or fences. Running as fast as you dare on walls is great.

"Coordination for rock running is also enhanced by practice. We can simulate specific and quicker foot-eye coordination on plenty of things near home. For instance, running up and down stairs at speed, sideways and backward. Running off trails in a forest is good. You can also practice proprioception at home—or the office when doing simple tasks such as talking on the phone, thinking, cooking, or watching TV—by balancing on one foot (for greater challenge, shut your eyes) or a wobble board."

up, or down. The receptors in the joint relay this information to the brain. When the joint is injured, sprained, or stretched, these receptors start relaying incorrect information. It they are not retrained properly, you will end up like many people and continue having recurrent ankle sprains."

Strengthening Exercises

Strengthening exercises for the foot and ankle can help prevent injuries and can speed recovery from an injury. Balancing exercises and the use of Thera-Bands are good to help strengthen the ankles. Thera-Bands can be used with many of the exercises. Stop any weight-bearing exercises if you experience pain. Here are some exercise options.

- Sit in a chair and write the alphabet with your toes to simulate ankle motion in all directions.

- Stand on one foot on a pillow or similar soft and unstable cushion and try to maintain your balance, first with one foot and then the other. As your ability to balance increases, move into short, controlled, up-and-down knee bends.

Supplements for Quick Recovery

Because ligaments and tendons do not have their own direct blood supply, their healing is slow. Ultrarunner Karl King found that the nutritional supplements of 1 gram glycine, 1 gram lysine, 0.5 gram buffered vitamin C, and one Aleve tablet is helpful in the healing process. Take this combination at breakfast and at bedtime. The supplements provide the major building blocks for connective tissue, while the Aleve is an anti-inflammatory.

Two dietary supplements, glucosamine sulfate and chondroitin sulfate, have been found to reduce joint pain. In 2005 the American College of Rheumatology announced a National Institutes of Health–funded study that showed using the supplements was effective at reducing moderate to severe knee pain due to osteoarthritis. Smaller European studies have made the same findings.

Glucosamine sulfate is a natural substance that helps build cartilage, the cushion at the ends of our bones, and maintain joint fluid thickness and elasticity. Chondroitin sulfate, also a natural substance, helps lubricate joints and gives tendons and ligaments their elasticity. Initial studies have found these over-the-counter supplements helpful in stimulating cartilage to grow and inhibiting the enzymes that break down cartilage. Many athletes have added this combination to their daily vitamin and supplement intake as a must-have. Drugstores, pharmacies, and health food stores typically offer these two supplements (often in one capsule) in an assortment of supplement formulas by different companies. Give these supplements time to work—a month or more.

- Use a wobble board to work the injured ankle as well your good ankle.

- Move the ankle up and down in a pumping motion to help decrease swelling.

- Rotate your feet up to 50 repetitions in each direction. Do four to five sets every other day.

- Strengthen your ankles by balancing with one foot flat on the ground and the other leg bent back at the knee, as if you were in the normal support phase of a running stride. Start at 30 seconds at a time and practice until you can hold your balance for several minutes. When you have mastered this step, close your eyes and do the same thing. Repeatedly losing your balance and then recovering gradually strengthens the ankles even more. Doing this exercise with your eyes closed retrains you to quickly react to changes as your nerve endings detect a twist or turn when the foot hits the ground.

■ Stand on one leg and slowly rise all the way up onto your toes and then slowly lower your heel to a flat foot. Balance yourself as necessary. Start with 25 repetitions and work up to 50 daily. This is another good proprioception exercise.

■ Walk on your heels for five steps, then walk five more steps on your tiptoes. For a more stable ankle, do this forward, backward, and side-to-side for a few minutes.

■ Stand with your forefeet on a raised surface (such as a book, low step, or block of wood), and rise up onto your toes and then back down again. Hold each, at the top and at the bottom, for 10–15 seconds. Repeat until both calves are fatigued.

■ An isometric exercise with the feet pushing against each other helps strengthen muscles without joint movement. When sitting on a chair, push down with one foot on top while pulling up with the other foot on the bottom. Then reverse feet. When sitting on the floor, you can also put your feet bottom to bottom, first pushing the big toes against each other and then the little toes against each other. Hold the motions for 6–10 seconds and repeat several times a day.

■ Hop on one foot and then change to the other foot. Practice forward and backward, and side-to-side movements.

Research at the University of North Carolina found that training your calf muscles can protect your ankles from injury. The study followed 20 athletes and found those who rolled or sprained their ankles had less range of ankle motion than healthy athletes. The two calf muscles—the gastrocnemius and soleus—limit the ankle range of motion. Cathleen Brown, MA, the lead study author, advises calf raises with knees slightly bent to strengthen the soleus. To stretch the gastrocnemius, use the familiar stretch where you lean against a wall with one leg in front of the other. Repeating this with the back knee bent stretches the soleus.

Ankle-Support Products

Weak ankles can be a problem, particularly on trails. After turning or spraining an ankle, an ankle support will provide the protection necessary for light training. Otherwise weak ankles can also benefit from an ankle support. Adhesive taping of the ankle can be helpful; however, for it to be effective, someone who is experienced must do the taping. While taping restricts extreme motion, the tape loses strength as it moves with the skin—40% of its strength can be lost within 20 minutes. Ankle supports are better at providing support.

Ankle supports are typically made from a compression-type sock. Some offer a figure eight–style stretch wrap, which gives additional strength and support. Some ankle supports can be found in drugstores and sporting goods stores. Cramer, DonJoy, Futuro, Mueller, and Spenco all make basic ankle supports. Many are simply a one-piece pull-on neoprene or stretch device with a hole for the heel and

Work Those Calves

Matt Mahoney, one of the proponents of barefoot running and running without socks, feels the most important ankle muscle is the calf: "This is what you use to take the weight off your heel and shift to the ball of your foot when your ankle starts to twist." He recommends the following calf exercises, emphasizing, "You will know you're doing these exercises right if your calves are sore for several days afterward."

- Run backward.

- Run barefoot in sand.

- Climb stairs, both up and down. Land on the ball of your foot as you descend.

- Do calf raises on a step, with weights, standing for the gastrocnemius and sitting for the soleus. Using machines is useful for these. Do the standing calf raises one foot at a time on a step with a weighted belt. Do the sitting raises on a machine with weight resting on a padded bar across the top of the legs.

---

toes. Ace wraps, or similar elastic wraps, are helpful after a sprain but provide little support against initially turning your ankle. Sue Norwood, who has an eversion problem, likes the ASO Ankle Stabilizer that her doctor told her to wear for the year after her surgery—it's supportive but lightweight and easy to use, and is one of the most popular.

All the ankle supports listed on the preceding pages are compact in size and fit easily into a fanny pack or backpack. Because the supports vary in fit and material, experiment wearing the support against the skin or over a sock to find the best fit on your foot. If you are prone to ankle injuries, consider carrying one as a preventive measure.

Fractures

Any bone in the foot can fracture; however, some are more prone to injury than others. The terms break and fracture are synonymous—both describe a structural break in the continuity of the bone. A fracture may occur from a fall, the twisting motion of a turned ankle, a blow from hitting your foot on a rock or tree root, or simply from a bad foot plant. The toes are the most likely bones to fracture in the foot—usually the first (big toe) and the fifth (little toe). The Jones fracture (breaking the fifth metatarsal on the outside of the foot) is common. This type of fracture is common with a fall or loss of balance where you put a sudden and undue amount of pressure on the outside of your foot. But there are many types of fractures.

Fractures usually manifest themselves with a great deal of pain and tenderness directly above the fracture site. When a soft tissue injury has occurred, there will

ANKLE-SUPPORT PRODUCTS

The **ANKLE STABILIZING ORTHOSIS (ASO)** is made to prevent or treat ankle sprains. It features an elastic cuff closure to decrease the degree of potential inversion, figure eight straps to replicate ankle taping, a low profile to allow it to fit in any type of shoe, and a lace-up closure. It is designed to keep the foot in a neutral position. A model is available with rigid side stays to increase stability. medspec.com

The convenient **ANKLEWRAP** differs from the typical Ace wrap. Made from a knitted blend of nylon and Lycra with a foam inner layer, it breathes to wick away perspiration, stays put with superior sticking power, and is fully adjustable. At 10 feet long by 1.5 inches wide, it is long enough to make a complete figure eight wrap with three heel locks. fabrifoam.com

CHO-PAT ANKLE COMPRESSION SLEEVES provide compression to the ankle with three types of sleeves. cho-pat.com

CROPPER MEDICAL'S BIO SKIN ANKLE BRACES are a compression support material made with four layers: a hypoallergenic Lycra knit outer layer, a SmartSkin membrane that absorbs moisture and wicks it from the skin, a Lycra knit/fleece inner layer, and a SkinLok layer against the skin. Bio Skin stretches with the body's movement, giving compression without bunching and binding, and it does not constrict the joints. Unlike neoprene, Bio Skin breathes. Three designs are offered with either plastic stays or gel inserts. bioskin.com

The **KALLASSY ANKLE SUPPORT** is a proven design for rehabilitation of severe ankle sprains. The support is made of nylon-lined neoprene that provides warmth and compression. A strap that wraps around the ankle provides stability, and a nonstretch lateral strapping system helps prevent inversion motions of the ankle. If you are prone to turned ankles, this support is one of the most stabilizing ankle supports available. It is often available in sporting goods stores or can be purchased online.

OPTP (ORTHOPEDIC PHYSICAL THERAPY PRODUCTS) has a wide range of devices for balance/proprioception, stretching, strength training, and more. optp.com

THE PERFORM 8 LATERAL ANKLE STABILIZER provides excellent external stabilization of the ankle's lateral (outer) ligaments, similar to ankle taping. While a lightweight elastic compression sock provides support to soft tissue, an elastic figure eight strap wraps around the foot. Pads protect and relieve pressure on the Achilles tendon. This support is excellent for athletes prone to chronic ankle sprains. brownmed.com

WOBBLE and **ROCKER BOARDS** can be used to improve balance and strength, retrain injured muscles, improve muscle memory, and build core strength. You can get a wobble board for both feet or two smaller wobble boards, one for each foot. **SIMPLY FIT BOARDS** (simplyfitboard.com), **FITTERFIRST** (fitter1.com), and **INDO BOARD** (indoboard.com) each offer wobble boards.

also be discoloration of the skin above the fracture. Fractures that are ignored can result in a malunion or nonunion of the pieces of bone as they heal. This could require surgery to correctly align the bone ends.

Emergency room physicians and sports specialists often use the Ottawa Ankle Rules[45] to determine the likelihood of an ankle fracture before an X-ray is taken (and to avoid unnecessary X-rays). The study takes two approaches:

- Pain in the malleolar (ankle bones) zone and either an inability to bear weight immediately and in the emergency room, or bone tenderness at the posterior (back) edge of either malleolus.

- Pain in the midfoot zone and either an inability to bear weight immediately and in the emergency room, or bone tenderness at the navicular (the bone at the top front of the foot at the curve up the ankle) or fifth metatarsal (the midfoot bone on the outside of the foot).

Treating Fractures

Treatment of fractures typically combines ice, immobilization, and elevation. Toe fractures are usually buddy taped, and the patient is advised to wear a firm-soled shoe or a wooden orthopedic shoe that restricts flexion of the foot. Buddy taping is done by lightly taping the injured toe to the toe next to it, with a piece of cotton or tissue between toes (never tape skin to skin). Buddy taping provides support and a limited degree of immobilization of the toe. A fracture of the big toe can warrant a

Types of Fractures

AVULSION—the tearing away of a part of the bone attached to a ligament or tendon

BUTTERFLY—a bone fragment that is shaped like a butterfly and part of a comminuted fracture

COMMINUTED—more than two fragments; may be splintered

COMPLETE—the bone is completely broken through

DISPLACED—bone fragments are moved away from each other

IMPACTED—fragments are compressed by force into each other or into adjacent bone

INCOMPLETE—the continuity of the bone is destroyed on only one side

NONDISPLACED—the bone pieces are still together in the correct locations and at the correct angles

SEGMENTAL—several large fractures in the same bone

SPIRAL—the fracture line is spiral in shape

full foot cast. A Jones fracture or any other fracture of the foot or ankle will require a cast and immobilization for four to six weeks.

Standard practice with fractures is to immobilize the joint above and the joint below the fracture. You may start with a non-weight-bearing cast, requiring the use of crutches, and later have it changed to a weight-bearing walking cast.

Refer to the chapter "Cold and Heat Therapy" for more information on making the most of icing techniques.

Stress Fractures

Stress fractures are a common sports injury. Sudden or repetitive stress, usually from overuse without proper conditioning; playing high-impact sports; increasing the time and intensity of one's activity too rapidly; or a change in running surfaces—from a softer to a harder surface, results in a small crack in the outer shell of the affected bone. Over time, if not treated, this crack will develop into a fracture of the bone. Often you will have no recollection of having injured the foot.

The most common foot bones to stress fracture are the second and third metatarsal bones in the forefoot—between the toes and the ankle. Some doctors will use an X-ray to make the diagnosis, but often a stress fracture does not show on an initial X-ray because the bone's callus formation has not yet taken place at the fracture site. A bone scan or MRI, which are different from an X-ray, is useful for a questionable diagnosis and will usually confirm whether you have a stress fracture.

Other possible causes of stress fractures include wearing worn-out or poorfitting shoes, or ill-fitting insoles; abnormal foot structure or mechanics (arch or pronation problems, or leg-length discrepancies); or tightness and inflexibility. Your medical specialist may recommend additional calcium in your diet and/or a DEXA scan bone-density test. Female athletes who have infrequent periods are most at risk for stress fractures.

At the point of the stress fracture, there is typically pain to the touch, often first felt as a dull ache or soreness. The pain usually becomes worse as the break grows. Swelling is common.

Treating Stress Fractures

After a confirming scan, a sports doctor, orthopedist, or podiatrist will usually recommend at least six weeks off. Follow their advice. To run or exercise heavily on a stress fracture is asking for more problems. Switch to more cushioned shoes and use this recovery time to focus on other non-weight-bearing exercises and cross-training: cycling, pool running, swimming, and weight training. Ask your doctor whether you can use a limited–weight-bearing exercise machine such as a stair climber or an elliptical trainer.

An Ace wrap or compression sock will help control swelling. An orthopedic or wooden shoe may be used to splint the foot. Anti-inflammatories are helpful. Elevation of the foot above the level of the heart will help reduce pain and swelling. Ice the area 20 minutes at a time three to four times a day and after any exercise.

The "Cold and Heat Therapy" chapter gives more information on making the most of icing techniques. Difficult cases may require splinting, casting, or surgery.

Dislocations

A dislocation is a complete displacement of bone from its normal position at a joint's surface, which disrupts the articulation of two or three bones at that junction and alters alignment. The dislocation may be complete, where the joint surfaces are completely separated, or incomplete (subluxation), where the joint is only slightly displaced. The dislocation may be caused by a direct blow or injury, or by a ligament's tearing.

In the foot, the most common dislocations are the toes. Any of the toes can be dislocated, but the most typical are the big or little toe. The ankle can be dislocated by any combination of fractures of the tibia (the big inner bone of the lower leg) or fibula (the small outer bone of the lower leg), resulting in a displaced talus. Ankle dislocations can be a major lower leg injury with severe consequences if the circulation to the foot is compromised.

Treating Dislocations

Dislocated toes are fairly simple to treat. Resetting dislocations is called reduction. With one hand, stabilize the ball of the foot with your thumb on the injured toe. With the other hand exert traction to the toe while pulling slowly and steadily on the displaced section of toe. Pull firmly enough that it clears the previous section of toe. The connecting ligament will then pull the toe back into place almost automatically. This reduces the dislocation. The toe then needs to be buddy taped to the toe or toes next to it for stabilization. A small piece of gauze, cotton, or tissue between the taped toes will prevent skin breakdown if the tape is on for any great length of time. A firm-soled shoe will help keep the toe in line and the foot-toe joint stable. Frequent icing and elevation in the next 48 hours is recommended.

To temporarily correct and stabilize an ankle dislocation and related fracture, an orthopedic trauma surgeon recommends straightening the foot by exerting traction in a straight and steady motion—so that as much as possible it is in its natural position and angled to the lower leg. The foot, ankle, and lower leg then need to be stabilized with a splint. Use any available materials to keep the extremity stable. Check the toes frequently for normal skin color and warmth, which indicate good circulation. A dislocated ankle needs to be treated by an emergency room physician or orthopedic surgeon as soon as possible.

If either a toe or ankle dislocation is an open dislocation, where the bone has come through the skin, extra care must be taken. This open, or complex, dislocation is usually associated with a fracture, and the bone may still be outside of the skin or may have pulled back inside. First, clean the wound, and then proceed with the reduction. Then, leaving the wound open, apply a sterile dressing, and splint the extremity. Check the end(s) of the extremity farthest from the body to be sure there is adequate circulation, adjusting the extremity as necessary. When the open dislocation is stabilized, seek out immediate medical attention.

Tendon and Ligament Injuries

The primary function of tendons is to transmit muscle force to the moving joints with limited elongation. Tendons are ropelike structures that attach muscles to bones. Ligaments are similar structures that attach bones to other bones. When muscles and bones move, they exert stresses on the tendons and ligaments that are attached to them. The foot is a complicated but amazing engineering marvel. With 26 bones, 33 joints, 107 ligaments, 19 muscles, and tendons to hold the structure together and allow it to move in a variety of ways, it offers all kinds of opportunities for tendon and ligament injuries.

Troy Marsh, an orthopedic physical therapist, describes tendon disorders as "a major problem among competitive athletes, often interfering with training and competition. Tissue damage may result from a sudden traumatic episode such as an ankle sprain, or it may arise with no apparent cause but usually due to cumulative trauma or overuse."

The terms *tendinitis, tendinosis,* and *tendinopathy* all refer to tendon injuries. These terms are commonly confused and misused:

TENDINITIS—The suffix *-itis* means inflammation. The term *tendinitis* should be reserved for tendon injuries that involve larger-scale acute injuries accompanied by inflammation. (Tendinitis is often spelled as *tendonitis*, but the preferred spelling used in most of the medical literature is *tendinitis*.)

TENDINOSIS—The suffix *-osis* implies a pathology of chronic degeneration without inflammation. Tendinosis is an accumulation over time of small-scale injuries that don't heal properly; it is a chronic injury of failed healing.

Rob Conenello, past president of the American Academy of Podiatric Sports Medicine, says chronic conditions such as tendinosis and fasciosis do not have an inflammation component, so ice is not helpful. Ice should be used for acute injuries.

When our muscles move in new ways or do more work than they can easily handle, our muscles and tendons can sustain damage. If the increase in demand is made gradually, muscle and tendon tissues will usually heal, build in strength, and adapt to new loads. It is this principle we use to build muscle and tendon strength.

Many athletes, however, participate in activities that injure a tendon on a microscopic scale and then do more injury before the tendon heals. If you continue the injurious activity, you will gradually accumulate these microinjuries. When enough injury accumulates, you'll feel pain. This kind of injury that comes on slowly with time and persists is a chronic injury; acute tendon injuries are sudden tears that cause immediate pain and obvious symptoms. Tendon injuries often require patience and careful rehabilitation because tendons heal more slowly than muscles.

Tendons are critical for converting the movement of muscle contraction to movement of the foot and/or ankle. The most common tendon injury is to the Achilles tendon, which connects the muscle of the posterior calf to the bottom of the calcaneus bone and mediates plantar flexion (toes down) function across the ankle. Injuries to other tendons that cross the ankle are usually the result of lacerations or direct trauma. Injuries to tendons can vary from mild (stretching) to moderate (tearing) to severe (rupture).

A common tendon problem affects the ankle flexors. These tendons are caught under the pressure of the shoe's tongue and laces across the front top of the foot. Walking or running steep hills can also cause this problem. Another common tendon injury is post-tibial tendinitis. This affects the posterior tibial tendon from the inside of the ankle and the foot. Major tendons and ligaments in the foot and ankle include the following:

- Achilles tendon
- Calcaneofibular ligament
- Lisfranc ligament
- Posterior talofibular ligament
- Tarsal canal ligaments
- Anterior tibial tendon
- Inferior talofibular ligament
- Peroneal tendons
- Sinus tarsi syndrome

Treating Tendon Injuries

There are multiple treatments for tendon injuries. Your podiatrist, sports podiatrist, or orthopedist is the best person to determine the treatment you need. In addition to the treatments below, sometimes a biomechanical assessment is needed. The following list is taken from tendonpain.org, a website devoted to tendon injuries (the following suggestions for tendinosis also work for tendinitis).

REST. By the time you feel pain from tendinosis, your injury has been gradually building for many weeks. Remember that tendons heal slowly.

PHYSICAL THERAPY EXERCISES can help heal tendinosis, as long as you are careful to progress gradually. Studies have shown that loading a tendon parallel to its length helps the collagen fibers grow with better parallel alignment and speeds the healing process. Find a physical therapist who has a lot of experience with tendinosis, and make sure he/she is willing to go as slowly as your body requires.

SHOCK WAVE THERAPY is a treatment for tendinosis. An extracorporeal ultrasound device delivers sound waves to a very focused area of the tendon.

ICE is a common treatment for tendinosis. Many physical therapists suggest that you use ice following your exercises or whenever you need some pain reduction during the day. Don't use it just prior to your exercises. It's hard to say if ice has any long-term beneficial effect on tendinosis, but it can be an excellent form of pain control that has no negative side effects (as long as you take care not to get ice burn from too much ice).

SUPPORTS AND ORTHOTICS are often used for ankle injuries. Some people find that supports can add stability during activity. These should not be worn all the time because you can lose strength and flexibility.

NUTRITIONAL SUPPLEMENTS are somewhat of an unknown area. There has been little scientific research to investigate the effects of nutritional supplements on the healing of tendinosis. Glucosamine sulfate and chondroitin sulfate are not likely to help tendinosis. Other supplements that claim to help heal tendons and ligaments contain the amino acids glycine, lysine, and proline.

BODYWORK is done by physical therapists. Massage and other techniques can help loosen up. Many practitioners try to help you with your posture and body mechanics, and some do hands-on soft tissue work.

SURGERY should be a last resort for tendinosis. Some athletes have a positive outcome, while others a negative outcome. Educate yourself about the surgical procedure before you consider it for yourself, and give your injury plenty of time to heal on its own before you resort to surgery.

CORTISONE injections are not recommended by tendonpain.org because of the possibility of an adverse reaction on the tissue in the area of injection if repeated injections are given.

If pain and injury persist after a course of treatment, ask for an MRI. A partial or full tendon rupture can only be diagnosed with an MRI. Troy Marsh reports that "chronic Achilles tendinosis sufferers, most often seen among male recreational runners between 35 and 45 years old, responded favorably to a 12-week training program of high-load eccentric calf muscle training and returned to full running activity. A comparison group with the same diagnosis, treated conventionally with anti-inflammatory drugs, orthotics, rest, and therapy modalities, was not successful and each subject ultimately was treated surgically."

Tendon and fascia pain may be helped with a quick and simple minimally invasive medical treatment. The TOPAZ MicroDebrider utilizes patented Coblation technology to offer a quicker return to daily activities with a significant improvement in patient outcomes. This can effectively work on plantar fasciitis. Small punctures in key areas of the heel are made to allow the insertion of a pencil tip–size wand device, the MicroDebrider. Radio frequency energy is transmitted through the wand for short 500 millisecond intervals. The Coblation technology forms a plasma that gently and precisely dissolves soft tissue at relatively low temperatures and increases vascular blood supply. Check with your orthopedic surgeon or podiatrist for more information about this treatment.

Platelet-rich plasma (PRP) injections have helped many athletes return to healthy activities after tendinosis injuries. Platelets contain powerful tendon-healing growth factors. Doctors remove a small amount of the patient's blood, spin it in a centrifuge, separate out the platelets, and then reinject these at the injury site. James Korak had tried everything for his severe plantar fasciitis before trying PRP. You can read his story in the "Plantar Fasciitis" section farther down in this chapter.

Marsh suggests "remembering to keep the proximal muscle groups such as the hips and thighs strong and responsive in all planes of motion. Integrating functional and sport-specific strength and balance exercises, such as single-leg heel raises, into your training will enhance performance and hopefully prevent any serious tendon disorders—and prepare you for the next athletic event."

Further information, including reports on medical studies, can be found at tendonpain.org.

Treatment Options: Trigger Point Therapy and ASTYM

If you receive treatment for tendon injuries and the pain, numbness, or other abnormal sensations continue, ask your health care practitioner about other treatment options. Two common options are trigger point therapy and ASTYM.

Trigger points are tiny contraction knots, a wad of muscle fibers staying in a hard contraction, never relaxing. A trigger point in a muscle could be painful or it could not manifest pain until touched. Often though, its pain is referred elsewhere. These muscle knots can send referred pain and numbness into the plantar fascia, Achilles tendon, toes, ankle, forefoot, heel, and arch. Referred pain from trigger points mimics the symptoms of many other common injuries—hence the relationship to tendons and ligaments. Massage or kneading of the trigger points is done to break up the knots.

Twyla Carolan, a kinesiologist and masseuse, says of trigger points: "You might not even realize that you have such a knot until you apply direct pressure to it and the resulting pain has you leaping to your feet in panic. One of the odd things about trigger points is that they are notorious for hanging out in one spot while sending pain to another. This means that it can be quite difficult to actually locate the source of a pain problem, unless you find it by accident."

Nathan Wilson, an ultrarunner, wrote, "I found that by massaging trigger points on my lower legs and feet for a couple of weeks, I was able to gain flexibility in my ankles, which I have not had in years. *The Trigger Point Therapy Workbook* really complemented *Fixing Your Feet*, as it helped highlight the anatomical

How Tendons Heal

Tendons have limited blood supply, and nutrition is often supported via synovial fluid within the presence of a tendon sheath. In other words, tendons are designed to transmit tensile loads, have limited elastic properties, and heal slowly compared to other, more oxygenated tissue. This is important to know as one begins to understand the basis of optimal healing after injury and repair. It is very important to understand if prevention and performance is in mind.

Optimal healing consists of three phases: inflammation, repair, and remodeling. The first three days after acute tendon injury sees inflammation. During this time tendons are most sensitive to mechanical load and are chemically irritated. Relative rest is indicated. Interestingly, after about three weeks, inflammatory cells are not present and medications may lose the desired effect.

Repair of damaged tissue lasts about four to six weeks and consists of the deposition of new collagen. Early mobilization is a key factor for strengthening the repairing tendon and begins the process of organizing the new collagen along the lines of functional stress. Prolonged rest may not provide the controlled loading stimulus necessary for maturation of the healing tissue and may actually set up a degenerative process—a condition referred to as tendinosis.

Remodeling is the process of reorganizing the "contracted and disorganized" collagen fibers. Effective remodeling requires a progressive return to normal loads and activity to prevent contractures and to promote strength and flexibility. This process may take up to a year to mature and should include all three planes of functional motion. The three planes of motion at the foot and ankle can be appreciated when running trails as the surface becomes uneven or pitched, or when sharp turn angles are required.

Targeting tendon tissue for early treatment should focus on aerobic training and has been shown to increase tensile strength and endurance. This means high repetitions (100–200 per set) with low loads and introducing eccentric loading as soon as tolerable. Eccentric loading, unlike its concentric counterpart, is the lengthening of muscle under load. For example, a single-leg heel raise using one's own body weight is concentric on the up phase and eccentric on the down phase. Standing toe raises are effective in strengthening tendons on the front of the ankle.

—Troy Marsh, an orthopedic physical therapist

structure of the feet and the connections between parts of the body and the feet, which are also mentioned in your book."

Trigger points can be treated by a specialist or through self-treatment. If your health care specialist has experience with trigger points, the points are easy to locate and treat. If not, ask for a referral to a physical therapist or other specialist. A couple of good sources of information about trigger point therapy include:

- *The Trigger Point Therapy Workbook: Your Self-Treatment Guide for Pain Relief,* 3rd ed., by Clair Davies (Oakland, CA: New Harbinger Publications, 2013).

- *TriggerPoint Performance Therapy* at tptherapy.com. It offers tips, charts, and products for trigger point pain relief.

ASTYM (A-stim) is a treatment process of soft-tissue injuries done by a physical therapist. Done properly, it can rejuvenate tendons, ligaments, and muscles by getting rid of scar tissue. An ASTYM treatment effectively stimulates scar tissue to be reabsorbed by the body and degenerated tendons to regenerate and heal. Following an ASTYM treatment, you will be given a stretching and strengthening regimen for the affected area. Compliance with these exercises is an important part of the treatment. On the feet, ASTYM can be used for plantar fasciitis, heel pain, Achilles tendinosis, and ankle sprains and strains. More information can be found at astym.com.

Achilles Tendinitis

The Achilles tendon connects the gastrocnemius and the soleus, the two major muscles of the calf, to the heel bone. It stabilizes the heel every time you take a step. The tendon makes it possible for you to rise up on your toes, run, and jump. Achilles tendinitis occurs when the sheath surrounding this cord becomes inflamed. There may be small tears in the tendon, or sudden and repeated stretching of the tendon causes an inflammation that is painful behind the heel, ankle, and lower calf while walking and running. The pain may be felt during the early part of your run or hike and then subside, only to worsen after stopping. This pain is your first warning, followed by swelling of the Achilles tendon and pain to the touch at the base of your heel.

A mild first-degree injury makes it difficult to rise up on your toes or walk on your heels. With proper treatment, you should be able to walk with little pain after about 48 hours. You should not resume normal athletic activity for several weeks. A second-degree injury is when there is partial tearing of the tendon from its attachment point. This injury will take six to eight weeks to heal, with an additional two to four weeks of stretching exercises before normal athletic activity can be resumed. In a third-degree

Achilles tendon

injury, an extreme case, the Achilles tendon ruptures. This requires immediate medical intervention, usually surgery, and a long healing and strengthening process. There is sudden calf pain and usually an audible snap if the tendon ruptures. The tendon will ball up in the calf with a related defect in the lower tendon. If the tendon is swollen, or you suspect a tear, usually a second- or third-degree injury, you should not risk running on it. You can further damage or rupture the tendon. If the pain is mild and goes away in five minutes with a warm-up, typically a first-degree injury, it is usually OK to continue.

Suddenly increasing your activity, increasing your mileage too quickly, or running steep hills or speedwork can lead to an inflamed Achilles tendon. To prevent Achilles tendon problems, increase your activity, mileage, and hill training gradually. Strengthening your ankles, as well as lower leg and calf muscle stretching, can also help prevent problems. Overpronators, whose arches collapse when walking or running, are more prone than others to Achilles problems. Wearing shoes that do not fit or support the foot can also lead to an Achilles tendon injury.

Rich Schick, a physician's assistant, adds the following:

> The Achilles tendon is not a simple structure. It is more correctly termed the Achilles complex. If it were as simple as we perceive it, there would be a straight pull from the calf muscle to the heel, and the tendon would be very prominent instead of following the contour of the leg. In reality the tendon passes through a series of little tunnels of very tough tissue that hold it close to the leg.
>
> In severe cases of Achilles tendinitis, calcium deposits can form in and on the tendon, preventing it from passing through these little tunnels and resulting in a permanent disability or the need for surgery. If you grasp the tendon between your thumb and forefinger, move your foot up and down, and feel a grating or bubble-popping sensation, this is a sign of serious tendinitis. The finding is called crepitus and represents severe inflammation. If not treated appropriately, it can lead to calcific tendinitis.

Ignoring the signs of Achilles tendinitis and not seeking treatment can lead to a chronic inflammation or even tendon rupture. The pain may occur when warming up and then ease up. The athlete continues to train and the pain returns after the session has ended. Over time, the periods of pain-free training become shorter and shorter. Eventually, training may become impossible and treatment mandatory. This can lead to the formation of a cyst in the tendon. As the cyst expands, the tendon thins out and becomes more susceptible to rupture if overstressed.

Treating Achilles Tendinitis

The major causes of Achilles tendon problems are a lack of strength and flexibility in the calf muscles, a weakness in the tendon, or a weak ankle joint. Treatment may include any or all of the following: icing as described on the next page, stretching and flexibility exercises, wearing flexible shoes or boots with a well-padded heel counter, and avoiding the ups and downs of hills.

If you suspect you have Achilles tendinitis, stop running—do not run through the pain. Ignoring the symptoms may cause the tendon to rupture, which usually requires surgery. Call your orthopedist or podiatrist if the pain persists. The doctor may put your foot in either a flexible or immobilizing cast to reduce movement and weight bearing. Once the cast is removed, you will need to do stretching exercises to strengthen the tendon before resuming normal athletic activity.

The treatment for a mildly injured Achilles tendinitis is the same RICE treatment used for ankle sprains and strains: rest, ice, compression, and elevation, with the addition of a *P* (PRICE) for protection—usually a heel lift to reduce tension on the tendon. The first 24 hours are the most critical for beginning treatment. Early treatment decreases swelling and lessens the risk of additional injury. Initial rest of the foot is also important. A lightly wound Ace wrap will provide compression to help keep swelling down while providing support. Apply the Ace wrap from the forefoot upward toward the calf. Do not wear the Ace wrap to bed at night. Apply ice for 20 minutes at a time up to six to eight times daily. Ice can be very helpful in the healing process. See the "Cold and Heat Therapy" chapter for more information on making the most of icing techniques. See also "Supplements for Quick Recovery" on page 265.

The injured area should be elevated above the level of the heart as much as possible during the first 48 hours. This keeps blood away from the injured area and reduces pain and swelling. The use of anti-inflammatory medications is usually warranted.

A small heel pad will alleviate the stresses on the tendon. For some individuals, wearing low-heeled shoes as often as possible will help keep the Achilles tendon stretched. An Achilles notch in shoes or mid- and low-top boots will accommodate the Achilles tendon in plantar flexion. The Achilles Tendon Strap made by Cho-Pat can provide relief from the discomfort of Achilles tendinitis.

Adding a small, thin, friction-reducing pad in the Achilles notch of the shoe's heel counter can reduce pressure on the inflamed tendon. Tamarack, the maker of the popular ENGO Patches, makes a thin ENGO Back of Heel Patch, perfect for protecting the tendon. Another option during an event is to cut a slit into the center of the shoe's Achilles notch in the heel counter.

A lightweight plastic night splint worn to bed can help to stretch the foot, limit contraction of soft tissues at night, and avoid morning stiffness. Night splints help avoid foot drop and accompanying muscle tightening. Night splints are proven as a treatment method for preventing the plantar fascia and Achilles tendon from contracting during the night. Many athletes swear by them. Check with your podiatrist, orthopedist, or medical supply store. Several night-splint models are available. If the pain persists, consult a medical specialist. He or she will need to rule out partial tears of the tendon, an inflammation of the tendon's sheath, or degenerative changes. Many physical therapists can apply a treatment called iontophoresis, which uses electrical current to apply a steroid medication over the inflamed tendon. Avoid cortisone injections into the area because they can cause tendon rupture.

Rupture of the tendon requires specialized care. If the rupture is fresh, within hours of the injury, surgical repair of the tendon is usually done. Older injuries

ACHILLES TENDINITIS PRODUCTS

The **ACHILLES HEALER** reduces stress on the Achilles tendon. The strap is made from ProWrap, a knitted blend of nylon and Lycra with patented foam lining. fabrifoam.com

CHO-PAT'S ACHILLES TENDON STRAP fits under the arch and around the ankle to relieve pressure on the Achilles tendon. Trials at the Mayo's Sports/Medicine Clinic have shown the strap effective as an addition to traditional treatments for Achilles tendinitis, particularly during the push-off phase of gait. The strap is available in four sizes based on ankle circumference at its widest point. cho-pat.com

ENGO BACK OF HEEL PATCHES can be applied to the shoe's heel counter for long-lasting protection of the Achilles tendon. Strong, latex-free adhesive prevents migration and movement, even through moisture and sweat. Scientific and field tests show ENGO's slippery surface significantly reduces rubbing, providing immediate relief. goengo.com

HAPAD THREE-QUARTER-LENGTH HEEL WEDGES provide the necessary heel lift to help reduce the pain associated with Achilles tendinitis. They are available in three thicknesses. The coiled, springlike wool fibers provide firm and resilient support as they mold and shape to the foot. hapad.com

The **N'ICE STRETCH NIGHT SPLINT SUSPENSION SYSTEM** is made for both Achilles tendinitis and plantar fasciitis. This night splint uses bilateral suspension straps to provide continuous nighttime stretching of the Achilles tendon and plantar fasciitis. The straps allow for independent bi-plane dorsiflexion adjustment. A removable Sealed Ice pack provides cold therapy coupled with stretching of soft tissues. The unit is hinged to fold compactly. brownmed.com

may also be treated surgically, though many patients will improve by casting the leg. Diminished strength and rerupture is more frequently seen in patients who are cast without surgery, so the preference is to surgically repair the rupture. Following surgical repair of Achilles tendon injuries, the patient is usually cast; then when the cast is removed, the patient receives extensive rehabilitation to regain strength and flexibility. Often a heel lift is required for six months to a year after the cast has been removed.

Earth shoes, with their heel depression, or a shoe with a heel drop lower than the forefoot can be helpful. This puts the foot into dorsiflexion so that your heel is below the front of your foot. One caveat: This works best as a preventive for mild, chronic Achilles tendinitis, and for walking only. They should not be used for moderate/severe acute cases, given that rest and heel lifts are usually the best course of treatment.

Exercises to Stretch the Achilles Tendon

Stretching helps athletes improve flexibility and counter muscular imbalances that put them at a greater risk of injury. Proper stretching of the Achilles tendon can help prevent an Achilles injury.

The **PROSTRETCH** is a popular tool that effectively stretches the Achilles tendon, the plantar fascia, and the calf muscles. It builds lower extremity strength, balance, and flexibility benefits in three minutes of use prior to activity, thus reducing the risk of injury. The ProStretch can also be used for hamstring and anterior tibialis stretching. prostretch.com

POWERSTEPS ULTRASTRETCH NIGHT SOCK is made with soft material and an adjustable strap that gently pulls the toes to stretch the calf muscles and tissues of the foot and ankle. powersteps.com

RUNNER'S REMEDY ACHILLES TENDONITIS SLEEVE is a foot sleeve with a small pocket on the side of the tendon to hold one of four supplied ice packs. runnersremedy.com

The **SLANT BOARD** from Fitter adjusts to three levels and folds flat for travel. It comes in two widths. fitter1.com

The **STRETCH-EZ** from OPTP cradles the foot for a comfortable stretch of the foot, heel, Achilles tendon, hamstring, quadriceps, and inner/outer thigh and calf. Made of poly laminate and webbing. optp.com

The **TP MASSAGE FOOTBALLER, BALLER BLOCK,** and **MASSAGE BALLS** were created to relieve plantar fasciitis, Achilles tendinitis, and heel pain. They work on the muscles and/or trigger points by applying pressure to the trigger point area. Also offered is a *Performance Therapy for Foot and Lower Leg* DVD, which shows a complete foot and lower leg exercise routine. tptherapy.com

One method of stretching is to stand far enough from a wall or heavy piece of furniture so that when you lean forward toward the wall or furniture, you can feel the tendons stretch in the back of your leg while keeping your feet flat on the floor. Lean forward and stretch only to the point of feeling the stretch, not to the point of feeling pain. Alternate a 20-second stretch with a 20-second rest standing straight; repeat 10–20 times. Continue this daily stretching until the Achilles stops hurting.

Les Appel, DPM, who designed the Powerstep Insole, recommends facing a wall with one foot flat on the floor and the other foot's heel on the floor and toes up on the wall 3–4 inches. Gently move your knee slowly toward the wall until you feel slight stretching on the bottom of your foot and the back of your leg. Hold this position for 30 seconds, and repeat five times per foot.

A Swedish study showed excellent results with a simple stretch. Stand on a step or ledge on the balls of your feet. Push yourself up with your good leg and slowly transfer your weight to the affected leg. Slowly lower yourself all the way down until the injured leg's heel is below the stair level and you feel the pull on the soleus calf muscle. Alternate this stretch with the injured leg's knee straight and then slightly bent. Repeat three sets of 15, twice a day. Additional strength can be gained by adding weight over time. Use dumbbells, a light barbell, or a weighted backpack.

The Prostretch, Stretch-EZ, and slant boards are popular tools to effectively stretch the plantar fascia as well as the Achilles tendon and the gastrocnemius and soleus musculature of the back of the lower leg. Studies have shown that utilization of the these tools can more effectively increase ankle dorsiflexion (toe-up motion of the ankle) than the conventional and commonly used wall stretch technique mentioned on page 281. Their use is recommended as both a preventive measure and a treatment technique.

Ankle Tendons

The ankle is surrounded by tendons. The main ones that concern us here are the two peroneal tendons and the posterior tibial tendon.

Peroneal Tendons

The peroneus longus and peroneus brevis tendons run behind and around the lateral malleolus (the outside ankle bone). The peroneus longus flexes the ankle downward and out while the peroneus brevis tendon flexes the ankle up and inward. The tendons, in a sheath, pass through a groove behind the lateral malleolus. The sheath forms a tunnel around the tendons and a band of tissue called a retinaculum reinforces it. Their function is to stabilize the foot and ankle and protect them from sprains.

When these are stretched beyond normal, as with a turned ankle, pain from the injury, swelling, and inflammation will occur. A forceful stretch can cause a tear in the tendons. When the tendons momentarily slip out of the groove, it is called a subluxation. Early treatment of a subluxation is critical since a tear or rupture is likely if left untreated. Degenerative tears are usually due to overuse over long periods of time. Having high arches puts one at risk for developing a degenerative tear.

Posterior Tibial Tendon

The posterior tibial tendon runs behind the medial malleolus (the inside ankle bone). It helps turn the foot inward when walking or running. Pain can be in the shin or down to the ankle and instep area.

Treating Ankle Tendon Injuries

A physical examination will help determine which tendons are involved and where they are inflamed, torn, or ruptured. An MRI may be ordered if a tear or rupture is suspected. Icing, a combination of cold and heat therapy, and anti-inflammatory medications are in order. Wrapping the ankle for support will help. In some cases immobilization may be necessary. Start a program of stretching and strengthening of the ankle and lower leg—especially calf stretches. You may be referred to a physical therapist.

For a posterior tibial tendon injury, your podiatrist may prescribe an orthotic. Otherwise make sure you have good arch support in all your shoes and do not walk barefoot (Green Superfeet insoles are recommended).

Bursitis

Bursa are small fluid-filled sacs found between areas of high friction such as where muscles or tendons glide over bone. The bursa acts as a shock absorber, allowing movement between neighboring structures, usually in opposite directions. The body has more than 150 bursa sacs. Bursitis is the formation of an inflamed fluid-filled sac from trauma or overuse. On the feet, bursitis may develop beneath a callus or a bunion, under the metatarsal heads, or at the heel.

Typical causes of bursitis in the feet can be repetitive motions or an injury or sustained pressure to a joint. As the usually slippery bursa sac becomes inflamed, it loses its gliding capabilities and becomes gritty and rough. Inflamed bursas are painful and irritating all the time. Bursitis in the heel can manifest itself with the same symptoms as plantar fasciitis, but the heel bursitis will persist with any weight-bearing activity, whereas with plantar fasciitis the symptoms are relieved after the fascia warms up.

Treating Bursitis

The first action is to stop or reduce the motion or action that is causing the bursitis. The use of NSAIDs will help reduce the inflammation. Heat will relax the joint and promote tissue repair. In severe cases, fluid may be drawn from the sac to relieve pressure. Gently warming up before strenuous exercise can help avoid bursitis. Switch to soft running surfaces, and increase stretching and strengthening exercises. If you experience chronic bursitis, ask your doctor about medications and treatment options to relieve the pain and discomfort.

Plantar Fasciitis

The plantar fascia is a band of connective fibrous tissue that runs from the heel to the ball of the foot, forming the foot's arch. The band helps in support and stabilization of the foot during hiking and running. The arch flattens when standing. As you begin a step, the heel lifts up and also the plantar fascia tightens to form the curve of the arch and provides a strong push off with the toes. An inflammation of the fascia, called plantar fasciitis, occurs most often with overuse. The stretching and tearing of some of the fibers in the plantar fascia as it inserts into the heel bone causes the inflammation. If you have flat feet or high arches, or if you overpronate, the plantar fascia is strained, mainly at the heel. The stresses of impact sports, running, and hiking may flatten, lengthen, and eventually cause small tears in the plantar fascia. Tears near the heel bone often cause a heel spur to develop. Plantar fasciitis is usually the top foot complaint among runners.

Athletes who are predisposed to plantar fasciitis injuries typically have increased their mileage too fast, increased the frequency and intensity of their workouts, increased the amount of hill work, and/or have a lack of flexibility and strength in their ankle and foot. They may also have a foot imbalance such as flat feet or high arches. Running on old or poorly supporting shoes, transitioning too quickly to minimalist shoes, and walking too long in sandals or barefoot may also be factors.

Plantar fascia

Plantar fascia pain is commonly felt in the morning or after long periods of sitting. The first steps at these times cause a sudden strain to the band of tissue that has started to heal itself during the night. The pain and stiffness is usually centered at the bottom of the heel, but symptoms may radiate into the arch. Although the pain may decrease somewhat with your initial activity, as the day progresses, it may return and be quite painful.

Consult your podiatrist or orthopedist if you are suffering from pain in the arch of your foot or suspect that you have plantar fasciitis. In some cases the fascia may involve a partial or full rupture, which will require more aggressive treatment. An aggressive, multidisciplined medical approach using medical, biomechanical, and physical therapy treatments can help to return you to action as soon as possible. The Achilles tendon may also be involved, causing pain under the foot as it stretches. Recovery time can range from three months to a year—and in severe cases, even more.

Treating Plantar Fasciitis

Generally prescribed treatments for plantar fasciitis include rest, moist heat and stretching in the morning or before activity, icing massage after activity, heel cups, taping of the foot or an arch brace, orthotics, foot exercises, and shoe modifications. Ice your heels and the bottom of your foot after exercise (see the chapter "Cold and Heat Therapy" for information on making the most of icing techniques). By all means, replace your worn-out shoes and insoles. Usually you need either to provide more support to the arch or lessen the amount of overpronation. An arch support or arch pad can provide pain relief. Motion-control shoes can help if you overpronate. In extreme cases, oral anti-inflammatory medications, cortisone injections, physical therapy, cast immobilization, and even surgery may be necessary. Because the plantar fascia has low vascularity and a lack of good blood flow, it is slow to heal.

The first thing any doctor or physical therapist should tell you is to stop all impact activities for a period of weeks or months and to always wear shoes. Going barefoot is one of the worst things someone suffering from plantar fasciitis can do. Keep in mind that the tiny tears need to heal, and it makes sense to stop the activity that caused them in the first place. With your doctor's approval, switch to cycling, using an elliptical trainer, pool running, or swimming to help maintain fitness while keeping pressure off your feet. Have shoes by your bedside in case you have to get up at night. Avoid sandals unless they have an arch support.

You also need to regain flexibility and elasticity in the soleus muscle/sheath to prevent the condition from occurring again. Stretching is the way to do that, but you have to start out slow and easy, that is, writing the alphabet with your foot in warm bathwater. (See the section on stretching on pages 288–289 for various useful exercises for increasing flexibility.) Once you've started to heal, you can move on to the more demanding stretches. The most common comment by those who have conquered plantar fasciitis is how stretching helped more than anything else. A physical therapist or chiropractor can help adjust muscle imbalances. Back issues and weak core muscles can lead to subtle changes in your stride that you'll feel in your feet—so work on strengthening your core.

A study by the American Orthopaedic Foot and Ankle Society looked at heel pain related to plantar fasciitis.[46] Dr. Glenn Pfeffer reported chronic heel pain as the most common foot problem, with up to 80% caused by proximal plantar fasciitis. The study compared a common polypropylene custom orthotic device, three over-the-counter heel pads (a ViscoHeel silicone heel cushion, a Tuli's Heel Cup, and a Hapad Comf-Orthotic), and stretching alone. After comparing the results of five control groups, they found that stretching and off-the-shelf shoe inserts were just as effective as stretching and the more costly orthotics. Their recommendation: "For the initial treatment of heel pain, stretching and a simple, inexpensive, off-the-shelf device is the best way to go." When wearing heel pads, be sure to use them in all your shoes. It is a good idea to check your insoles in all your shoes to see whether they provide good support.

In an interesting article, "Plantar Fasciitis—A New Perspective,"[47] Robert Nirschl, MD, makes a case for plantar fasciitis as a painful degenerative plantar tendinitis, not an inflammation problem. His research found no inflammatory cells in injured plantar fascia—meaning that anti-inflammatory medications and cortisone

Cortisone Injections

While the inflammation for which corticosteroids are given can recur, corticosteroid injections can provide months to years of relief when used properly. These injections also can cure diseases (permanently resolve them) when the problem is tissue inflammation localized to a small area, such as bursitis and tendinitis. However, tendons can be weakened by corticosteroid injections in or near tendons. Tendon rupture as a result has been reported. Unique side effects of joint injections involve injury to the joint tissues, particularly with repeated injections. These injuries include thinning of the joint cartilage, weakening of the ligaments of the joint, increased inflammation in the joint (arthritis) due to a reaction to a corticosteroid that has crystallized, and introduction of infection into the joint. Source: medicinenet.com will not have curative potential. For plantar tendinitis Dr. Nirschl recommends stretching and strength training all areas of the leg to restore strength, endurance, and flexibility. Also recommended is the use of a night splint, arch bracing or a soft orthotic, and footwear with good midfoot flexibility. In extreme cases, surgery may be indicated to remove painful tendinitis tissue. If your plantar fascia pain does not respond to prescribed treatment, consider asking your podiatrist or orthopedist to look into this study.

Orthotics will often help relieve plantar fascia pain. AliMed Rehab and Aetrex make orthotics for plantar fasciitis. Gary Buffington recommends trying inexpensive orthotic shoe inserts before you have expensive orthotics made. Gary suggests you "wear them always until you are better—even in your bedroom slippers if you go to the bathroom at night. I think it would be best if you never took a step without them under your foot for a month." He also recommends contrast baths of two buckets of water, one at 68°F and the other at 103°F. He says, "Put your feet in for 5 minutes in hot, 2 in cold, 2 in hot, 2 in cold, and then 5 more in the hot for a total of 19 minutes twice a day or more." An alternative method is to ice the sole of the foot for 10 minutes; then place the foot on a hot water bottle (as hot as you can stand it) for 10 minutes. Repeat for three or more rounds, twice a day, for at least a week.

It is possible to tape the plantar fascia area under the foot for support, though doing so can be hard to manage. The tape, however, loses strength as it moves with the skin—40% of its strength can be lost within 20 minutes. Using one of the supports listed below will work better over time. An arch brace wraps around the arch to provide support and decrease the pull of the plantar fascia on the calcaneus heel bone. The Count'R-Force Arch Brace and the PSC wrap are two wraparound supports that provide relief from plantar fasciitis pain. The Hapad Longitudinal-Metatarsal Arch Pads or Comf-Orthotic 3/4 Length Insoles may also be used to relieve pain.

Lightweight plastic night splints are proven as a treatment for preventing the plantar fascia and Achilles tendon from contracting during the night. Many athletes swear by them. The splint helps stretch the foot, limit contraction of soft tissues at night, and avoid morning stiffness. Night splints also help avoid foot drop and accompanying muscle tightening. Check with your podiatrist, orthopedist, or medical supply store. Several night splint models are available. The Strassburg Sock and the Powersteps Ultrastretch Night Sock are two alternative-style night splints that can be worn at night or while resting to lightly stretch the plantar fascia. Before getting out of bed, curl your toes downward 8–10 times to loosen the plantar fascia.

If the problem persists after trying some of these measures, make an appointment with a podiatrist or orthopedist. Advances in medical technology have resulted in the use of shock waves to reduce the troublesome inflammation and help jump-start blood flow, which in turn reduces pain and encourages healing. Common sense should tell you to try other conservative treatments before moving to the shock wave treatment or surgery.

Orthotripsy and extracorporeal shock wave therapies use high-energy shock waves similar to those used for treating kidney stones. Shock wave therapy is indicated for use with patients suffering from chronic plantar fasciitis and heel-pain syndrome who fail to respond to the traditional and conservative treatments. The sound shocks cause microtears that heal with new blood vessel growth, allowing the plantar fascia to mend pain free. This noninvasive procedure is worth checking out before considering surgery. Recent studies show an 83% success rate after one treatment and 97% after two. Check with your podiatrist to find a specialist in your area who is trained in this new technology.

Robert Conenello, a podiatrist and past president of the American Academy of Podiatric Sports Medicine, says the most promising treatment is EPAT (shock wave). EPAT stands for Extracorporeal Pulse Activation Technology and is noninvasive. He suggests three consecutive weeks of treatment, which utilizes an acoustic wave that causes a localized tissue inflammation, which in turn allows the tendon of fascia to regain flexibility. EPAT offers a cure, and the athlete can continue to train while receiving treatments.

Endoscopic plantar fasciotomy is an invasive procedure in which a specialized camera is inserted into the heel area. Using the camera, the surgeon can see the plantar fascia through a very small incision, less than 0.5 inch, and release the extreme tension on the plantar fascia.

Plantar fasciitis pain can sometimes be helped with a quick and simple, minimally invasive medical treatment. The TOPAZ MicroDebrider utilizes patented Coblation technology to offer a quicker return to daily activities with a significant improvement in patient outcomes. Small punctures in key areas of the heel are made to allow the insertion of a pencil tip–size wand device, the MicroDebrider. Radio frequency energy is transmitted through the wand for short 500-millisecond intervals of treatment. The Coblation technology forms a plasma that gently and precisely dissolves soft tissue at relatively low temperatures and increases vascular blood supply. Check with your orthopedic surgeon or podiatrist for more information about this treatment.

Another new cutting-edge treatment is platelet-rich plasma (PRP). Platelets contain powerful tendon-healing growth factors. Doctors remove a small amount of the patient's blood, spin it in a centrifuge, separate out the platelets, and then reinject these at the injury site. James Korak finally resorted to PRP for his severe plantar fasciitis. He shares his story.

> We first tried a cortical steroid injection directly into the plantar fascia, but it provided minimal to no relief. After two months another injection was done with MRI guided imaging. No relief was gained. The PRP was next, and they drew 15cc of my blood and spun it in a special centrifuge that separated the platelets that are enriched with stem cells. The resulting plasma was injected in the previous location using MRI guided imaging.
>
> I had to wear a boot for three weeks followed by physical therapy. No running for a month. Within three days of the procedure, I noticed there was no pain and my plantar fasciitis felt 100% healed. Insurance didn't cover the procedure because it is so new.

Many athletes get so frustrated trying to resolve their plantar fasciitis that they try different things that others tell them about. Jayne Cassedy wrote, "Two things helped me recover from plantar fasciitis. The first is a homeopathic ointment called Traumeel. It's an anti-inflammatory and an analgesic from Germany. It works! I usually get it in health food stores. Second, lessons in Feldenkrais, a movement therapy. I also used professionally made orthotics from a podiatrist."

Stretching Exercises for Plantar Fasciitis

Athletes can improve their flexibility and counter muscular imbalances that put them at a greater risk of injury by following a simple stretching program. The best results may come from a combination of plantar fascia and Achilles tendon stretching in multiple directions.

New Stretch Relieves Pain from Plantar Fasciitis

A new stretch is proving quite effective to help treat and potentially cure plantar fasciitis. In a study recently published in *Journal of Bone and Joint Surgery*, researchers found that patients suffering from the painful heel spur syndrome had a 75% chance of having no pain and returning to full activity within three to six months of performing the stretch. In addition, patients had about a 75% chance of needing no further treatment.

The study was a two-year follow-up on 82 patients with plantar fasciitis, all of whom were part of an original clinical trial of 101 patients in 2003. The patients were taught a new stretch, specifically targeting the plantar fascia, which was developed by Benedict DiGiovanni, MD, associate professor of orthopedic surgery at the University of Rochester and author of the study, and Deborah Nawoczenski, PT, PhD, professor of physical therapy at Ithaca College.

The stretch involves sitting in a chair with one leg crossed over the other knee. Then stretch the arch of the foot on the crossed leg by taking one hand and pulling the toes back toward the shin for a count of 10. The exercise must be repeated 10 times, and performed at least three times a day, including before taking the first step in the morning and before standing after a prolonged period of sitting.[48]

Morning Stretches

■ Before getting out of bed, lie on your stomach, put your toes and forefoot against the mattress, and straighten your leg so your heel stretches your calf muscle. This can make your first steps less painful.

■ Also before getting out of bed, slowly stretch the toes upward toward the head at least three times, holding the stretch for at least 15 seconds.

■ The stretch described in the "New Stretch" section above is good for mornings.

■ Another effective morning calf stretch is to stand facing a wall with your hands on the wall. Extend one foot behind you about 24 inches, while bending the other leg at the knee. Keep the heel of the back foot flat on the floor for two minutes and keep the knee straight—you will feel the calf muscle stretch. Repeat with the other foot.

Other Effective Stretches

■ Toe curls can strengthen your arch to prevent pronation. Sit down, take your shoes off, and curl your toes under as hard as you can and as many times as you can. In the beginning, you might get a cramp. Just walk around and try the curls again. Picking up marbles off the floor with your feet and dropping them into a bowl is another good toe exercise.

■ Les Appel, DPM, who designed the Powerstep Insole, recommends facing a wall with one foot flat on the floor and the other foot's heel on the floor and toes up on the wall 3–4 inches. Gently move your knee slowly toward the wall until you feel slight stretching on the bottom of your foot and the back of your leg. Curl your toes to raise the arch and transfer your weight to the outside of your foot. Uncurl your toes, hold for 30 seconds, and again curl your toes. Hold each position for 30 seconds, repeating five times per position per foot.

■ Rolling a tennis ball back and forth under the arch of the foot or simple self-massage across and along the arch can also help. Ice massage can be done using a small frozen juice can rolled under your arch.

■ Better than a tennis ball is the TP Massage FootBaller. Apply pressure with the FootBaller by using the floor, a table, or any hard surface to allow slight movement of your foot on the device. As pressure is applied, the material will slightly change shape in about five to seven seconds. As the materials change shape, roll the FootBaller to and fro, covering the entire affected area of the foot so that the trigger point or spasm is relieved.

■ The Prostretch, Stretch-EZ, and slant boards are popular tools to effectively stretch the plantar fascia, as well as the Achilles tendon and the gastrocnemius and soleus musculature of the back of the lower leg. Studies have shown that utilization of these tools can more effectively increase ankle dorsiflexion (toe-up motion of the ankle) than the conventional and commonly used wall stretch technique previously mentioned.[49] Its use is recommended as both a preventive measure as well as a treatment technique.

Plantar Fibromas

Occasionally a plantar fibroma (fibrous nodule) may form in the plantar fascia. These will usually not go away without treatment. There may be pain from the insole pushing against the nodule. Steroid injections may help and an orthotic can be made, but often surgical removal will be necessary.

PLANTAR FASCIITIS PRODUCTS

ACCOMMODATOR ORTHOTICS provide relief from heel pain and plantar fasciitis. The **HIGH-IMPACT ACCOMMODATOR** offers the benefit of an Impact Plus energy-absorbing poromeric polymer pad in the heel. The **VISCOELASTIC ACCOMMODATOR** combines accommodator and three-quarter–length design with the proven attributes of a pure, supple, viscoelastic polymer. Each offers a shaped longitudinal arch to relieve fatigue while supporting the arch, and a mild metatarsal arch, which supports and reduces unnecessary pressure from the metatarsal heads. alimed.com

BUNGA GEL HEELCUPS are made from a medical-grade polymer material. bungapads.com

The **COUNT'R-FORCE ARCH BRACE,** an alternative to taping, is ideal for running and hiking. Designed by Robert Nirschl, MD, an orthopedic surgeon/sports medicine specialist, it has a curved shape that allows a wide distribution of the abusive forces causing the heel and plantar fasciitis pain. Two tension straps allow for personal adjustment. countrforce.com

HAPAD ARCH PADS can relieve the discomfort of plantar fasciitis. The **LONGITUDINAL-METATARSAL ARCH PADS** provide a corrective action that strengthens the longitudinal and metatarsal arches without restricting the natural flexibility of the foot. These pads may also help flat feet. The **COMF-ORTHOTIC 3/4 LENGTH INSOLES** are an all-in-one Longitudinal-Metatarsal Arch Cushion and heel cushion that relieve plantar fasciitis and foot fatigue by supporting the arch, cushioning the heel, and distributing pressure across the ball of the foot. It helps support flat feet. hapad.com

HAPAD HEEL PADS AND CUSHIONS are useful in treating heel pain associated with stone bruises, heel spurs, leg-length discrepancies, and Achilles tendinitis. The **HORSESHOE HEEL PADS** relieve heel pain, and the **MEDIAL/LATERAL HEEL WEDGES** help correct misalignment of the heel and ankle. hapad.com

The **LYNCO BIOMECHANICAL ORTHOTIC SYSTEM** is a ready-made, triple-density orthotic system that comes in enough variations to accommodate 90% of foot disorders, including plantar fasciitis. Each model has either a neutral-cupped heel or a medial posted heel, and comes with or without a metatarsal pad. **ADDITIONAL REFLEX** self-adhesive pads can be added to the orthotics to relieve pain from Morton's toe, sesamoiditis, and leg-length discrepancy. aetrex.com

The **N'ICE STRETCH NIGHT SPLINT SUSPENSION SYSTEM** is made for plantar fasciitis and Achilles tendinitis. It uses bilateral suspension straps to provide continuous nighttime stretching of the plantar fasciitis and Achilles tendon. The straps allow for independent bi-plane dorsiflexion adjustment. A removable Sealed Ice pack provides cold therapy. The unit is hinged to fold compactly. brownmed.com

OS1ST FS6 PERFORMANCE COMPRESSION FOOT SLEEVE is a socklike sleeve that uses compression zone technology to provide support. os1st.com

The **PF NIGHT SPLINT** comes in multiple models to relieve the pain of plantar fasciitis. The **ORIGINAL PF NIGHT SPLINT** is a lightweight plastic splint designed to lessen morning pain caused by contractures and muscle tightening while sleeping. The **FREEDOM PF NIGHT SPLINT II** is a low-profile, lighter-weight splint, and the **SOFT PF NIGHT SPLINT** is made for sleeping but allows ambulation. All splints fit both right and left feet and include a liner and straps to protect the leg and instep from pressure. An extra-wide model of the PF Night Splint is offered for those individuals with larger calves and ankles. alimed.com

POWERSTEP INSOLES BY DR. LES APPEL offer a unique four-phase design to relieve heel and arch pain. Made with a strong prescription-like arch support, it has a strong heel cradle that prevents the foot from pronating (rolling inward) and the arch from flattening—eliminating strain on the plantar fascia. powersteps.com

POWERSTEPS ULTRASTRETCH NIGHT SOCK is made with soft material and an adjustable strap that gently pulls the toes to stretch the calf muscles and tissues of the foot and ankle. Its **PF SUPPORT SLEEVE** can be worn under socks for daytime use. powersteps.com

The **PRO-TEC SOFT SPLINT** combines the benefits of a compression sock with the stability of a traditional night splint. pro-tecathletics.com

The **PROSTRETCH** effectively stretches the plantar fascia, the Achilles tendon, and the calf muscles. It builds lower-extremity strength, balance, and flexibility in three minutes of use prior to activity, thus reducing the risk of injury. It can also be used for hamstring and anterior tibialis stretching. medi-dyne.com

The **PSC–PRONATION/SPRING CONTROL STRAP** can treat plantar fasciitis, chronic heel pain, heel spur syndrome, and shin splints. This reusable strapping device is made of ProWrap, a knitted blend of nylon and Lycra with patented foam lining. It wraps around the arch to provide superior support to the plantar fascia, while also wrapping around the heel to reduce the force of heel strike and biomechanically move the foot's midline to a more neutral position. fabrifoam.com

RUNNER'S REMEDY PLANTAR FASCIITIS SLEEVE is a foot sleeve with a small pocket in the arch to hold one of four supplied ice packs. runnersremedy.com

SPENCO CUSHIONS are made from a noncompressible, viscoelastic material to relieve heel pain associated with heel spurs, thinning heel pads, and plantar fasciitis. They reduce shock to the joints and evenly distribute pressure throughout the cushion. Available at sporting goods stores and some drugstores. spenco.com

The **STRASSBURG SOCK** is easy to use at night or during extended periods of rest. A good alternative to the typical night splint, this system can be easily used and carried while backpacking. A standard over-the-calf tube sock uses two adjustable straps: one around the calf just below the knee; the other attached to the toe of the sock and passed through a D ring on the upper strap. Tension on the toe strap keeps the plantar fascia in a neutral to slightly stretched position, reducing or eliminating pain under the heel during initial weight bearing in the morning. thesock.com

(continued on page 292)

PLANTAR FASCIITIS PRODUCTS (continued)

The **STRETCH-EZ** from OPTP cradles the foot for a comfortable stretch of the foot, heel, Achilles tendon, hamstring, quadriceps, and inner/outer thigh and calf. Made of poly laminate and webbing. optp.com

THERMOSKIN PLANTAR FXT is a low-profile alternative to cumbersome night splints. The Thermoskin material helps increase skin temperature several degrees for the optimal level of heat therapy. Made with soft materials, it maintains the plantar fascia in a comfortable and flexed position during sleep. swedeo.com

The **TP MASSAGE FOOTBALLER, BALLER BLOCK,** and **MASSAGE BALLS** were created to relieve plantar fasciitis, Achilles tendinitis, and heel pain. They work on the muscles and/or trigger points by applying pressure to the trigger point area. Also offered is a *Performance Therapy for Foot and Lower Leg* DVD, which shows a complete foot and lower leg exercise routine. tptherapy.com

23

Heel Problems

The heel bone, called the calcaneus, is the largest bone in the foot and absorbs most of the shock and pressure from walking and running. The most common cause of heel pain is incorrect movement of the foot during running, hiking, or walking. With every heel strike, pressure up to four times the body's weight is placed on the heel, flattening the heel's fat pads and sending shock and stress to the bones of the foot and the arch. Some of the shock and stress travels on up the leg. As we age, the thickness of the heel's fat pads and the fat pads under the balls of our feet decreases; our natural shock absorption is reduced, pressure is increased, and we become more susceptible to injury. Heel pain may also be caused by heel-pain syndrome, heel spurs, plantar fasciitis, or Haglund's deformity.

Heel-Pain Syndrome

Heel-pain syndrome is usually caused by overuse of and repetitive stress on the foot's heel. This can be caused by a sudden increase in athletic activity, by shoes with heels that are too low or that have lost their cushioning, or by the thinning of the fat pad on the bottom of the heels. This can be resolved by increasing activity level slowly, by wearing shoes with good cushioning, or by using a heel pad or cup.

Heel Spurs

Heel pain may also be caused by heel spurs or plantar fasciitis, which arise from the heel bone and attached soft tissues being stressed. Achilles tendinitis may also be a cause of heel pain. This type of heel pain is often the worst in the morning after getting out of bed and putting your feet on the floor—sometimes it improves after a few minutes. The section on plantar fasciitis in the preceding chapter should be considered mandatory reading for any athlete experiencing heel pain. Heel spurs and plantar fasciitis are closely related, and those with heel pain can benefit from many of the same treatments, stretches, and products. After reading about

PRODUCTS FOR HEEL SPURS

ACCOMMODATOR ORTHOTICS provide relief from heel pain and plantar fasciitis. The **HIGH-IMPACT ACCOMMODATOR** offers the benefit of an Impact Plus energy-absorbing poromeric polymer pad in the heel. The **VISCOELASTIC ACCOMMODATOR** combines Accommodator and three-quarter–length design with the proven attributes of a pure, supple, viscoelastic polymer. Each offers a shaped longitudinal arch to relieve fatigue while supporting the arch, and a mild metatarsal arch, which supports and reduces unnecessary pressure from the metatarsal heads. alimed.com

BUNGA GEL HEELCUPS are made from a medical-grade polymer material. bungapads.com

HAPAD ARCH PADS can relieve the discomfort of plantar fasciitis. The **LONGITUDINAL-METATARSAL ARCH PADS** provide a corrective action that strengthens the longitudinal and metatarsal arches without restricting the natural flexibility of the foot. These pads may also help flat feet. The **COMF-ORTHOTIC 3/4 LENGTH INSOLES** is an all-in-one Longitudinal-Metatarsal Arch Cushion and heel cushion that relieves plantar fasciitis and foot fatigue by supporting the arch, cushioning the heel, and distributing pressure across the ball of the foot. hapad.com

HAPAD HEEL PADS AND CUSHIONS are useful in treating heel pain associated with stone bruises, heel spurs, leg-length discrepancies, and Achilles tendinitis. The Horseshoe Heel Pads relieve heel pain, and the Medial/Lateral Heel Wedges help correct misalignment of the heel and ankle. The coiled, springlike wool fibers provide firm and resilient support as they mold and shape to the foot. hapad.com

The **HEEL HUGGER** is designed to treat heel pain and inflammatory problems of the heel. The neoprene sock surrounds the foot from the heel to the midfoot, providing support, stabilization, and compression to control edema. Therapeutic Gel pads with Sealed Ice provide additional stabilization and cold therapy on either side of the calcaneus heel bone. The Heel Hugger provides relief from heel spurs, plantar fasciitis, Achilles tendinitis, heel contusions, narrow heels, and rear-foot instability. brownmed.com

treatments for these injuries, make sure that you also read "Treatment Options: Trigger Point Therapy and ASTYM" in the preceding chapter.

Heel spurs are small points of calcium buildup sticking out and downward from the calcaneus heel bone, touching and irritating your plantar fascia. (Painful protrusions on the back of the heel are called Haglund's deformity; see page 296.) Stresses to the plantar fascia where it inserts into the calcaneus cause heel spurs to develop. A heel spur can usually be seen on an X-ray. A heel bruise or stone bruise is pain felt directly under the calcaneus. This pain is usually tenderness at a small site just forward of the heel's pad on the bottom of the heel.

Achilles tendinitis, flat feet, and excessively high arches are common conditions that make one prone to heel spurs.

POWERSTEP INSOLES BY DR. LES APPEL offer a unique four-phase design to relieve heel and arch pain. Made with a strong prescription-like arch support, it has a strong heel cradle that prevents the foot from pronating (rolling inward) and the arch from flattening—eliminating strain on the plantar fascia. powersteps.com

The **PSC–PRONATION/SPRING CONTROL STRAP** is designed to treat plantar fasciitis, chronic heel pain, heel spur syndrome, and shin splints. This reusable strapping device is made from ProWrap, a knitted blend of nylon and Lycra with patented foam lining. It wraps around the arch to provide superior support to the plantar fascia while also wrapping around the heel to reduce the force of heel strike and biomechanically move the foot's midline to a more neutral position. fabrifoam.com

SPENCO CUSHIONS are made from a noncompressible, viscoelastic material to relieve heel pain associated with heel spurs, thinning heel pads, and plantar fasciitis. Check their website to see their current product line. They reduce shock to the joints and evenly distribute pressure throughout the cushion. Available at sporting goods stores and some drugstores. spenco.com

The **TP MASSAGE FOOTBALLER, BALLER BLOCK,** and **MASSAGE BALLS** were created to relieve plantar fasciitis, Achilles tendinitis, and heel pain. They work on the muscles and/or trigger points by applying pressure to the trigger point area. Also offered is a *Performance Therapy for Foot and Lower Leg* DVD, which shows a complete foot and lower leg exercise routine. tptherapy.com

TULI'S makes different versions of heel cups with a waffle design. The standard design is single-ribbed, the **PRO HEEL CUP** has a double-ribbed waffle design, and the **GEL HEEL CUP** is double-ribbed with gel polymer. For those with weak ankles, the **CHEETAHWRAP FIT** ankle support incorporates a standard heel cup with a neoprene ankle sock-type support. medi-dyne.com

Treating Heel Spurs

Proper conditioning of the feet and gradually working up to longer distances can help minimize heel pain. Many stretches can help prevent and also treat heel spurs, as well as plantar fasciitis (see section on stretching on pages 288–289).

Resting your feet and using ice is helpful when you first experience pain—ice 20 minutes up to six to eight times a day for several days. The "Cold and Heat Therapy" chapter gives more information on making the most of icing techniques. As pain subsides over time, warm soaks can help.

Tom Noll found his solution to heel pain by experimenting with different running shoes and using arch supports. By participating in discussions on an e-mail listserv, Tom began to see similarities as some people mentioned that they too had problems with the same model shoe he was wearing. He changed shoes and determined that he needed the arch support in all his shoes.

One very basic but important recommendation is to never walk in bare feet until you are pain free—especially in the morning getting out of bed. Keep a pair of shoes with an arch support at your bedside. Use sandals only if they have an arch support.

The use of orthotics in resolving heel pain has been proven. The biggest issue with custom orthotics is their cost. Many athletes first try an inexpensive over-the-counter orthotic. If that does not work, the more expensive custom-made orthotic may be necessary (see the "Orthotics" chapter, page 154, for detailed information on common types of orthotics).

The products listed on the following pages are quite varied. Some heel cups have a waffle design or special-density material on the bottom of the cup; others have a U-shape cutout at the bottom of the heel. Most heel cups simply cup the heel, while others are incorporated into a sock design. The viscoelastic materials in some heel pads provide excellent cushioning. Heel pads are small and fit easily into a shoe to provide cushioning. Try several to find a design that works best for your pain or injury. Heel cups and pads are small and can easily be carried as preventive measures if you are prone to heel pain. The Count'R-Force Arch Brace and the PSC strap are alternatives to heel cups and pads.

Haglund's Deformity

Haglund's deformity is a bump in the form of an enlargement of the back of the heel bone (calcaneus) at the area of the insertion of the Achilles tendon. Sometimes it has the appearance of a square, shelflike bump. When wearing shoes irritates the bump, it becomes red, swollen, and painful. The enlarged bone may also irritate the Achilles tendon, resulting in pain with motion of the ankle joint and foot. Shoes with a rigid heel counter rub up and down on the heel bone. A bursa sac between the Achilles tendon and the heel bone can become irritated, and over time bursitis may develop.

Haglund's deformity is also called pump bump or retrocalcaneal bursitis. It may be a bone deformity present from birth, or it may be acquired by injury over an athlete's lifetime. It is most often present in women and those who wear hard-shelled ski or cross-country boots with rigid heels or heel counters. Individuals with a prominent protrusion of the heel bone are also susceptible to an inflammation in the heel area.

John Gale wrote, "I have been diagnosed with Haglund's deformity on my right foot. For the most part, street shoes and running shoes do not bother it. Hiking and mountaineering boots do, particularly on steep uphills. In particular, plastic mountaineering boots are a problem due to the stiffness of the boot. Unless I am very careful with fit and proper padding, boots will irritate it, remove the top layer of skin, and leave me limping about for a few days. I have had some success creating a doughnut out of Molefoam, which pads the bump and distributes the pressure from the heel cup around the whole heel rather than just the bump."

The primary symptom of Haglund's deformity is pain at the back of the heel. The tissues also may thicken over the bone bump, forming a callus. The callus can grow quite thick and become inflamed while you are wearing shoes.

Treating Haglund's Deformity

The focus of treatment should start with reducing the painful pressure on the bump. In mild cases, a change of shoes will solve the problem and allow the irritation to heal. Changing to shoes with a lower or softer heel counter or a heel counter that is notched for the Achilles tendon can help. A heel pad can lift the heel up above the part of the heel counter that is rubbing on the bump. Pads around the bump may help. Moleskin, or Molefoam, as John Gale mentioned, is not very thick and compresses with wear. A better choice is a pad made from the familiar Spenco green insole foam. These are flat insoles and you can easily cut them to make a pad with a hole in the center. Hold this pad on with a layer of tape. Be careful when applying the pad that this does not make the shoes/boots tighter and cause other problems. An ENGO patch or ENGO's Cushion Heel Wrap, which adheres to the heel counter, will also reduce friction to the area. Icing the painful area, followed by warm water soaks, can help. Anti-inflammatories can be taken to reduce the pain. If this condition becomes unbearable during an event, cutting a notch or slice into the heel counter can relieve some of the pressure off the bump.

Surgery to remove the excess bone may be necessary in extreme cases. Cortisone injections are not recommended due to the area's proximity to the Achilles tendon.

Toe Problems

"**W**hile we all have toes, some are better than others," says Herb Hedgecock, humorously relating the anatomy of his feet.

"I have ugly feet. My mother and father stuck me with an 'ugly foot gene,' which was a cruel thing to do. Sometimes I look at the perfect feet that others were blessed with and wonder what the hell I did to deserve Morton's toe and double-wides. The first place I get blisters is on my short fourth toe that curls under the long third monster. And the right foot does this even more. The second place is on the big toe, and this seems to happen because the second toe is so damned long and the big toe curves in, causing them to rub. Because the second and fourth toes are so out of proportion, this seems to cause toes one, three, and five to also get in on the act. Ergo, toe blisters near the toenails, but who needs ten toenails?"

Just as varied as the many shapes and types of toes are problems associated with them. This chapter will cover the whole gamut of common toe ailments. But first, a word about strengthening your toes.

Strengthening Your Toes

Strengthening exercises can help keep toes flexible. Practice picking up marbles off a carpeted floor with your toes. Release and repeat 20 times. Put a large, sturdy rubber band around all five toes. Spread your toes outward and hold for five seconds, then release. Repeat 10 times. To work on toe flexibility, pull on each toe, gently twisting it to the right and then the left. Then push each toe up and down, while doing the opposite to the next toe. Yoga Toes (yogapro.com) and Correct Toes (correcttoes .com) are made from gel and fit over all five toes with spaces to separate each toe. The gentle stretching may help relieve pain from many foot conditions.

The Basics: Toenail Trimming

I mentioned earlier that I have three absolutes. The first is wearing moisture-wicking socks, the second is wearing gaiters for trails, and the third is properly trimming toenails. How hard can it be to trim your toenails? I guess for a lot of folks, it's a huge deal and something they have a hard time doing. In all the years I have been patching feet, I have observed that untrimmed toenails are the number one cause of problems leading to toe blisters and black nails. Socks will catch on nails that are too long or that have rough edges. This puts pressure on the nail bed, leading to blisters under the toenails or at the tips of the toes or painful toenails, as they are pushed back into the cuticle. Nails that are too long are also prone to pressure from a toe box that is too short or too low.

Ultrarunner Joe Kallo wrote, "I followed your directions regarding using an emery board on the edges of my nails to smooth them, and it worked like a dream! This was the first ultra I've run that I've finished with no loose or painful toenails! And it was 100 miles!"

TIP: The True Meaning of Buff

Elisabeth Archambault has a great toenail tip: "Consider getting a nail buffer (available for a couple of bucks in drugstore cosmetic departments) and buffing them to a shine. Smoothing out the natural ridges is one more way to reduce friction. I'm convinced this helps socks to last longer too."

Toenails should be trimmed regularly, straight across the nail—never rounded at the corners. Leave an extra bit of nail on the outside corner of the big toe to avoid an ingrown toenail. After trimming toenails, use a nail file to smooth the top of the nail down toward the front of the toe and remove any rough edges. If you draw your finger from the skin in front of the toe up across the nail and can feel a rough edge, the nail can be filed smoother or trimmed a bit shorter. Remember though, the shorter you trim your nails, the greater the likelihood that you will experience an ingrown toenail. Conversely, nails that are too long can rub against the front of your shoes and catch on your socks, which can lead to a black toenail, wear holes in your socks, cut into other toes, and crack the nail when you run downhill. Shoes that are too tight in the forefoot or too short can cause the nail to press into the sides of the toe.

Use an emery board nail file from your drugstore. Better yet, invest a few bucks in a nice metal file that will last a long time and serve you well. To trim your nails, there are regular nail clippers, nippers, and scissors made exclusively for thicker toenails. If your local drugstore or pharmacy doesn't have them, check out footsmart. com for a great selection.

A little bit of care in toenail trimming goes a long way in preventing toe blisters and black toenails, and in making your socks last longer.

Black Toenails

The technical name for the runner's black toenail, subungual hematoma, describes simply a blood-filled swelling under the nail. This common occurrence is caused by the trauma of the toe or toes repetitively bumping against the front of the shoe.

Blood pools in the space between the nail plate and nail bed as they separate or compress from repeated trauma. Individuals with Morton's toe are most susceptible to experiencing black toenails. The nail becomes discolored and usually has associated pain. Most often the nail bed turns dark, almost black or blue because of the blood.

Subungual hematomas are quite common in races of 50 miles or more and especially in multiday events. An article in the April 2014 *Sports Medicine* noted that these occur in approximately 3%–10% of runners in multistage events.[50]

A nail drill makes a clean hole to relieve pressure.

Some athletes tell of losing their nails after the nail bed has turned a whitish color. Vince Gerber wrote, "After finishing the Javelina Hundred my big toenail was floating on a giant blister. This was the first time I ever had white toenails, as opposed to the many black toenails I've experienced. The blister had no blood, just clear fluid. The first couple of days I used a safety pin to puncture and drain the blisters, which would seal and fill back up within a few hours. For the next few days, I would puncture and drain the blister once every day or two. Again, the blisters would slowly fill up again. After about ten days the blisters were totally deflated and the skin dried and started to peel off. Catching an edge of the nail while putting on a sock is what tore the first one halfway off. Then it was a matter of just pulling it off . . . no pain involved at that point. Caught the next one on a bed sheet, then snipped off the remaining side."

Vince makes a good point. Unless you want to tear the nails off, make sure to wrap a Band-Aid around the toe, covering the edges of the nail. Tearing a nail off before it is ready to fall off can be quite painful.

Many runners are simply prone to black toenails. The best means of preventing black toenails is to wear shoes with a generous toe box and with the proper length for your feet. Some runners cut slits in their shoe's toe box or cut out a portion of the toe box to gain relief.

Ultrarunner Nancy Shura-Dervin tells how she has resolved blood blisters under toenails: "Beginning about three months before the big race, I use an emery board to file down the thickness of the nails (I do all ten). You just sand the entire toenail surface . . . slowly. I perform this as a nightly ritual! This should be done gradually and gently, taking several weeks to get the entire nail paper thin! As new nail grows out, just sand it down. I also gently file over the end of each nail to take off any new growth. I came upon this idea based on the fact that several runners have had their toenails surgically removed. The thinner the nail bed, the more pliable it is to pressure. The end result is that my toes feel nailless to the touch. I stop sanding about three days before the event just to be sure the nail is not tender. As the nails get thinner, at first they can be a little tender (just like immediately after losing a nail) but the sensation soon diminishes." This greatly reduces the occurrence of toenail blisters caused by toe box pressure against a rigid toenail.

Black toenails can come from toenail trauma caused by clenching your toes. This curling downward of the toes can also lead to toe blisters. A small pad under the ball of the foot can help relax the toes, but many athletes have to mentally will themselves to uncurl their toes.

Treating Black Toenails

If there is no pain from the black toenail, no action may be necessary. If the pain and pressure increases, the pressure must be relieved. To relieve pressure from a black toenail, use one of the following methods, depending on the look of the toenail. The treatment may have to be repeated several times. Although the methods below might sound painful, they are usually not. The blood has separated the nail from the nail bed and is a barrier between the nail and the live skin underneath. Here are three ways to drain the fluid. In all three methods, holding slight pressure on the nail bed will help expel the blood.

■ If the discoloration does not extend to the front of the toenail, swab the nail with an alcohol wipe, and use a small nail drill, drill bit, or hypodermic needle to gently drill a hole in the nail with light pressure and rolling the needle/bit back and forth between your thumb and fingers. The blood will ooze through the hole. Keep slight pressure on the nail bed to help expel the built-up blood. Stopping too soon will cause the blood to clot in the hole and the problem will reoccur. I purchased a small nail drill through eBay and like its ease of use.

■ An alternative method is to use a match to heat a paper clip and gently penetrate the nail with the heated point. The heat in this method can cauterize the blood and stop the flow of blood out from under the nail. Press on the nail to expel the blood.

■ If the discoloration extends to the end of the toenail, use a sterile pin or needle to penetrate the skin under the nail and release the pressure.

Care must be taken to prevent a secondary bacterial infection through the hole in the nail or at the end of the nail by using an antibiotic ointment and covering the site with a Band-Aid. If the hole seals up, use the drill, needle, or paper clip to open it up again. Loss of the nail usually follows in the months ahead. The new nail will begin growing, pushing up the old nail, and may come in looking odd. Do not be concerned about the process unless an infection develops. Remember, it can take six to nine months for a new nail to grow in completely.

You may find relief by wearing a metatarsal pad, a small circular pad that pushes up the ball of the foot and drops the toes down, which takes pressure off the toenails. Contact Hapad (hapad.com) for information on these pads.

Once your toenail has come off, a new nail will grow in. Sometimes though, the new nail may grow in odd or wavy looking, thicker, or any other unusual appearance. Richard Schick suggests applying petroleum jelly or an ointment of your choosing to the nail bed a couple of times a day to keep it from becoming dry and stiff. Second, as Nancy Shura-Dervin suggested, use a nail file to keep the newly emerging nail as thin as possible until it is fully regrown. This keeps the nail flexible and without the structural strength to cause problems.

Athletes who have frequent problems with black toenails often choose to have them surgically removed. Tim Jantz, a podiatrist, describes the process of removing a toenail:

> After the toe is numbed, the nail is removed and the growth plate is treated with 89% phenol (some use sodium hydroxide) to destroy the growth plate. The area is then rinsed with alcohol and dressed with an antibiotic and dressing. The usual postoperation care is daily soaks and dressing with a topical antibiotic and a Band-Aid for approximately four weeks, sometimes longer. The toe has endured a chemical burn and so heals by draining. It can have a raw feeling for a week or so, and I wouldn't want to stub it or have anyone step on it for a few weeks. You may also want to wear roomy shoes or sandals for a week. The procedure is about 95% successful.

Kevin O'Neall wrote, "I was plagued with ingrown nail pain for most of my life. By the time of high school I had learned to grit my teeth and dig them out using an X-acto blade and tweezers. Ten years ago I submitted to surgery. As I watched, the podiatrist removed the ingrown nails and then treated the toes so they wouldn't regrow. The surgery was painless, took 15 minutes, and cost around $200. The toes were sore for less than a week, feeling as if I'd stubbed my toes walking barefoot into a heavy chair. I've never had a recurrence of the ingrown nails."

If you are prone to black toenails and have tried all the options to prevent them, consult a podiatrist about nail removal.

Big Toe Problems

Big toes are susceptible to problems in their joints. Hallux limitus is a decreased range of motion in the joint located at the base of the big toe. This condition can progress into hallus rigidus, wherein the joint becomes rigid. There can be pain in the big toe when it is pushed upward, as happens when we walk, run, or stand on our toes. The joint can become inflamed and swell. As the condition progresses, the pain can become more constant. There can be crepitus, or a grinding feeling in the joint with movement, and sometimes a bump can be felt on the top of the joint. Because the inflammation is on the top of the joint, it should not be confused with a bunion, which is on the side.

A premature wearing down and tearing of the joint's cartilage causes hallux limitus and rigidus. Without the cartilage, the bones rub together, and new bone growth occurs, often leading to bone spurs. The deterioration of the cartilage can be caused by repetitive injuries, age-related changes, and hereditary defects.

If there is pain when the toe moves and it seems to be underneath the toe or at the ball of the foot, it could be sesamoiditis. Read the "Sesamoiditis" section in the next chapter on forefoot problems.

Treating Big Toe Problems

Early treatment is best to avoid long-term problems. Make sure your shoes are wide enough and long enough to prevent pressure on the toe. A shoe with as rigid a sole as possible is preferred. Use a soft-gel pad to cushion the ball of the foot and reduce pressure on the big toe joint. Resting the foot, warm water soaks, and gentle massage with topical pain relievers can help. Custom-made orthotics will help stabilize the foot.

Hammertoes, Claw Toes, and Mallet Toes

Hammertoes are toes that are contracted at the toe's middle joint, making the toe bend upward at its center and forcing the tip of the toe downward. The ligaments and tendons have tightened and are forcing the toes to curl. This can lead to severe pressure and pain. Blisters or corns may form at the top bend in the toe and calluses at the ends of the toes. Hammertoes can occur in any toe, except the big toe. There are two types of hammertoes: rigid and flexible. A rigid toe has no ability to move, but in a flexible toe, the joint can be moved. Hammertoes are typically the result of a muscle imbalance that causes the ligaments and tendons to tighten. Individuals with flat feet, high arches, and Morton's toe are prone to hammertoes.

Al Czecholinski relates his experience with surgery for hammertoes:

> I had hammertoe surgery on two toes on my right foot about four years ago. I'm very happy with the result. Prior to the surgery the foot was always swollen and sore where the toe joints were being rammed back into the foot. The podiatrist said that eventually these joints would be very damaged and arthritic, making even walking difficult. That being said, do not take the surgery lightly and try all conservative measures before getting the surgery. I lived with a sore foot for years and got a second opinion before I had the surgery. The surgery involved sawing out a section of bone to make the toe shorter so the tendon would become relatively longer. The sawed bones plus the pins that were inserted to hold the bones while healing hurt quite a lot. I spent about six to seven weeks in a big rigid foot immobilizer. Then it took a few more weeks to be able to walk fairly normally. If the hammertoes are only causing blisters due to rubbing and there's no swelling or joint damage, the surgery is probably not worth it. First try orthotics and modifying your shoe's toe box.

Claw toes are similar to hammertoes except they are contracted down at the middle joint and up at the joint at the ball of the foot. Mallet toes are contracted at the end joint only. Causes and treatments are the same as for hammertoes.

Treating Hammertoes, Claw Toes, and Mallet Toes

Be sure your footwear has a high and broad toe box. This usually allows the other toes additional room so there is less friction against the individual toes. For toes that are flexible, toe crests or splints that straighten the toe can sometimes be used. Gel caps or toe shields that slide over the toes can protect the toes from friction.

PRODUCTS FOR HAMMERTOES, CLAW TOES, AND MALLET TOES

Assorted products are available in your local drugstore and pharmacy, among them **DR. SCHOLL'S HAMMERTOE PADS** and **GEL TOE SHIELDS** or **TOE CAPS** for cushioning the toes. Other products include the following.

FOOTSMART carries the **SILICONE TOE CREST** that fits over one toe and nestles under the hammertoe for support while relieving pressure and friction. The **TOE STRAIGHTENER** properly aligns hammertoes (also available in a double toe model). The **GEL TOE SEPARATOR AND SPREADER** may also provide relief. footsmart.com

HAPAD offers **VISCO-GEL TOE CAPS, HAMMERTOE CUSHIONS, TOE CUSHIONS,** and a **TOE SPREADER.** hapad.com

PRO-TEC'S TOE CAPS, made from custom-grade silicone, are soft and stretchable to fit all toes. Locate a reseller through their website. pro-tecathletics.com

Strengthening exercises can help keep toes flexible. Refer to the "Strengthening Toes" section earlier in this chapter.

Pamela Adams, a chiropractor, offers another alternative:

Chiropractors who specialize in sports rehab and extremity adjusting may be able to help. Even yoga for feet or a course of Rolfing (which eliminates scar tissue) may help. Tendons can shorten; tendons can lengthen. Why not try conservative approaches while saving up for surgery? You may be pleasantly surprised. I've had patients with bunions; hammertoes; and overlapping, curly, or otherwise misaligned toes. Unless the problem is congenital, or due to an injury such as a fracture, most toe problems come from faulty alignment and biomechanics, poor shoes, and poor form during activity. I always suggest surgery as a last, not first, choice. Meanwhile, go barefoot at home and wear shoes that allow your toes to spread out when you toe off.

Adventure racer Steve Daniel's three outer toes on each foot curl up under the others—toward the big toe. When he did the Primal Quest 2003, he decided to go with what he thought was the best combination for his feet—Injinji toe socks and pretaping each toe at the joints and around any blister-prone areas with Leukotape. Even with these measures, his little toe felt as if it had been beaten with a hammer. That's obviously because it was pounded the whole time under the other toes. Steve talked to his podiatrist and was told surgery was his best option.

My wife had a problem toe that turned into a hammertoe. To help her, I used a thin strip of Kinesio Tex tape. I applied the tape to the underside of the toe, then up and over the tip, stretching it as I applied it to the top of the toe under tension. That helped straighten the toe and worked for her until she finally had surgery.

Corrective surgery may be the best option, but as Steve found out, it is expensive. There are often three surgical choices: cut the tendons on the bottom of the toes; cut the tendons, fuse the joints, and put titanium pins through the toes; or cut the tendons and then add some tendons on the top side of the toe to draw the toe up and out. Each has its pros and cons. Your orthopedic surgeon is the best person to explain each procedure and help you make an intelligent choice.

Ingrown Toenails

Ingrown toenails, most common to the big toe, may cause infection and require medical attention. One or both sides of your toenail may grow into the flesh of the toe. The result is a reddened, irritated, and swollen toe that is sensitive to any degree of pressure. These are usually very painful and require immediate attention. Increased redness, pain, and tenderness to the touch can indicate an infection. Toes are typically in a warm and moist environment, and bacteria can quickly take hold. The most common cause of an ingrown toenail is improper nail trimming (see "The Basics: Toenail Trimming," page 298).

Sometimes trauma from a stubbed toe or someone stepping on your toe can cause the nail to be jammed into the skin. Repeated trauma, such as the pounding to which athletes typically subject their feet, also can lead to ingrown toenails. The medical term for an ingrown toenail is onychocryptosis. Ingrown toenails can cause a break in the skin, which can lead to infection.

Treating Ingrown Toenails

Soak your foot in warm water or Epsom salts two to three times a day to reduce the infection. Do not poke at the ingrown nail. If you cannot trim the nail yourself, check with your orthopedist or podiatrist. An ignored ingrown toenail can become seriously infected. Apply a layer of antibiotic cream to help reduce inflammation and cover with a Band-Aid.

Rich Schick, a physician's assistant, recommends the following method to care for an ingrown nail:

> File the entire top surface of the nail from near the cuticle to the tip until you get it as thin as possible. A regular nail file will work, but a medium-grade metal file is much quicker. This weakens the nail. Then soak the foot in hot water for about 30 minutes to soften the nail, further weakening the nail. Then use a cuticle trimmer (available in most drugstore beauty departments) to free the ingrown portion. Do not attempt to work from the tip toward the base. Come from the side, and a little toward the base of the toe and use the "wings" of the instrument to lift and free the ingrown segment. As you continue forward, the trimmer will often cut the piece off. If not, snip it with a nail clipper. I prefer a small pair of wire cutters for the task.

Assorted products are available in your local drugstore and pharmacy. In addition to ingrown toenail files and toenail softening cream, here are a few specialty products:

- The Barrel Nipper, long-handled nail clippers made for thick, tough, curved nails (footsmart.com)

- Dr. Scholl's Ingrown Toenail Relief Strips

- Viso-Gel Toe Protectors from Hapad (hapad.com), Bunga Toe Pads (bungapads.com), or Bunheads and Jelly Toes (capezio.com) to cover and protect the nail

Morton's Toe

Morton's toe, often called Morton's foot, is a common problem in which the second toe (next to the big toe) is longer than the big toe. In the 1930s, podiatrist Dr. Dudley Morton discovered that many people had a short first metatarsal bone. He concluded that this condition impacted their gait, causing their foot to hyperpronate—a dysfunction of the foot causing your ankles to roll in when you stand, walk, and run. Estimates for Morton's toe range from 15% of the population to as high as 50%–60%.

Those with Morton's toe have a second toe that extends beyond the big toe.

The first metatarsal (of the big toe) is shorter than normal, and this makes the second toe appear longer than it actually is. This is usually a hereditary condition. The constant pressure placed on the longer second toe while walking or standing can lead to callus formation under the second metatarsal head. The repeated pressure of the longer second toe against the front of the shoe or boot may traumatize the nail. If a hematoma develops under the nail, the nail will change color and may fall off. Because of the excessive pressure on the second metatarsal head in the forefoot, Morton's toe is often associated with metatarsalgia.

Morton's toe makes buying shoes harder. It is important to fit shoes to this longest toe. Your toes need space and breathing room and your longer toe is no exception. In addition, make sure you trim your nails and file them smooth. Good toenail care, especially of this long toe, will prevent the nail from hitting on the front of the shoe—jamming the nail back into the nail bed. If you are bothered by toe pain, gel caps could help. These are a gel tube that covers the toe, and many are reusable.

Treating Morton's Toe

To get a good fit, look for shoes or boots with a high and wide toe box. It may be necessary to use a shoe or boot a half size to a size larger than normal in order to have space for the longer second toe. The use of orthotics can align the foot by providing arch support. A metatarsal pad under the metatarsal heads of the forefoot can relieve pressure on the second metatarsal head. (A good source of metatarsal pads is hapad.com.) The use of a nonslippery insole will keep the foot from sliding forward. Look for an insole with a good heel cup, an arch that fits your foot, and a surface material that grips the foot and sock. Some runners will cut a slit in the top of their shoes over or on either side of the toe to relieve pressure. Another option is to cut out a small piece of the toe box over the toe. Orthotics may also provide relief. Surgery is usually a last resort.

If you find a blister or corn starting at the top of the toe, use a gel cap or tape to protect the area. If you begin to experience pain at the base of the toe, a pad might help. Use a U-shaped pad and position the cutout area at the site of the pain. To find the right position, first make a mark at the sore area with a marking pen. Then slide your foot inside your shoe and step down to transfer the ink onto the insole. Stick the pad to the insole with the opening toward the toes.

FOOTSMART carries Gel Toe Caps and Digi-Cushions to cushion the toe, and Felt and Silicone Callus Cushions for the base of the toe. footsmart.com

Overlapping Toes

Sometimes toes will overlap other toes. This can occur with any of your toes and cause extreme irritation. Overlapping toes typically involve one toe lying on top of an adjacent toe. The fifth toe is the most affected digit. Overlapping toes usually involve the fourth and fifth toes. The cause of overlapping is unknown. Many experts suspect that they are caused by an imbalance in the small muscles of the foot.

Peter Fish wrote, "I was quite interested in the material about toes that curl under, as I have a similar problem and have also considered surgery. In my case, it's mostly the little toes that get squeezed under the others, and taping them only contributes to the problem by increasing the pressure. I wear soft orthotics, and I have gotten a degree of relief by just making a cutout on the edge of the orthotic to make a depression for my little toe to fit into. These toes develop a sharp callus on the side of the toe, which I treat frequently, then sand it down with a callus file. The next toes in get blisters on the bottom, also from curling under, and these I tape, using one strip of tape over the end and another wrapped around perpendicular. As I've been doing longer races, I've felt that these solutions were not quite adequate." Sometimes Peter will use two thin Spenco green flat insoles, one over the other. He makes a cutout in the two insoles, which allows a deeper space than using one insole. The bottom insole has a small cutout where the toe will drop while the upper insole has a larger cutout. Start with small cutouts and make them larger until they work for your feet. Make sure the added insole volume will fit OK in your shoes.

Treating Overlapping Toes

Custom-made orthotics may help align the toes. Off-the-shelf orthotics commonly found in drugstores and sports stores will generally not help this condition. A podiatrist can make the correct type of orthotic. Shoes with a high and wide toe box can give toes the space they need. Gel toe straighteners, toe caps, and toe combs can be used on and between toes. A strip of 0.5-inch tape applied to the inside of the pinky toe and then over the tip, and applied to the side of the foot under tension, can straighten it a bit. Pamela Adams, a chiropractor, offers an option worth considering in the section on hammertoes. Chiropractic toe adjustments may be of help as well. If the condition is painful and causes problems when participating in sports, consult with your podiatrist to determine your options.

Nancy Shura-Dervin has a good tip to help manage these curling or overlapping toes. A good preventive measure is to cut the little toe out of the insole. This measure allows the little toe to ride on the shoe bottom while the foot and other four toes ride higher up on the shoe insole. It effectively prevents one toe from riding on top of another toe. This measure can be used for any of the five toes and can also be used for more than one toe as well. Here's how:

- Remove the insole and stand barefoot on the insole.

- Use a narrow marker pen to outline the space between the fourth and little toe, then mark a bit toward the little toe where the toe meets the foot.

- With scissors, cut the little toe part out of the insole, making the cut smaller than the marks at first.

- Put the insole back in the shoe and try it on, noting that your little toe should ride on the bottom of the shoe.

- Continue removing the insole and trimming as needed to make the toe opening comfortable; you shouldn't feel the cuts at all.

Surgical correction sometimes involves releasing the tendon and the soft tissues around the joint at the base of the fifth toe. In severe cases, a pin may need to be surgically inserted to hold the toe in a straight position. The pin, which exits the tip of the toe, may be left in place for up to three weeks.

FOOTSMART carries the Gel Toe Separators and Spreader. footsmart.com

Making Overlapping Toe Separators

This is an idea to help runners, adventure racers, and hikers with the problem of overlapping toes. You will need Injinji toe socks, ENGO Blister Prevention Patches (large ovals), and removable insoles. There are two types of separators you can make.

Toe Separator Number 1

I use an ENGO Blister Prevention Patch as the toe separators. They make

An ENGO patch used on a sock as a toe separator

a small and large oval, but I like the large because of its size.

The first toe separator is easy to make and use—and it uses one large ENGO patch. Take a scissors and cut a long oval into a strip, about 0.75 inch wide and 1.75 inches long. If you are cutting this for a middle toe or for large toes, it may have to be 1–1.25 inches wide and a bit longer. Round all corners. Cut one of the remaining sections into a small strip, 0.25 inch wide and 1.25 inches long. Take the large oval and

An ENGO patch used as a toe separator

remove half the backing from one end. Wearing Injinji socks, put the large oval between the two affected toes. Put the end of the large oval with the exposed adhesive over the toe next to the toe that goes under it. The blue side will go from the top of one toe, run between the toes, and under the toe that normally goes under the other one. What you have is an S-shaped patch from the top of one toe, between them, and then under the next toe. Take the small strip and remove the backing, and put one end of the adhesive on the white backing that is underneath the toe at the bottom of the S. The other end of the strip can be stuck onto the top of that toe's sock. The small strip is needed to hold the bottom of the S under the toe when you put your foot in your shoe. The S-shaped patch will keep the toes apart. Obviously, these are single use. If the patch seems too weak, use two strips to make the S patch stronger.

Toe Separator Number 2

This toe separator is more complicated to make and apply. It uses a large or small oval, depending on the size of the toes. The idea is to pinch the patch into an upside-down T where the base of the T goes between the two problem toes. The patch is stuck to your insole in a position where it keeps the two toes apart. The slippery surface of the ENGO patch will prevent rubbing, and the upward base of the upside-down T will keep one toe from going under the other toe.

How to Make Your Own Toe Separator Number 2

Using a utility knife, score two cuts, about 1 inch apart on the back side of the patch. Make them only deep enough to cut through the paper backing—do not cut through the patch itself. Try to have the 1-inch-wide space in the middle of the patch. Make the cuts wide enough so the folded separator will be tall enough to match the height of the toes it will go between. This is important—a separator used between middle toes will have to be taller than ones used for pinky toes. Men's toes may also require taller separators. Using the tip of the knife, remove the 1-inch strip. Fold the patch in half so the sticky sides match to each other. The two ends of the cut backing should meet in the middle. You can now open the two ends and cut the patch into the needed shape based on where the patch will go on the insole and the length of your toes.

Separator Number 2 Height and Length

Separators for pinky toes need to be shorter in height and length than ones for the middle toes. You may have to make more than one separator based on the size you need to find the right fit.

How to Use Separator Number 2

To use the separator in your shoe, remove the insole for the foot with the overlapping toes. The smoother the insole the better the patch will stick. Clean the surface of the insole of all lint, dust, or other things that could interfere with the patch adhering. Make sure the insoles are dry. Put the insole on the floor and stand on it so your foot falls into any indentations. Usually, an insole will have indentations under the heel, ball of the foot, and some of the toes. Using a pen, make a mark between the two affected toes. Put on a pair of Injinji socks and make sure the marking is still in the right place.

Once the placement has been confirmed, with sock on, place the separator between the two toes to make sure it fits. The best way to do this is with your foot on the insole. The height should come up to the top of the toes with the sock on. If the height is too high, trim it with a scissors. If it's too low, make another separator where the pinched section is higher.

The length needs to be long enough to cover the body of the toe—without hitting the crease between the toes. If the separator touches the crease, it could rub and cause problems, especially if the foot moves forward in the shoe. If it's too long, trim it with a scissors.

Once the fit has been checked, you can place the separator on the insole. Line it up so the upward part is in the correct place. Then remove the protective backing to expose the adhesive and place the patch on the insole with the upward part over the line on the insole. Rub the separator to make sure it is firmly secured to the insole. Use scissors to trim any part that extends over the sides of the insole.

If the patch does not stick, you probably have an insole with a surface that is not smooth enough or too soft with too much fabric that does not allow the adhesive to hold. In this case, you may want to try another insole with a better surface. They can be peeled off the insole if they are placed wrong, but will probably not stick as well if you try to reattach them. The patches will not stick to a wet insole. For easier removal, use a blow dryer or heat gun to heat the patch.

If the Separator Number 2 is Too Weak

It's possible that the pinched section of the ENGO patch will be too weak or thin to keep the toe from going under the next toe. If you can tell the toe is going under, here's an idea to make it stronger. Take another ENGO patch and cut a strip the width of the top of the separator, remove the adhesive backing, and pinch it over the existing separator so it reinforces the upward part of the separator and extends onto the base. This will strengthen the part between the toes and make it stiffer and better able to keep one toe from going under the other.

Stubbed Toes

Occasionally we stub our toes badly, and this can result in a hematoma, a bruise, or even a fracture. Stubbed toes are more common in running shoes than in hiking boots. Stubbing a toe on a rock or tree root can be very painful. Check the toe for discoloration that can indicate a deep bruise or a fracture. There may be a laceration into the nail bed or into the toe itself.

Treating Stubbed Toes

Treatment includes buddy taping, icing the toe (a cold stream will also work), elevating the foot, and wearing a firm-soled shoe or boot. Buddy taping provides support and a limited degree of immobilization to the toe.

Buddy taping as seen from the front

It involves lightly taping the injured toe to the toe next to it after placing a piece of cotton or gauze between toes (never tape skin to skin). See the chapter "Cold and Heat Therapy" for information on making the most of icing techniques. For elevation to be effective, the injured toe should be above the level of the heart and iced. A firm-soled shoe will keep the toe from bending, providing additional immobilization.

If it heals in a few days, it is probably not fractured. On the other hand, if the injury does not respond to treatment, medical treatment and an X-ray may be necessary (see the section on fractures, page 267). A doctor may have you wear an orthopedic shoe, a wooden-soled shoe that does not allow the foot to bend. If the toe is fractured, expect a healing time of four to six weeks.

If you stub your toe and the nail is bent backward, it's important to prevent the toenail from catching on your sock and tearing off. Wrap either a Band-Aid or tape around the toe to hold the toenail in place. The use of an antibiotic ointment under the nail will help prevent infection. Trimming off any loose parts of the nail will help prevent the nail from lifting off further.

Toenail Fungus

Toenail fungus is a major problem affecting many athletes. As I have patched feet over the past years, I have mentioned toenail fungus to many athletes and find most are in denial about this medical problem. John Mozena, DPM, podiatrist and marathon runner, says, "Because nail fungus can seriously impact your running as well as your general foot health, we urge runners to practice prevention and seek medical care at the first sign of the problem."

Toenail fungus

Nail fungus, also known as onychomycosis, is a persistent fungal infection of the nails that occurs when fungi called dermatophytes invade the nail bed. The fungus lives within the nail bed, making it difficult to reach and treat. Toenails infected with a fungus usually become thick and deformed. The infection may cause the nail to have a brown, white, or yellowish discoloration. The nail may become brittle and give the appearance of debris under the nail. As the fungus progresses, the nail thickens, which can cause pressure inside footwear. Toenail fungus more often affects men and the chance of its occurring increases with age—but it can affect anyone regardless of age and gender. In spite of these symptoms, many people live with a nail fungus for years because it seldom causes discomfort.

Athletes are at greater risk of developing toenail fungus because of their exposure to specific risk factors.

- Nail trauma can make the nail bed more susceptible to fungal growth.

- Sweaty socks and tight shoes promote a warm, moist environment that can contribute to the growth of the fungus.

- Because nail fungus is contagious, warm and moist environments such as communal showers and locker rooms are places where the fungus can be contracted.

The following steps can reduce your chances of getting toenail fungus:

- Wash and dry feet daily, especially between the toes.

- Wear moisture-absorbing socks.

- Make sure that shoes are completely dry before putting them on.

- Wear shower shoes or flip-flops when showering in public areas.

- Don't apply nail polish to nails that are suspected of infection.

- Wear shoes that breathe and rotate shoes every day.

- Use an antifungal powder or spray.

- Inspect feet regularly and have a doctor check for nail fungus during office visits.

Treating Toenail Fungus

Because the fungus starts in the nail bed and spreads, it is important to stop the progression when symptoms of infection are first seen. Usually doctors will prescribe a strong medication to destroy the fungus. Prescription medications may include oral antifungal medications or topical medications. If you are prescribed an oral medication, be sure to discuss its side effects with your doctor. Because nails grow slowly, treatment can take at least six months to a year or more. This allows the medication to eliminate every last fungal agent around the affected area while a new nail grows in healthy and strong. Podiatrist Christine Dobrowolski, the author of *Those Aching Feet*, talks about treatments for toenail fungus.

The most aggressive and effective treatments are with oral antifungal medications. The most common oral antifungal medications are Sporanox and Lamisil. The most effective topical medication is Penlac lacquer. Another prescription topical is a urea-based medication called Carmol. To increase the effectiveness of the treatment, I recommend combination therapy. If you choose to take an oral medication, make sure you use a topical antifungal agent as well. Nail removal is also an option. Once the nail is removed, the topicals can reach the nail bed and become more effective. The nail will grow back in over a period of eight to ten months. Permanent nail removal is reserved for those with chronic ingrown nails, ulceration under the nails, or pain from the fungal nails. (Other medications are worth considering too, for example, Jublia, Nizoral, and Diflucan.)

Robert Conenello, a podiatrist and past president of the American Academy of Podiatric Sports Medicine, says most athletes struggle with toenail fungus. He says, "It can be caused by some sort of trauma to the nail plate that allows a separation from the nailbed. This creates an ideal environment for opportunistic organisms, like fungus, to flourish. Newer prescription topical medications such as Jublia and Kerydin have proven to be as effective as the orals; however, they do require patient compliance for at least a year. Over-the-counter topicals might be helpful when used with topical Urea, which improves the permeability of the antifungal. My suggestion is to keep toenails short and utilize a prescription antifungal."

Another treatment option that is widely advertised is the use of a laser to shine through the nail and destroy the specific pathogens embedded in and under your nail causing the infection. The treatment takes about 30 minutes for all 10 toes, without pain and no damage to healthy tissue. In the first clinical study, 88% of the treated patients grew out a normal nail after one treatment. Costs average $1,100 for both feet or $800 for one foot. Ask your podiatrist about this treatment or do an online search to find where it is offered. Dr. Conenello reports that these laser treatments are very costly and their long-term efficacy as a "cure" has been disappointing.

There are several home remedies that many people try, often successfully. If these do not work for you, do not hesitate to consult a doctor. First, tea tree oil, manuka oil, or eucalyptus oil is often used for nail fungus. For best results, apply a few drops to the affected nail and skin around the nail two to three times daily. Dab it on with a cotton swab or ball. Hold it in place with a bandage or tape. As well as killing the fungi, it helps relieve the associated itching. Test a drop or two on your skin to be sure you are not allergic to the oil. The oils can be found in your local drugstore or pharmacy.

Another nail treatment that has been used with success is Vicks VapoRub. Trim the nail back as far as possible and scrape out as much of the loose nail as possible. Apply a thin coat of VapoRub over the nail and in the space underneath. Cover the nail with a Band-Aid. Repeat every morning and evening, and over a few months the fungus will die out and a new nail will grow in. Soaking your toes twice daily in Listerine and/or Listerine and white vinegar (1:1 solution) has worked for some people. One pedorthist recommends putting a capful of rubbing alcohol on your toenails after showering each day. He says that the icky part of the nail will dry out and flake off, and a new nail will grow in normally.

Vinegar can be helpful for toenail fungus. Do a foot soak with one part apple cider vinegar to two parts water, soaking for 15 minutes at a time. Adding a dash of Listerine can be helpful for its healing proprieties. Do not use this soak if you have scratches, open sores, wounds or cuts on your feet. If a rash, redness, or itching develops, discontinue the soaks.

If you use tea tree oil, manuka oil, eucalyptus oil, or Vicks VapoRub, you must apply it twice daily for at least 90 days (and 180 days is better). Dr. Dobrowolski emphasizes, "With any home remedy or nonprescription topical, you must understand that the effectiveness of the treatment is fairly low, less than 10%. If you do try one of these therapies, make sure to use it every day. File the top of the nail down to roughen up the surface and apply the medication with a cotton swab. We really don't have effective, affordable, safe medications available right now for the treatment of toenail fungus. So, when patients have failed other conventional treatments, I'll recommend trying almost any affordable and safe treatment that has helped others in the past, but I just wouldn't expect much."

The bottom line, Dr. Dobrowolski adds, is that "treating toenail fungus is very difficult. If you have fungal toenails that cause pressure, pain, or infection, consider talking to your doctor about prescription medications, nail removal, or laser treatments. Make sure you take precautions to prevent re-infection and take multiple approaches to eradicate the problem. If your fungal toenails are only unsightly and don't cause any discomfort, try a weekly application of an over-the-counter topical along with methods to prevent re-infection." Be forewarned that many oral or other strong treatments may cause liver damage, so exercise caution and follow your doctor's instructions.

Check your local drugstore for over-the-counter medications such as Miranel. Online searches will also give you additional options. Two of these are Fungi-Nail at funginail.com and Funginix at funginix.com, treatments aimed at the cuticles and nail beds. If over-the-counter medications do not resolve the fungus, consult with your doctor.

Turf Toe

Turf toe is pain at the base of the big toe where it connects to the ball of the foot—a sprain of the big toe metatarsophalangeal joint. It is usually caused from either jamming the toe or hyperextension (bending back) of the big toe. There may also be an associated stiffness and swelling. This injury is especially common among athletes who play on the hard surface of artificial turf. Football and soccer players are most susceptible to it because of all their running and jumping.

The injury is actually a tear of the capsule that surrounds the joint at the base of the toe. Tearing this joint capsule can be extremely painful. It can lead to instability and even dislocation of the joint at the base of the toe. An X-ray is in order.

Robin Fry, a physician's assistant, remembers that during an ultramarathon in 1993, he was "running away from the fire-tower aid station. Suddenly, a terrible pain shot out from my left foot and a swear word or two shot out from my mouth. I had slammed my left great toe into an unseen remnant of a small shrub or tree, barely protruding from the rough trail surface." Years later in 2001, his podiatrist performed surgery to repair the toe, which by then was very deviated laterally, and was crowding the second toe and pushing it into the third toe. After a period of recovery, Robin reports, "I do get some occasional aching in the repaired toe, but it generally stays at a tolerable level and only hurts after some very long, hard efforts. The long-crowded toes of my left foot are gradually resuming a normal alignment. I rarely take any NSAIDs. I have been taking daily Cosamin DS, a glucosamine and chondroitin-sulfate supplement. And I am back to my old training ways."

Treating Turf Toe

The common treatment consists of resting the sore toe, icing the area, and elevating the foot. Your doctor may prescribe an anti-inflammatory medication and recommend not bearing weight on the affected foot. Avoid playing your sport for about three weeks to allow the joint capsule to heal. When returning to play, you may have to wear a special toe support to protect the joint capsule. Like many injuries, the condition can recur and the rate of rehabilitation can slow with each occurrence. As Robin found out, surgery may be necessary in extreme cases or when the initial injury heals incorrectly.

HAPAD DANCER PADS fit under the ball of the foot with a cutout encompassing the big toe joint to relieve the pain under the first metatarsal joint. The coiled, springlike wool fibers provide firm and resilient support as they mold and shape to the foot. hapad.com

25

Forefoot Problems

Four conditions commonly affect the front of the foot (the forefoot): bunions, metatarsalgia, Morton's neuroma, and sesamoiditis. Any of them can be bothersome and painful, but when they happen to an athlete, they can make enjoying your sport more challenging.

Bunions

Bunions, or hallux valgus, are one of the most common deformities of the forefoot. A bunion is a bump caused by enlarged bone and tissue at the outer base of the big toe where the joint angles inward toward the other toes. A displacement of the first metatarsal bone toward the midline (center) of the body and a simultaneous displacement of the big toe away from the midline (and toward the smaller toes) cause this bump to appear. Over time, the big toe can come to rest under, or occasionally over, the second toe. The bony bump is a form of arthritis.

The deformity gives you a wide foot and causes a weakening and sagging of the arch. The motion of the joint and shoe pressure can cause pain. There may be corns on the adjacent sides of the first and second toes. A callus may develop over the bunion, and bursitis can form between the skin and the bunion bone.

A similar bump at the outer base of the fifth (little) toe is called a bunionette. These are formed when the little toe moves inward toward the big toe. Bunionettes are sometimes called tailor's bunions.

Bunions are caused by various factors. An abnormal pronated foot that rolls inward is one of the most common causes. Other causes include a family history of bunions, wearing shoes that are too narrow-toed, and limb length discrepancy. Individuals with flat feet are more prone to bunions, calluses, and hammertoes.

Treating Bunions

Be sure that your shoes are wide and deep enough in the forefoot and toe box. If you overpronate, try an arch support or orthotic to reduce the overpronation.

Bunion discomfort may be relieved with wider shoes, pads between the big and first toes, arch supports, and warm soaks. Wearing shoes or boots that are tapered in the toe area can cause bunions to worsen. Check the foot-care section of your local drugstore for a current selection of bunion relief products. If there is an inflammation of the bunion, take an anti-inflammatory medication, elevate the foot, and apply ice three times a day, 15 minutes at a time. For information on cold and heat therapy techniques, see page 337.

A full-service shoe shop or a pedorthist should be able to modify a boot to soften a pressure point or stretch a portion of the leather. This may relieve pressure on bunions, corns, and calluses.

To relieve pressure on the painful area, try one of these lacing techniques. Skipping the first set of eyelets is the easiest method to try. Or use two laces per shoe. Lace one through the bottom half of the eyelets, and tie it loosely. Lace the other through the top half of the eyelets, and tie it more tightly than the bottom lace. A third technique is to lace the first few loops loosely, tie a knot, and then lace the rest of the way up the shoe. Both methods allow a looser fit in the forefoot.

Bunion (top) and
bunionette (bottom)

Two simple big toe stretches can help relieve big toe discomfort associated with bunions.

1. Sit with your foot flat on the floor and then with the heel flat, raise the foot. Gently pull your big toe outward to the side and hold for several seconds. Repeat 10 times.

2. While in the same position, raise your foot on its heel, curling your toes tightly downward. Gently push down on your toes. Repeat 10 times.

When conservative measures don't provide relief, surgery may be necessary in extreme cases. A bunionectomy removes the bony prominence. In severe cases, an osteotomy procedure realigns the toe joint. In these surgeries, screws, plates, or wires hold the bones in position while they heal. The Mini Tightrope procedure, developed by George Holmes, MD, a foot and ankle surgeon with Rush University Medical Center, offers a less invasive alternative. In this procedure, one hole is drilled through the bone leading to the big toe and another through the bone leading to the second toe. A special type of wire, called FiberWire, is fed through the holes, with tiny buttons on each end keeping the wire from slipping out of the bones. The wire is tightened, pulling the outer bone toward the second bone into a better alignment. The surgeon then rebalances the associated ligaments, tendons, and nerves in the toe. Because no bones are cut, healing is faster and with fewer complications.

BUNION PRODUCTS

Assorted bunion products are available in your local drugstore and pharmacy, among them **DR. SCHOLL'S BUNION CUSHION PADS** and **HAPAD'S DAYTIME BUNION CUSHION.**

BUNION AID is a flexible splint that realigns the big toe while reducing bunion pain. One size fits all and it can be worn on either foot. While it is meant for 24-hour use, it is too bulky for use during running events. It can be worn in wide shoes or barefoot. bunion-aid.com

ENGO PATCHES are low-friction patches uniquely applied to areas of footwear and insoles—not skin—for easier, long-lasting bunion protection. Several sizes are available: small ovals for toes or large ovals for the ball of foot. goengo.com

FOOTSMART carries multiple products to help with bunions. footsmart.com

Metatarsalgia

Metatarsalgia is pain underneath the metatarsal heads of the foot. It typically occurs when one of the metatarsal heads collapses and points downward. Usually the second metatarsal head is affected, but it can also be at the third or fourth metatarsal heads. You may feel as if there is a small stone in your shoe, or you may feel pain, a burning sensation, or swelling at the ball of the foot. By pressing up slightly on each metatarsal head, you can usually identify the painful area. Typically the metatarsal head that is lower than the others is causing the pain and pressure. There will often be a callus at the pressure point. As we age, the fat pads on the bottoms of our feet tend to thin out and our feet become more susceptible to this problem. Metatarsalgia is often associated with Morton's foot.

Shoes that are too narrow in the forefoot or laced too tightly over the forefoot area can cause all of these problems. To see how the pressure in a narrow shoe affects the metatarsals, try this simple test. Grasp your foot around the base of the toes and squeeze gently. You'll see how it forces the metatarsals downward (on the bottom of the foot) and results in increased impact to the area with each step. For proper prevention, start with shoes that fit correctly and use good lacing techniques (for more on these topics, see the chapters "The Magic of Fit," page 42, and "Lacing Options," page 167).

Treating Metatarsalgia

Start by reducing your mileage and run on softer surfaces, or switch to a lower-impact activity. Icing can be helpful, especially in the first 24 hours. Take anti-inflammatories as needed. Strengthen the forefoot by picking up marbles with your toes (try using all your toes) and placing a washcloth on the floor and scrunching it up with your toes. Repeat each these three to five times.

A cushioned metatarsal pad can provide relief from metatarsalgia. If a pad does not help, try cutting a small hole in the insole under the painful metatarsal head.

Some metatarsal pads are made in a sleeve that wraps around the foot, and this design may cause problems during sports. To find the right position for a pad, first make a mark at the sore area with a marking pen. Then slide your foot inside your shoe and step down to transfer the ink onto the insole. Stick the pad to the insole.

Wearing shoes with a wide forefoot and high and wide toe box is also recommended. An orthotic may be necessary. If all else fails, ask your podiatrist about a cortisone injection.

Morton's Neuroma

Morton's neuroma is pain associated with a nerve inflammation usually affecting the third and fourth toes. It will sometimes be felt between the second and third toes. The nerves running between the metatarsal heads and the toes have become inflamed and irritated as they are squeezed at the base of the toes. The painful, swollen nerve is called a neuroma. There is typically tingling or a pins and needles sensation that radiates to the end of the toes—often progressing to a burning sensa-

Inflammation of a nerve, indicating Morton's neuroma

tion with sharp pain. Some people describe the sensation as walking on a pebble. If you press with your thumb at the base of your fourth toe and feel pain, you could have a neuroma. If untreated, scar tissue forms around the nerve and it becomes more painful.

This condition can be caused by a shoe's tight toe box that compresses the forefoot or by the nerves being pressured by the metatarsal heads and the bases of the toes. Sports that place a significant amount of pressure on the forefoot area can cause inflammation of the nerves. As we walk or run, we come up onto our toes, and this motion can cause the ligaments supporting the metatarsal bones to compress the nerve between the toes. Limiting your activities for a few days may be enough to allow the inflammation to subside.

Treating Morton's Neuroma

Treatments include applying ice to the pain area, an injection of anti-inflammatory medication, wider shoes, a more cushioned insole, and metatarsal pads that take pressure off the metatarsal heads. The pad reduces forefoot pressure and spreads the toes, which can relieve the pain. To find the right position for a pad, first make a mark at the sore area with a marking pen. Then slide your foot inside your shoe and step down to transfer the ink onto the insole. The site footsmart.com has a number of pads and insoles to help relieve the pain.

Massaging the foot usually helps to relieve the pain. Using icing techniques from the "Cold and Heat Therapy" chapter can help reduce pain and inflammation.

If you overpronate, the metatarsal bones have more movement, which can irritate the nerves running between the metatarsal heads. In this case, wearing firm motion-control shoes may help. Relief may also be gained by inserting a piece of lamb's wool between the toes. The use of an orthotic may be indicated. Bursitis, bunions, or arthritis may also cause metatarsal pain.

When a neuroma has not responded to conservative treatments, cortisone injections can provide relief for months or years. Alternative treatments include alcohol sclerosing injections and surgical excision.

Christine Dobrowolski, a podiatrist and author of *Those Aching Feet*, advises wearing shoes with a low heel to reduce excessive pressure on the ball of the foot, wearing rigid shoes, and using contrasting soaks to reduce inflammation. The soaks start with 5 minutes of heat followed by 5 minutes of ice/cold for 20–30 minutes.

Bob Agazzi's bout with Morton's neuroma over several years led him to study treatment options. He learned of the following treatments, from the least invasive to the most. When he wrote the list, he was down to the last step before surgery.

- Try shoes with a roomy toe box in both height and width, and make sure your socks aren't too tight.

- Try off-the-shelf orthotics.

- Try a metatarsal pad.

- Try deep-tissue massage.

- Try a cortisone injection.

- Try custom orthotics.

- Surgery is the last resort.

TIP: Strengthening Exercises

Toe exercises help to strengthen and tighten the metatarsal arch and stretch the tendons on top of the toes. Practice picking up marbles off a carpeted floor with your toes. Or put a towel on the floor and use your toes to scrunch up the towel and pick it up.

Your podiatrist or orthopedist can help identify the cause of the pain and make recommendations on how to treat the problems. A course of oral anti-inflammatory medication may be suggested. Cortisone injections are sometimes used to control the pain. Serious neuromas may require surgery to release or remove the affected nerve. Try to find a surgeon who goes in from the top of the foot to lessen recovery time and allow you to be more active during recovery.

To relieve pressure on the metatarsal heads and forefoot, try different lacing techniques (see the methods described in the "Bunions" section on page 316). With these methods the metatarsal heads are not squeezed by the pressure of normal lacing. The "Lacing Options" chapter describes other lacing techniques.

Sesamoiditis

Sesamoiditis is an inflammation of the two little bones beneath the ball of the foot under the joint that moves the big toe. These two sesamoid bones can become bruised and inflamed, resulting in either sharp, constant pain or pain that occurs with movement of the big toe. The bones can also fracture, resulting in sudden, intense pain and the inability to bear weight on the foot.

Athletes involved in sports that place repetitive and excessive pressure on the forefoot area can experience sesamoid pain. The increasing emphasis on minimalist-style footwear and landing on the ball of the foot might lead to sesamoiditis. Shoes with poor cushioning that offer inadequate protection against rocks can cause trauma to the sesamoid bones.

Rich Schick, a physician's assistant, points out that the sesamoid under the first metatarsal is often composed of several small bones:

> If the bones on an X-ray were smooth, appearing with no rough or jagged edges, it's likely inflammation. Even if it is a fracture, these bones only act as shock absorbers in the first place. One can continue to run with nothing to fear but pain. I high-centered on a sharp rock some years back and fractured mine. On X-ray there were two pieces like half moons with the round side smooth and the straight sides jagged as one would expect if you broke a round object in half. The literature said that these fractures could lead to chronic pain and the fragments could need to be surgically removed. As this worst case didn't seem all that frightening, I opted to

train and race as normal. The thing bothered me for about a year, but for the last several years has given me no pain at all.

These two little bones can became a major problem. The ball of Lyal Holmberg's left foot became painful during a short 5-mile run. An X-ray showed the sesamoid bone was broken into three pieces. Lyal reports, "As I continued running, the foot was killing me and caused a tilt toward the right, putting a strain on my left hip." A walking-type boot and an anti-inflammatory were prescribed for two weeks, followed by the use of a small dancer's pad behind the ball of his foot. Lyal said, "If I can walk and run without pain, then the problem is solved. If not, I may need surgery to correct the problem."

Treating Sesamoiditis

The use of soft pads or insoles can help. You can also cut a small hole in your insole under the sesamoid bones. Loosely lacing the forefoot of your shoes, as described in the "Bunions" section on page 316, can help relieve pressure on the sesamoid area. Using icing techniques from the "Cold and Heat Therapy" chapter can help reduce pain and inflammation.

Buddy taping the big toe to the second toe or toes next to it for stabilization will limit movement of the toe. A small piece of gauze, cotton, or tissue between the taped toes will prevent skin breakdown if the tape is on for any great length of time. A firm-soled shoe will help keep the toe in line and the foot–toe joint stable. Nonimpact activities are recommended until the injury has healed.

HAPAD DANCER PADS fit under the ball of the foot with a cutout encompassing the big toe joint to relieve calluses and the painful irritations of sesamoiditis. The coiled, springlike wool fibers provide firm and resilient support as they mold and shape to the foot. hapad.com

26

Numb Toes and Feet

Numb feet are usually caused by either transient paresthesia or peripheral neuropathy. Though both are bothersome, the first is usually temporary while the second can be very debilitating. Another form of numbness that is fairly common is Raynaud's syndrome.

If you are diabetic or even prediabetic, pay close attention to any changes in your feet. Neuropathy is a common diabetic foot problem. Likewise, cuts, sores, bruises, and toenail issues can lead to medical problems.

Transient Paresthesia

Transient paresthesia is a temporary nerve compression that can be caused by a gradual buildup of fluids in your feet during extended on-your-feet activity. As the feet swell and blood flow decreases, nerves become compressed. During the compression, the nerves do not receive the oxygen-rich blood they need, resulting in numbness and/or tingling. Tight shoes and/or tightly laced shoes contribute to the problem. Shoes with poor cushioning, coupled with a heavy, pounding gait, can also be a factor.

Numb toes can also be caused by chronic repetitive motions and stresses leading to interdigital neuritis, commonly called Morton's neuroma. Inflammation of the nerves between the metatarsal bones can radiate into the toes.

Ultrarunner and adventure racer Ginny La Forma has battled this numbness in her toes on many occasions. After the Hardrock 100-Mile Run, it lasted a few weeks, but after the Eco Challenge, it lasted over a year. She also suffers from Morton's neuromas.

If the problem continues after your activity has stopped, consider changing to more cushioned shoes and/or wider shoes, and changing insoles and arch supports. There may be some lymph system breakdown in the foot caused by microtrauma. If the problem persists, consult a sports specialist.

Information Resources for Transient Paresthesia and Peripheral Neuropathy

THE NEUROPATHY ASSOCIATION foundationforpn.org

NUMB TOES AND ACHING SOLES is a must-read for anyone experiencing peripheral neuropathy. Written by John A. Senneff, who suffers from peripheral neuropathy, the book deals with this disorder from the patient's perspective. Published in 1999 by MedPress.

PERIPHERAL NEUROPATHY: WHEN THE NUMBNESS, WEAKNESS, AND PAIN WON'T STOP, by Norman Latov, published by American Academy of Neurology and Demos Medical Publishing in 2006.

THE NUMB FOOT BOOK, by Drs. Marc Spitz and Alexander McLellan, offered at footpaincenter.com. Published in 2008 by MedPress.

THE OFFICIAL PATIENT'S SOURCEBOOK ON PERIPHERAL NEUROPATHY, edited by James N. Parker, MD, and Philip M. Parker, PhD; published by Icon Health Publications in 2002.

Peripheral Neuropathy

Peripheral neuropathy is a painful nerve condition that can manifest itself as a burning sensation in the feet but that sometimes will appear as a cold sensation. It may start as a mild tingling in the toes and progress to searing pain. It can spread upward in the body, even to the thighs. Other symptoms might include tingling, prickling, or numbness; the sensation of having invisible socks on your feet; a sharp jabbing or electric-type pain; extreme sensitivity to touch; muscle weakness; and a loss of balance or coordination.

The pain results from damage to peripheral nerves that can come from myriad causes. A partial list of causes includes poor blood flow to the feet caused by diabetes, kidney, or liver disease; an underactive thyroid; viral and bacterial infections; vitamin deficiencies; and pressure on a single nerve, although often, no cause is identified. It is called neuropathic pain because it occurs in the absence of dangerous stimuli, does not prompt protective reflexes, and does not subside when the danger has passed or the injury healed.

Ken Reed, an ultrarunner who discovered that he had peripheral neuropathy, shares this story. His condition started with a tingling in three of his left foot toes in the summer of 1998 that later turned to numbness. That fall, when the numbness progressed to shooting pains and aches, he sought medical advice. By the spring of 1999 it had progressed to pains in his lower legs, with the numbness also moving upward. Ken reports that when his feet are cold, they constantly ache, buzz, and feel numb. He has resolved to manage the pain and discomfort and hope for a miracle cure.

Treating Peripheral Neuropathy

Treatment often depends on the cause and symptoms of the neuropathy. It can be frustrating to treat, particularly if no reversible cause is identified. Typical treatments include over-the-counter or prescribed pain relievers for mild symptoms, tricyclic antidepressants for burning pain, antiseizure medications for jabbing pain, or other drugs. There is no one mediation or therapy that can reverse the nerve damage.

Self-care treatments include changing one's activity until the pain subsides, NSAIDs, steroid injections, changing your shoes, modifying your running form, physical therapy, proper care of your feet with loose socks and padded shoes, a semicircular hoop in bed to keep the cover off your feet, cold water soaks and skin moisturizers, massage to improve circulation and stimulate nerves, staying active, and reducing stress levels.

Ask your physician whether Neuragen could help your symptoms. This homeopathic topical medication works directly at the site of nerve pain and is available without a prescription. Your physician may know of additional medications to try.

Neuro-Reflex Therapy, Bentley Method (NRT) provides a holistic, natural treatment for pain relief and increased circulation for suffers of peripheral neuropathy. Do an online search for Neuro-Reflex Therapy to find a practitioner near you.

Raynaud's Syndrome

Raynaud's syndrome affects 5%–10% of the population. The discomfort is caused by a decreased blood supply to the fingers and toes. Attacks are precipitated by exposure to cold and stress.

Although the severity, duration, and frequency of attacks vary both between individuals and over time, the primary symptom of Raynaud's syndrome is changes in skin color. The affected areas turn white from the lack of circulation, then blue and cold, and finally numb. When the attack subsides, the affected parts may turn red and may throb, tingle, or swell.

Those affected by Raynaud's syndrome are more susceptible to cold and wet conditions, which can lead to trench foot. Severe itching and burning—more than normal or that doesn't go away—needs to be checked by your doctor.

Treating Raynaud's Syndrome

Keeping your whole body warm is a good prevention strategy. Wear wind- and water-resistant gloves and socks. Wool or wool-blend socks that retain warmth are good, as are SealSkinz socks (sealskinz.com) to block moisture. Shoes that block wind and moisture are also recommended. Be sure to allow space in your footwear for thicker socks. Constriction caused by tight socks and footwear can be harmful. Keep fingers and toes dry with powder. If you feel an attack coming on, get inside and warm your hands and feet.

Be careful not to injure the skin in affected areas, and treat injuries without delay. Even minor cuts and scrapes take longer to heal and may be more susceptible to infection when circulation is impaired.

If you suspect you have Raynaud's syndrome, see your physician. Doctors sometimes recommend medications to help combat this condition. The Raynaud's Association (raynauds.org) can offer help and support for this painful and frustrating condition.

Skin Disorders

Five skin disorders commonly affect the feet: athlete's foot, calluses, corns, fissures, and plantar warts. Dealing with these conditions when they first develop will help prevent more serious problems later.

Athlete's Foot

The facts are startling: 70% of people will be affected by athlete's foot in their lifetimes, 45% of people with athlete's foot will suffer from it in episodes for more than 10 years, and 7 out of 10 people with athlete's foot are male.

Athlete's foot, technically called tinea pedis, is a skin disease caused when normally occurring bacteria, especially yeast, mold, or fungi, grow out of control. The hot weather and foot perspiration that athletes typically encounter can make athlete's foot a common problem. The combination of a warm and humid environment in the shoes or boots, excessive foot perspiration, and changes in the condition of the skin combine to create a setting for the fungi of athlete's foot to begin growing. Athlete's foot usually occurs between the toes, but can occur on the soles and heels. Typical signs and symptoms of athlete's foot include itching, dry and cracking skin, inflammation with a burning sensation, and pain. Blisters and swelling may develop if left untreated. When these blisters break, small, red areas of raw tissue are exposed. As the infection spreads, the burning and itching will increase. Complications are rare, but secondary bacterial infections are possible. If your feet become swollen, warm to the touch, or have red streaks, call your doctor right away.

Another type of tinea infection is often called moccasin foot. In this type, a red rash spreads across the lower portion of the foot in the pattern of a moccasin. The skin in this region gradually becomes dense, white, and scaly. The use of a prescription-strength antifungal cream may be required to treat this infection.

Fungus under and around the nails should be treated promptly with antifungal medications. See the "Toenail Fungus" section (page 311) for information on treating fungal infections.

Preventive measures include washing your feet daily with soap and water; drying them thoroughly, especially between the toes; wearing moisture-wicking socks; regularly changing your shoes and socks to control moisture; and using a good, moisture-absorbing foot powder. Because athlete's foot is contagious, if you use a communal shower or bathroom after an event, or use a gym to train, avoid walking barefoot in these areas. Use flip-flops, shower booties, or even your shoes or boots.

Treating Athlete's Foot

Treatment includes keeping the feet clean and dry, frequent socks changes, and over-the-counter antifungal medications and foot powders (see the "Powders" section, page 128, for more information on choosing a foot powder). An antiperspirant may also help those with excessive foot moisture (see the "Antiperspirants for the Feet" section, page 137, for more information about these products). Because wet socks can create an ideal environment for fungal growth, the use of high-quality socks is essential. Moisture-wicking socks can still leave the feet damp. Drymax socks, with their inner fibers that repel moisture, are even better. Check your local drugstore or pharmacy for a complete line of athlete's foot antifungal ointments, creams, liquids, powders, and sprays.

See your doctor if your feet do not respond to treatment with over-the-counter medications. If the fungus returns, alternate medications because the fungus can sometimes build up a resistance to a particular fungicide.

To treat athlete's foot or a case of foot fungi, give tea tree oil, manuka oil, or eucalyptus oil a try. For best results, apply a few drops to the affected areas two to three times daily. Dab it on with a cotton swab or cotton ball. Hold it in place with a bandage or tape. As well as killing the fungi, it helps relieve the associated itching. Test a drop or two on your skin to be sure you are not allergic to the oil. The oils can be found in your local drugstore or pharmacy. Plain rubbing alcohol works for some people. After showering, rub your toenails with an alcohol-soaked cotton ball. If using alcohol or one of the oils, make sure to continue twice a day. Maintain this regimen for at least 90 days.

Many people swear by a vinegar foot soak for athlete's foot. Use apple cider vinegar in a mixture of five cups to one gallon of water. Soak at least 10 minutes a day for 10 days. When removing your feet from the mixture, wipe the affected areas with a cotton ball dipped in the vinegar. Do not use this soak if you have scratches, open sores, wounds or cuts on your feet. If a rash, redness or itching develops, discontinue the soaks.

Swabplus's Fungus Relief liquid-filled cotton swabs offer an easy way to carry athlete's foot medications. Bending one end of the swab releases the liquid medication. Check your local drug store or pharmacy (unidose.com).

Other over-the-counter antifungal creams or solutions commonly available in your local drugstore and pharmacy include Dr. Scholl's Fungal Nail Revitalizer System, Clotrimazole, and Lamisil. Lotrimin, Micatin, Swabplus, Tinactin, and Tolnaftate are all common. Zeasorb-AF is available as a powder and a lotion/powder combination. Stronger prescription medications are available through your doctor or podiatrist.

Whether using an over-the-counter or a prescription medication, use according to the directions. Continue several weeks after the fungus has cleared to ensure it doesn't return.

Calluses

Calluses are one of the most controversial foot-care subjects. For every athlete who bemoans their calluses, there are two or three others who love them. I have become passionate in telling athletes about the problems that calluses cause when blisters form underneath the hardened skin.

A callus is an abnormal amount of dead, thickened skin caused by recurring pressure and friction, called hyperkeratosis, and is usually on the sole of the foot, most often on the heels, the balls of the feet, or the bottom of the toes. It may be yellowish in color, layered, or even scaly due to excessive dryness. Calluses can form over any bony prominence. Calluses are never normal—they are signs of poor biomechanics or ill-fitting footgear. If it is a footgear problem, this needs to be identified and remedied. Unfortunately most biomechanical problems are things that we need to learn to live with. In many cases, there is nothing wrong or bad about calluses. They can protect against friction and act as a cushioning pad. Calluses become a problem when they become thick enough to interfere with the normal elasticity of the skin or act like a foreign body on the foot.

A common callus is called intractable plantar keratosis (IPK); this is a localized callus buildup at or near the metatarsal heads on the ball of the foot. An IPK often has a hard central core, which can cause pain when it is in a pressure area. Calluses are caused by a number of factors: poorly aligned metatarsal bones in the forefoot, an abnormal gait, flat or high-arched feet, excessively long metatarsal bones, and a loss of the fat pads on the underside of the foot. Individuals with flat feet are more prone to calluses, bunions, and hammertoes.

Unless the calluses are troublesome, most people tend to forget about them. Your body has made the callus as protection from pressure at those points with little natural fat or padding. To keep painful calluses from returning, you must correct the biomechanical problem that prompted their growth in the first place. Some calluses may have a deep-seated core, called nucleation, which can be painful to pressure. These are often known as corn kernels.

Calluses will continue to grow as they toughen. This can interfere with the fit of your shoes—which in turn can cause a blister—one way or another. Some degree of toughened skin is fine, but be careful of too-callused skin. The time to treat calluses is before an event. Should you develop blisters underneath the tough, hardened surface of a callus, it will usually form deep in the foot, which makes it hard to treat. Once you have experienced a deep blister, you are likely to work hard to rid your feet of their thick calluses. It is hard to drain these blisters. There is fluid underneath the callus, but finding the right depth and location is almost impossible. The section "Deep Blisters" (see page 252) discusses treating these problem blisters.

Am I a stickler about calluses? You bet. I've seen the grimaces on the faces of athletes who have deep blisters that cannot be repaired without a lot of pain. I've seen them hobble off, knowing it won't get any better. When I work at an event patching feet, I encourage athletes to rid their feet of calluses or at least reduce the size and thickness of their calluses. This will leave a smaller and thinner layer of callus, which will still protect the skin but may not cause as many problems if blisters form underneath.

Treating Calluses

Gently grasp some normal skin on your foot and roll it between your thumb and forefinger. Notice how supple it is. Now attempt to roll the callused area in the same manner. If it is too stiff or causes discomfort, the callus is too thick and is likely to cause pain or blisters. You need to thin it down.

Soak your feet a mixture of equal parts of white vinegar and hot water to soften calluses. After soaking, buff with a pumice stone or callus file to remove any dead skin. After the callused skin is dry, apply your choice of cream, lotion, medication, or pads. If your skin is particularly callused, at night after applying the cream, wrap your feet with plastic wrap to hold in the moisturizer. Over several weeks, simply keep working at it until all areas are as supple as normal skin.

For many athletes, calluses become rough with edges of skin poking up. These edges can catch on socks and lead to the start of a blister. They can also open up into a fissure, a crack in the skin.

Specialized tools are now available to reduce calluses. The Amope Pedi Perfect, Dr. Scholl's Express Pedi, and similar products make quick work of hard calluses. These are battery operated and use a wide roller head with micro-abrasive particles to remove excess hard skin. They excel at removing calluses on the heels, bottoms, and sides of the foot. Refill roller heads are available for all models. All models are designed to stop when too much pressure is placed on the skin, preventing overexfoliating, which can damage the skin. The downside to these tools is the roller style has limited value on toe calluses.

The Heel Smoother Pro is the perfect tool for reducing calluses on toes. This two-speed, battery-operated pedicure appliance smoothes calluses and removes dry skin anywhere on your feet. The shape of their DuraCrystal Power Tips is the perfect size to work on toes, but also works well on other areas of the foot. Even though this company has closed, you can often find these by searching online.

Check your local drugstore for a callus file. These are usually 8–9 inches in length with a rounded, cupped shape to effectively file rounded parts of your feet. Some have a fine file texture on one side and a coarser texture on the other side. If you can't find them locally, check out footsmart.com. The as-seen-on-TV PedEgg is an inexpensive alternative to files and can be easily found on many websites. The problem with these tools is that the skin is left with a roughened surface.

Never file too deeply into a corn or callus and do not cut into them with sharp objects. A pumice stone will work as well as a file.

A cushioned insole with a good arch support can help equalize the weight load of the foot, while pads around or near the callus can relieve pressure. To relieve heel discomfort from calluses, try a heel cup or heel pad that will distribute body weight evenly across the heel. Orthotics can help relieve pressure in the callused areas of your

CALLUS PRODUCTS

The important tip to remember is to use the lotions below daily or according to the package's directions. Using these lotions once or twice a week will not allow them to work their healing magic on your skin.

AMOPE PEDI PERFECT ELECTRONIC FOOT FILE uses a roller to quickly reduce calluses. amope.com

ANGELFEET PEDICURE FILES are made from surgical stainless steel with a revolutionary smoothing surface that will never wear out. Available in fine, medium, and coarse styles. angelfeetfile.com

DR. SCHOLL'S makes the **EXPRESS PEDI FOOT SMOOTHER, ULTRA OVERNIGHT FOOT CREAM,** and **ROUGH SKIN REMOVING FOOT CREAM.**

ENGO PATCHES are low-friction patches uniquely applied to footwear, insoles, socks, and athletic equipment—not skin—for easier, longer-lasting protection from calluses. Ultrathin patches leave footwear volume virtually unaltered. Strong, latex-free adhesive prevents migration and movement, even through moisture and sweat. Scientific and field tests show ENGO's slippery blue surface significantly reduces rubbing, providing immediate relief. Several sizes are available: small ovals for toes; large ovals for the ball of foot, arch, and heel areas; rectangles for custom trimming. goengo.com

FOOTSMART carries a complete line of skin-care products made for calluses. These products will help your feet feel softer and smoother while eliminating calluses. **CALLEX CALLUS OINTMENT** and polymer cushions and pads may also prove helpful. footsmart.com

HAPAD offers several options for callus control. Metatarsal pads and metatarsal bars, **METATARSAL COOKIES, DANCER PADS** with a cutout encompassing the big toe joint, and **HORSESHOE HEEL CUSHIONS** all reduce pressure on areas of calluses. The **IPK PAD** is made for intractable plantar keratosis. The coiled, springlike wool fibers provide firm and resilient support as they mold and shape to the foot. hapad.com

The **HEEL SMOOTHER PRO BY ARTEMIS WOMAN** is the best tool made for callus control. With two speeds, it stops when too much pressure is put on the skin. The DuraCrystal Power Tips do quick work on heel, toe, and other calluses. Comes with two tips for all shaped areas of the foot. Choose between a battery-operated and rechargeable model.

KATHY'S FAMILY FOOT BALM, FOOT SCRUB, and **FOOT BATH** are made with 100% natural and organic ingredients. kathysfamily.com

SKINMD NATURAL is a shielding lotion that enhances the skin's own natural protective factor by hydrating the skin. It also forms an invisible, protective barrier that helps prevent blistering and irritation, while keeping natural moisture in. skinmdnatural.com

ZIM'S MAX CRACK CREAM helps to moisturize, soothe, and soften dry, cracked, painful skin. There are three formulas: nighttime liquid, daytime cream, or with hydrocortisone. Look for Zim's in your drugstore or pharmacy. zimsusa.com feet. While a variety of callus pads are sold, they are only temporary fixes. The regular use of skin moisturizers will help keep the skin soft and eliminate the thick calluses. To relieve pressure on the painful area, make sure your shoes are sized right and fit well, and try different lacing techniques (see the lacing discussion in the "Treating Bunions" section, page 317). While there are over-the-counter plantar wart removal compounds available that can also be used on corns and calluses, care must be taken in their use. These products contain salicylic acid. Follow the product's directions to avoid damaging good tissue. Do not use these products if you are a diabetic.

Neil Olsen, an MD from Oregon, wrote that he tried prescription Lac-Hydrin: "I've had several cases of really nasty, hyperkeratotic, fissured feet soften up and smooth out with this." Other products are available at your local drugstore and pharmacy. Refer to "Skin Products" on page 176 for additional products that can be used on calluses.

Corns

Corns

A corn is a hard, thickened area of skin, generally on the top of, on the tip of, or between the toes, usually caused by friction and pressure. A corn is usually like a kernel of corn, round and yellowish in color. Corns on the outer surface of the toes are usually hard, while those between the toes are usually soft. The larger the corn and the more it rubs against your shoe, the more painful it becomes. Typically the corn is an inverted cone shape with a point that can press on a nerve below, causing pain.

Corns can be caused by tight-fitting socks and footwear, deformed toes, or the foot sliding around the shoe. Soft corns, caused by prominent, irregularly shaped bones and bumps, occur between the toes—soft from the perspiration in the forefoot area.

Treating Corns

Weekly warm water and Epsom salt soaks will help soften corns. Following the soak, apply a moisturizing cream and cover them with plastic wrap for 15 minutes. After removing the wrap, gently buff off any dead tissue with a pumice stone.

To relieve the discomfort of corns, start with properly fitting shoes with extra room in the toe box. You can also pad around the corn with corn pads, small pieces of one of the tapes previously mentioned, or Spenco 2nd Skin. There are many types of corn pads and toe sleeves. Lamb's wool can be wrapped around the toe for cushioning.

Check the foot-care section of your local drugstore for a current selection of corn relief products. These may include pads and creams to remove the corns. If your corns persist, consult your podiatrist.

To control corns, the pressure and friction must be eliminated, usually from improperly fitting shoes. To relieve pressure on the painful area, try the lacing techniques described in the "Treating Bunions" section (page 317). Both methods allow a looser fit in the forefoot.

PRODUCTS FOR CORNS

Assorted corn relief products can be found at your local drugstore and pharmacy. These include **BAND-AID CORN REMOVER, DR. SCHOLL'S CORN CUSHIONS, MOISTURIZING AND CORN REMOVER KIT,** and **ONE-STEP CORN REMOVER PADS.**

BUNGA OVAL PADS and **GEL PADS** are made from a medical-grade polymer material. bungapads.com

HAPAD has **METATARSAL COOKIES** that provide simple metatarsal arch cushioning. These can relieve the pressure that causes corns and calluses. hapad.com

PEDIFIX VISCO-GEL CORN PROTECTORS cushion and absorb pressure around corns. pedifix.com

Fissures

Fissures often develop in the thickened, callused skin on our heels, but they also occur on callused skin on the balls of the feet. These fissures can become infected, may bleed, and can split open into the deeper underlying tissues. Like many foot conditions, fissures can lead to infection if left untreated.

Wearing sandals and going barefoot can contribute to fissures. On vacation one summer, I wore Tevas every day. My feet were in and out of water all day. After several days of being in the hot, drying sun, I had several deep fissures on one heel. I discovered how painful these cracks can become.

Treating Fissures

Using a moisturizing cream and reducing calluses on your feet will help prevent fissures. If wearing sandals or going barefoot, use the cream morning and evening. The preceding "Calluses" section has information and products that will help in the elimination of fissures. The "Skin Care" section (see page 172) also has a list of products that keep your skin soft and callus free—thus preventing fissures.

Monty Tam, a thru-hiker, has a remedy for deep, dry, cracked heels. At night, rub on lots of petroleum jelly, slip a plastic produce bag over it, slip a sock over the bag, and then elevate your feet and sleep. In the morning your heels will be moist and flexible and won't feel as if you are walking on razor blades.

Rod Dalitz offers a tip on heel cracks or fissures: "Last year I suffered from heel cracks due to wearing sandals in New Zealand in November and December. I fixed them by sanding with some coarse waterproof emery paper glued to a board—more rugged and coarse than what you buy from your local store—and Neutrogena Formula Unscented Hand Cream, which seems a lot more durable than most creams. You don't need much. The sandpaper is so much quicker and more effective than pumice or flimsy commercial boards."

Gail shares how she managed fissures: "The most effective way my husband and I have dealt with these when they occur is by supergluing them together. They heal quickly and the pain is gone immediately. The hardest thing is reaching back to glue them (it's easier to have someone else do it for you). And of course you have to be careful not to glue your fingers to the feet and to let the glue dry completely before stepping down or putting socks on." So if you are bothered by these cracks in the skin, make a note to buy a tube of Gorilla Super Glue, Instant Krazy Glue, or SuperGlue.

Plantar Warts

Plantar wart

Plantar warts occasionally rear their ugly heads on the sole of the foot (the *plantar* surface) and cause foot pain. They can appear and then disappear suddenly, without any effort on your part, and may not recur for years. Usually painful from the pressure of standing and walking, plantar warts can become more painful due to sports activities. These warts are typically small, hard, granulated lumps on the skin that can be flesh-colored, white, pink, brown, or gray. They can also feel spongy, thick, and scaly. You may feel as though you have a small stone in your shoe when a wart appears.

Plantar warts are benign tumors caused by common viral infections, usually the human papillomavirus. They generally enter the sole of the foot through cuts and breaks in the skin. The period of time between contact and the wart making its presence known may be several months. There are three types of plantar warts. The first is a single, isolated wart. The second is one wart, often called the mother, surrounded by any number of smaller daughter warts. The third type is a cluster of many warts grouped together, usually on the heels or the balls of the feet. Plantar warts are irregular in shape. While usually small on the skin's surface, they penetrate deep into the foot, where they can cause deep pain.

Moist, cracked skin and open or healing blisters leave one susceptible to the virus. To avoid getting a virus, do not walk barefoot in communal showers or bathrooms. Use flip-flops, shower booties, or even your shoes or boots. Plantar warts thrive in the warm, moist environment found in sports shoes, so be sure to air your feet when able and change into fresh shoes and socks after participating in sports.

Treating Plantar Warts

Most warts disappear without treatment in four to five months. Sometimes, though, when the wart is bothersome or has not gone away on its own, treatment is necessary. While over-the-counter plantar wart removal compounds are available, care must be taken in their use. Many products contain salicylic acid. Follow the product's directions to avoid damaging good tissue. Usually the treatment consists of applying the medication and covering the area with a bandage—repeating daily until the problem is resolved. Check your local drugstore or pharmacy for a complete line of products. These include Compound W Wart Remover Gel, Liquid and Freeze Off, Dr. Scholl's Clear Away Plantar Salicylic Acid Wart Removal System for Feet, DuoFilm Liquid Salicylic Acid Wart Remover, and Wartner Cryogenic Wart Removal System. Do not use these products if you are a diabetic. Some individuals report success simply

Duct Tape for Wart Removal?

A study reported in the *Archives of Pediatrics & Adolescent Medicine*[51] identified duct tape, the all-purpose household fix with hundreds of uses, as an effective wart remover. Researchers say over-the-hardware-counter duct tape is a more effective, less painful alternative to liquid nitrogen, which is used to freeze warts. In the study, patients wore duct tape over their warts for six days. Then they removed the tape, soaked the area in water, and used an emery board or pumice stone to scrape the spot. The tape was reapplied the next morning. The treatment continued for a maximum of two months or until the wart went away. If you have stubborn warts, this duct tape treatment may be worth a try.

The duct tape irritated the warts, and that apparently caused an immune system reaction that attacked the growths, said researcher Dean Richard Focht III, MD, of Cincinnati Children's Hospital Medical Center. He said that researchers did not test other kinds of tape, and so they cannot say whether there is anything special about the gray, heavy-duty, fabric-backed tape.

The study was conducted at the Madigan Army Medical Center near Tacoma, Washington. It began with 61 patients between the ages of 3 and 22, but only 51 patients completed the study. Of the 26 patients treated with duct tape, 85% got rid of their warts compared with 60% of the 25 patients who received the freezing treatment.

Pediatric dermatologist Anthony J. Mancini, MD, of Children's Memorial Hospital in Chicago said he uses a form of duct tape therapy for warts. He combines duct tape with a topical, over-the-counter wart remover for nightly treatments. "The whole point of this is a nonpainful approach," said Dr. Mancini, who was not involved in the study.

---

covering the wart with a piece of duct tape until the wart falls off. You can use moleskin with a hole cut out to relieve painful pressure on the wart. Most drugstores or pharmacies have a selection of pads with cutouts for this purpose.

Kevin Corcoran suffered from plantar warts and used these patches. Each day when he removed the patch, he'd carefully remove the affected layer of skin with a handled razor knife, so that the next patch could further penetrate the skin. He attributes this to greatly reducing the time for the wart to disappear.

Occasionally, it is not a plantar wart but something else. It could be a plugged sweat gland (porokeratotic cyst) or a deep callus with a central core. Check with your doctor if your treatments don't work.

A home remedy is to soak your feet in a mixture of equal parts of white vinegar and hot water. You can also apply a cotton ball soaked in vinegar to the wart. Tape it with a Band-Aid and leave it overnight.

The treatments may put sports activities on hold until after the spot heals, generally in about a week. The common medical treatment by podiatrists for plantar warts involves the use of liquid nitrogen to freeze off the wart. Other treatment options include electrical burning, minor surgery, or laser surgery. Bill Johncock, DPM, recommends trying the simple remedies first, and if those don't work, see a professional. Check with your podiatrist to determine your treatment options.

Rashes

Capillaritis is a common rash that affects the legs of athletes. Presenting as a funky rash, it simply seems to come out of nowhere and without any related injury. The rash is a harmless skin condition in which reddish-brown patches are caused by leaky capillaries. As the capillaries become inflamed, tiny red dots appear on the skin. The dots form into a flat red patch, which becomes brown and then slowly starts to fade away. Its cause is often unknown, but it tends to develop after exercise. Many times the rash will appear under the socks and gaiters, often in extreme heat conditions. The rash may be caused by a reaction to Lycra, a common sock fabric, or other fabrics that irritate your skin. It could also be a heat rash from the combination of trapped sweat and hot temperatures. In extreme cases it will present with fluid-filled blisters. It can reoccur and even persist for years.

Delayed pressure urticaria is a form of swelling or hives, edema, or redness of the skin due to some form of pressure upon the skin. It can occur under the elastic of socks or gaiters and can be caused by tight shoes. The rash and pain can last 3–72 hours. Topical applications of Benadryl ointment might help, but usually a more potent corticosteroid is required.

Prickly heat rash is caused by a blockage of sweat glands in areas of heavy sweating, usually beneath clothing. This rash appears as red, itchy, inflamed bumps.

Other possible rashes include poison oak or poison ivy, or rashes that develop because of sensitivity to soap, lotion, or fabrics. These can be ruled out by a physician if they persist.

Treating Rashes

Capillaritis will disappear on its own over a few weeks. The use of a hydrocortisone 1% cream will help control the rash and any related itching. A dermatologist or general physician can be consulted if it does not go away on its own.

Maddalena Acconci, better known to adventure racers as MA, has a mix of ingredients that she uses for athletes' rashes. She will often mix a batch based on what she sees on feet and ankles. Her basic concoction is a triple antibiotic, hydrocortisone, Bag Balm, and either tea tree oil or manuka oil (studies have shown manuka oil is 20–30 times more active than Australian tea tree oil for gram-positive bacteria, and 5–10 times more active for fungi). MA says:

> If [the rash] is really bad, I use 1% hydrocortisone and manuka oil. If it's not so very bad, I use 0.5% hydrocortisone and tea tree oil. Sometimes I find people who react badly to antibiotic creams, so I use Burt's Bees Rescue Ointment, which also works great for a whole plethora of race ailments. I don't know if anything I do is unique. I just do what I think will work. For example, I had a racer develop a very mysterious redness

on the soles of his feet. None of us could figure out what it was—just red, nothing else. He really wanted to race but his soles were sensitive. I mixed Benadryl cream with Rescue ointment, rubbed it in, cut a layer of Molefoam to shape, and topped it off with a layer of moleskin. I taped it with Leukotape to hold it together. He wore his slightly larger pair of shoes and a thin double-sock combo. It worked, he raced, and the rash went away.

If you are often affected by rashes, try different socks, apply powder under your socks, or wear a thin sock liner made from silk. Prickly heat rash usually lasts for a few days and then disappears on its own, although it may last longer if hot and humid conditions continue.

28

Cold and Heat Therapy

Injuries can be helped through the use of cold and heat therapy. Each has its place in the rehabilitation phase of an injury, as they help healing by reducing swelling, reducing pain, and promoting circulation. The rule of thumb is to start with cold and switch to heat or a cold/heat combination later.

Do not use cold or heat therapy on an area where the skin is broken. First treat the wound. Individuals with known or suspected circulatory problems or cold hypersensitivity, paralysis, areas of impaired sensation, or rheumatoid conditions should consult a physician before using cold or heat compression therapy.

Cold Therapy

Cold therapy, generally referred to as cryotherapy, is an essential part of rehabilitation after an injury, as well as a preventive measure to avoid problems. Icing is usually done in combination with all the other RICE components: rest, compression, and elevation. Remember that all four are important and should be used together for faster recovery from an injury. Cold therapy is effective for sprains and strains, contusions and bruises, muscle pulls, and postexercise soreness. Those with Raynaud's syndrome or former frostbite sufferers should not use ice on affected body parts.

Icing progresses through four stages—cold, burning, aching, and finally numbness—usually taking about 20 minutes in all. The numbness stage should be reached in order to receive the full benefits of icing; when the area goes numb, stop applying ice. The duration of icing depends on the type and depth of the injury. Body areas with less fat and tissue should be iced for less time than fatty or dense areas (for example, a bony area less than a hamstring). After an injury, soft-tissue damage can cause uncontrolled swelling. This swelling can increase the damage of the initial injury and increase the healing time. The immediate use of ice will reduce the amount of swelling, tissue damage, blood clot formation, muscle spasms, inflammation, and pain.

Cold therapy works by decreasing the tissue's temperature and constricting the blood vessels in the injured area. This decreases blood flow, venous/lymphatic drainage, and cell metabolism, reducing the chance of hemorrhage and cell death in an acute injury. Once the fourth stage of icing, numbness, is reached, light range of motion can be started. Avoid strenuous exercise during cold therapy.

Rob Conenello, past president of the American Academy of Podiatric Sports Medicine, reminds us that the use of ice is indicated for acute injuries, but not chronic conditions such as tendinosis and fasciosis, which do not have an inflammation component.

Cheap Freeze

Homemade ice packs can be made with three parts water and one part rubbing alcohol. Mix in a freezer-grade zip-top bag, and keep one or two in the freezer. The result is a hard slush. If the mix is too hard, let it melt and add a little more alcohol. If it is too liquid, add a little more water. The right consistency will allow the bag to be formed around your foot, ankle, or other body part. Use a towel between the ice bag and your skin. Care must be taken not to get an ice burn from these packs because the alcohol can make them colder than over-the-counter packs.

Do not place ice directly on the skin unless you are using an ice cup or similar delivery system. For these, slide the ice over the area in a slow but steady motion. Ice until the area becomes numb. Otherwise, always use a thin towel, washcloth, or T-shirt between the ice bag and skin. If you have an Ace wrap on the injured part, apply the ice directly over the wrap. Ice cubes in a plastic bag will work, but crushed ice conforms better to the body. When at home, use a bag of frozen peas or corn, which conforms nicely to the curves of the foot or ankle. Use an Ace wrap or other type compression wrap to hold the ice against the injured area. This type of icing is perfect for deeper tissues.

The most effective way to use ice is to ice for 20 minutes, wait 10 minutes, and then reapply the ice for another 20 minutes. Repeat this up to six to eight times a day for three days after an injury

Can you ice too much? As long as you follow the rules of icing, you can ice as many times as you like and as long as it feels helpful. By allowing the skin to warm before re-icing, you can ice over and over—especially for chronic overuse injuries.

TIP: The Ice Masseur Cometh

Ice massage can be done by freezing water in a paper, foam, or plastic cup. When the water has frozen, remove part of the cup and rub the ice around the injured area. Because it cools the area faster than normal icing, limit the massage to 6–8 minutes at a time, usually three to four times a day. Ice massage is effective when used with range-of-motion exercises and stretching.

Heat Therapy

Heat therapy is used less often than cold therapy. Heat therapy is recommended only after swelling and inflammation have subsided (usually at 48–72 hours after an injury). If the skin is hot and red, swollen, or sensitive to touch, do not use heat. The heat increases blood flow to the injured area, allowing the blood's nutrients to help in the healing process, aid in the removal of waste products from the injured site, and promote healing. Heat can help reduce muscle spasms and pain. Stiffness decreases as tissue elasticity increases. Heat should not be applied for longer than 15–20 minutes at a time and should not be applied to areas of broken skin.

Combination Cold and Heat Therapy

A combination of cold and heat therapy, often called contrast hydrotherapy, can be used 48–72 hours after an injury. This can be easily accomplished by alternating the use of cold and heat packs, 10 minutes at a time. An alternative is a contrast bath. Fill two buckets or basins, one with cold water and some ice and the other with tolerable hot water. Alternate your soaking in each for two minutes. With combination therapy, the cold keeps the swelling down while the heat keeps the blood and its nutrients circulating through the injured area.

Avoid contrasting areas that are injured because the heat may aggravate the inflammation more than the cooling phase can control. The heat cycle should be at least one minute and as long as five minutes. Always finish the session with cold. If possible, increase the heat and cold as you work through the contrast cycles.

Dave Barrows, an experienced marathon runner, developed a serious case of bilateral tendinitis. A sports medicine doctor recommended a regimen of contrast baths. Dave had success by following the recommendation:

> Once or twice per day I followed a routine of soaking 5 minutes at a time for 30 minutes per session, first in an ice bath, then immediately into a 105°F hot bath, and back and forth 5 minutes at a time until I had done 15 minutes in each per session. I used a plastic tub for the cold with 10 pounds of crushed ice and water (anything less melts too much before you get to the end of the session). For the hot I filled the bathtub or if at the gym I used the hot tub, which is kept at 104°F. I bought a thermometer for checking the temperature of the hot bath at home. Also, a stopwatch is important to keep you honest about the time. As you might expect, this contrast bath surges blood in and out of the feet with good results. It's time-consuming but well worth it. Twice a day for ten days resulted in remarkable improvement for my very serious case.

There are many cold and heat packs available. The list on page 340 includes options proven to work well for athletes. Along with cold and heat packs are the many topical creams and gels. Products such as Biofreeze (biofreeze.com), IcyHot (icyhot.com), and Flex-Power Sports Cream (flexpower.com) can be used for localized muscle pain. Check out your local sports store, drugstore, or pharmacy for more options.

COLD AND HEAT PRODUCTS

ACTIVEWRAPS provide heat and cold compression therapy to specific areas of the foot and ankle. They are specifically designed and patented for the unique curvatures of these areas. Each ActiveWrap system includes a comfortable plush medical compression wrap and hot/cold (microwave- and freezer-safe) packs that can be assembled in any position within the wrap. The pack wraps around the foot and stays soft and flexible when cold so it molds comfortably in place. activewrap.com

ARTIC EASE makes reusable wraps that combine instant cold and compression for therapy for injuries. articeasewrap.com

ICEWRAPS.COM is a website that carries all types of ice wraps and packs. icewraps.com

CRYOCUP is a reusable ice massage tool that you fill with water and freeze. cryocup.com

CRYO-MAX REUSABLE COLD PACKS contain Cryo-Max fluid-filled modules that remain cold for 8 hours. The packs can be found in your local drugstores or pharmacies. lifeweartech.com

PRO-TEC ICE-UP PORTABLE ICE MASSAGER is a small go-anywhere ice massage device that remains frozen up to 10 hours. pro-tecathletics.com

RUNNER'S REMEDY offers icing and compression products, such as a **PLANTAR FASCIITIS SLEEVE** and an **ACHILLES TENDINITIS SLEEVE.** runnersremedy.com

THERMACARE AIR-ACTIVATED HEATWRAPS are made of comfortable, wearable clothlike material that conforms to your body's shape to provide therapeutic heat. Each wrap contains small discs made of natural ingredients that heat up when exposed to air, providing at least 8 hours of low-level therapeutic heat on the site of pain. Various sizes are available. Look for these wraps in your drugstore or pharmacy. thermacare.com

TOREX PREMIUM THERMAL MEDICAL DEVICES makes **TOREX FOOT SOLUTIONS FOR UPPER FOOT, ARCH, HEEL** and an **ANKLE SOLUTIONS MALLEOLAR CRYO-COMPRESSION** to provide maximum pain and swelling relief deep into joints and tissue. torexhealth.com

Foot-Care Kits

There are probably few of us who have run, hiked, fast-packed, thru-hiked, or adventure raced who have not needed a foot-care kit—at least if the outing was for a day or longer. Limping home or back to camp with a blister on your heel that will bother you for days does not make you smarter. The only way to look smarter is to plan for the next time with a foot-care kit.

Consider making three types of foot-care kits. The first is a basic self-care kit for keeping your feet healthy at home. The second is to carry with you in the field or wherever your sport takes you. The third is an event kit for long-distance or multiday activities. Each is equally important.

In chapter 18, "Providing Foot Care for Athletes," I make the case for race directors of multiday events to require mandatory foot-care gear. Kits made from the list in chapter 18 are more complete than the fanny pack kit described on page 343. In multiday events, such a kit, with knowledge on how to use the contents, could help lead to higher finishing rates.

The website backpackinglight.com asked me whether I could put together a 2-ounce foot-care kit. I made a small kit that weighed 1.5 ounces and fit in a small plastic bag. It contained a few Spenco Sport Blister Pads, alcohol wipes, compound tincture of benzoin swabs, a pin, a strip of adhesive felt, several feet of tape around a straw, and a small tube of lubricant. Nothing more. Not enough for an expedition-length adventure race but enough for about a week of general use.

You can easily carry a few things just in case you need them. The space and weight are minimal. It could make the difference between being able to continue on foot the next day if you are by yourself. If you are with friends, it could make the difference between holding up the group or continuing on.

Even a minimalist could benefit from carrying a blister patch, an alcohol wipe, a foot of tape, and a pin. A small 2-by-3-inch bag could easily carry these four items. Too many fail to plan and leave open the door to pain from the unexpected but waiting-to-pounce blister.

You can make your own blister kit or purchase a general first aid kit or a blister medical kit. Most general first aid kits contain items for basic first aid care and can be used for blister care by adding a few more specific items. The kits mentioned in the product section on page 346 are made specifically for blister care. No matter what each kit contains, you should customize the kit to suit your needs and stock it with sufficient equipment for your outing.

A 2-ounce foot-care kit

Dave told me, "I have carried a small kit in my pack for years. I have not used it on myself but have patched many a runner or hiker met on the trail. I still carry it for that day I'm in need. It's homemade with moleskin patches, and there is a salve made with one-third Vaseline, one-third diaper rash cream to keep the area dry, and one-third witch hazel. I stir it using a Popsicle stick and keep the salve in a little travel plastic jar. And there are individual alcohol patches. It's all real 'high tech' and kept inside a zip-top bag."

Spend a bit of time preparing your feet before your trip, and reduce the chances of needing many of the supplies in a kit. Pretrip preparation includes three steps: reducing calluses with a callus file or creams, getting the skin on your feet in the best possible condition, and trimming your toenails correctly.

If you make a foot-care kit, make sure it is stocked with the right materials and you and/or your crew know what's in it and how to use it. Lisa Bliss, a former Badwater medical director, relates, "Runners have come to the medical HQ with blisters asking for our help in treating them so that they can continue their run. I would ask them what they had in their foot-care kit and get blank stares in response: 'Foot-care kit?' Then their crews would get a clue and scrounge frantically around through some supplies and pull out—Band-Aids!—even those little circle ones! Just insane!"

Some people have asked about my foot-care kit. On the following page is a picture of the yellow toolbox that carries all my supplies for an event such as Badwater or Western States. I like the removable top tray that holds the stuff I always use. The box is made by Flambeau and is about 20 by 9 by 7.5 inches. It is available through flambeaucases.com in several sizes. It has a lock tab, which is handy. I have shipped this box to events all over the world. When I do, I wrap the top tray in plastic wrap to hold the contents in place, padding the inside with foot-cleaning cloths.

The author's foot-care kit for events

Basic Self-Care Kit for Home Use

A basic self-care kit for good foot treatment does not have to be large. The following items are recommended; add to the kit as necessary for your particular foot conditions.

- Toenail clippers for trimming nails
- File or emery board for smoothing nails after clipping
- Foot powder for absorbing moisture
- Moisturizer cream for softening dry skin, calluses, and corns
- Callus file or pumice stone for removing calluses and dead skin
- Antiseptic ointment for treating cuts and scrapes

Fanny Pack Kit

If you are an athlete who finds yourself continuously bothered by foot problems, or who often covers long distances without crew support, consider making a small foot-care kit to carry in a fanny pack. Hikers should carry a kit as part of a larger overall first aid kit because of their remoteness from assistance. The following items are recommended.

- Compound tincture of benzoin swab sticks or squeeze vials
- Alcohol wipe packets
- A fingernail clipper or pin and matches for draining blisters
- Foot powder in a small container
- A small container with your choice of a lubricant
- Your choice of tapes wrapped around a pencil or straw
- A plastic bag with your choice of blister patching materials and several pieces of toilet paper or tissues
- Several ENGO Blister Prevention Patches
- A small pocketknife with built-in scissors

Depending on your personal needs, you might consider adding a lightweight ankle support; pads for metatarsal, arch, or heel pain; and a heel cup.

Event Kit

If you participate in events in which you or your crew will be providing foot care, a larger kit is necessary. The kit should contain material based on the length and type of event. Do not rely on medical personnel or aid stations to have the materials you need. The following materials form the core of the kit. Add or eliminate materials based on your personal preferences and experience. Look in the tool section of your local hardware stores for a plastic toolbox with trays in which to store the materials.

This same kit list can be used by medical teams to plan for coverage of all types of events. Simply modify the quantity of items for the number of participants and the length of the event in distance and days. Medical teams should have one or more hydrocolloid dressings to treat open blisters (refer to the "Beyond Blisters" section of the "Blisters" chapter).

- Lubricant of choice
- Powder of choice
- Blister patches of choice in various sizes (example: Compeed and Spenco Blister Pads)
- Spenco 2nd Skin or GlacierGel
- Tapes of choice in a variety of widths
- An assortment of ENGO Blister Prevention Patches
- Compound tincture of benzoin or other tape adherent
- Adhesive removal pads or nail polish remover

- Alcohol pads
- One large sterile hydrocolloid blister dressing
- Tube of Desitin Maximum Strength Ointment or zinc oxide
- 10-cc syringe (for Desitin or zinc oxide)
- 18-gauge needle (for Desitin or zinc oxide), blunt if possible
- Supply of 25-gauge needles for draining blisters
- Several #11 scalpels for lancing blisters
- Tube of 2% Xylocaine jelly
- One container of all-purpose first aid salve or ointment like Green Goo
- Gauze pads (2-by-2-inch and 4-by-4-inch) for draining blisters
- Toenail clippers
- Nail file
- Callus file
- Sharp-pointed scissors
- Utility scissors for cutting tape and shoes
- Sewing needles and dental floss to stitch damaged shoes
- Nail drill
- Tweezers for pulling blister skin to cut a hole in it
- Shoehorn
- Betadine for cleaning dirty wounds/blisters
- Antiseptic ointment
- Extra socks
- Self-adhering wrap
- Ace wrap
- Ankle support
- Pads for metatarsal, arch, or heel pain
- Latex gloves
- Antibacterial hand wipes
- Small basin for soaking feet
- Small soft sponge for cleaning feet
- Nail polish remover to get rid of tape reside on skin
- Hand towels for drying feet

- Plastic bags for garbage
- Sharps container or clear water bottle labeled as such

FOOT-CARE KIT PRODUCTS

ADVANCED BLISTER KIT is from podiatrist and blister expert Rebecca Rushton from Australia. Contains materials used by professionals: toe sleeves, dressings, tape, swabs, ENGO patches, and more. blisterprevention.com.au

ADVENTURE MEDICAL KITS offers a **BLISTER MEDIC KIT** plus a wide array of kits for any type of activity, any length of event, and any number of people. adventuremedicalkits.com

BRAVE SOLDIER ANTISEPTIC HEALING OINTMENT was developed by a dermatologist as an effective treatment to keep abrasion wounds moist and protected, Brave Soldier helps heal blisters, road rash, minor cuts, and burns. It's made with tea tree oil as a natural antiseptic, aloe vera gel for its natural healing properties, jojoba oil as a natural moisturizer, vitamin E for rebuilding collagen and skin tissue, shark liver oil for reducing scarring, and comfrey for stimulating skin-cell growth and wound resurfacing. bravesoldier.com

GREEN GOO is one of those salves that are good for everything. It's 100% natural with antibacterial and antiseptic herbs to help heal and repair wounds and chafing. sierrasageorganics.com

SPENCO'S BLISTER KIT contains six 2nd Skin 1-inch squares, one sheet and six strips of Adhesive Knit, and one sheet of Pressure Pad ovals. The kit comes in a resealable pouch. Look for this kit in backpacking or sporting goods stores. spenco.com

SUPER SALVE is an antioxidant, antibacterial, and antifungal salve that helps soothe and heal dry and cracked skin, abrasions, and skin conditions common to harsh environments. It's made with a combination of herbs, including chaparral leaf, echinacea flower, hops flower, and usnea moss. supersalve.com

Part Five

Sources and
Resources

Appendix A: Product Sources

Rather than use this book as a definitive source for products, use it as a guide to the wide variety of foot-care products available. New products are always being developed. Remember, too, that your local stores are an excellent source for what is current in the foot-care marketplace.

When products are mentioned in the text, the company name and website (if available) are provided. Generally, your first source for most of these products should be your local stores. Ask at your sporting goods store, running store, backpacking or camping store, pharmacy or drugstore, medical supply store, or orthopedic supply store for the products mentioned. While they may not stock all the products, they may be willing to place a special order. Please be aware that not all companies listed in this book sell retail and therefore their products may have to be ordered through a retailer or medical professional. Please respect their sales policies.

The following companies are sources of many of the products listed in this book:

THERATAPE.COM (theratape.com) stocks all brands of kinesiology tapes, taping tools and supplies, and videos and instruction on using the popular tape. Professional discounts are available.

ZOMBIERUNNER (zombierunner.com/fixingyourfeet) is a US web-based company run by ultrarunners that provides equipment and supplies for trail runners, ultrarunners, and other outdoor enthusiasts. They stock hard-to-find items such as tapes, blister patches, lubricants, powders, gaiters, electrolyte caps, and so on.

FOOTSMART (footsmart.com) carries a wide assortment of products for flat feet, arch problems, plantar fasciitis, Achilles tendinitis, toenails, bunions, hammertoes, corns, calluses, and skin disorders.

MEDCO SPORTS MEDICINE (medco-athletics.com) has products including tapes; self-adhering wraps; tape adherents and skin-toughening agents; various grades of moleskin; lubricants; powders; antifungal sprays and powders; first aid equipment; alcohol and compound tincture of benzoin prep pads; hot and cold therapy equipment; physical therapy equipment; ankle supports; Achilles tendon and plantar fasciitis straps; insoles and heel cups; most Cramer, Johnson & Johnson, Mueller, and Spenco products; and more.

MEDI-DYNE (medi-dyne.com) offers a number of brands for athletes: 2Toms, Cho-Pat, ProStretch, Skin-on-Skin, Tuli's, and more.

In the United Kingdom, check out Dr. Foot's website for a complete line of foot-related products (drfoot.co.uk).

Appendix C lists medical specialists and companies that often offer products related to their services and business. Check it out for additional options for many of the foot problems and disorders in this book.

You may find products similar to those mentioned that are only available in your area. Watching other athletes and their foot-care habits will often alert you to new products they have found to be useful. Do not hesitate to ask questions when you see new products.

Appendix B:
Shoe and Gear Reviews

The print magazines and websites listed below often offer formal reviews of shoes and foot-related gear and sometimes have additional content on their websites. Check out the magazines and websites to see the extent of their coverage. Many also post their editorial calendars online, allowing you to see which issues cover shoes and boots. The Fixing Your Feet blog has reviews and information about new foot-care products. You can subscribe at fixingyourfeet.com/blog.

Backpacker **magazine** backpacker.com

Outside **magazine** outsideonline.com

Runner's World **magazine** runnersworld.com

Trail Runner **magazine** trailrunnermag.com

UltraRunning **magazine** ultrarunning.com

Wear Tested **Gear Reviews** weartested.org

Appendix C:
Medical and
Footwear Specialists

American Academy of Orthopaedic Surgeons aaos.org

American Academy of Podiatric Sports Medicine aapsm.org

American Chiropractic Association acatoday.org

American Massage Therapy Association amtamassage.org

American Orthopaedic Foot and Ankle Society aofas.org

American Orthotic and Prosthetic Association aopanet.org

American Physical Therapy Association apta.org

American Podiatric Medical Association apma.org

International Chiropractors Association chiropractic.org

National Athletic Trainers' Association nata.org

Pedorthic Footcare Association pedorthics.org

Appendix D:
Foot-Related Websites

A free blog about feet, foot-related products, and foot-care issues is offered at fixingyourfeet.com. It also helps athletes learn about new foot-care techniques and products between editions of the book.

Websites related to barefoot running and minimalist footwear are listed at the end of the "Barefoot and Minimalist Footwear" chapter.

About Walking walking.about.com

The Ambulatory Foot Clinic—Podiatric Pain Management Center footcare4u.com

Blister Prevention blisterprevention.com.au

Dr. Pribut's Running Injuries Page drpribut.com/sports/sportframe.html

Dr. Todd's Relief for the Feet Products drtodds.com

Eneslow Foot Comfort Center eneslow.com

Footcare Direct—Target In on Your Foot Care Solution footcaredirect.com

Foot Express—Footcare Home Health Products and Treatments footexpress.com

Foot Health Network foot.com

Foot Store—Specializing in Foot and Heel Pain Treatment footstore.com

Foot Web—Footcare Treatment Information Resource footweb.com

Healthy Feet Store—Your Online Source for Footcare healthyfeetstore.com

My Foot Shop—Your Source for Healthy Feet myfootshop.com

Sports Injury Clinic sportsinjuryclinic.net

Notes

Please see chapter 9, "Blister Prevention: The New Paradigm," for a list of 21 additional resources and studies in blister prevention.

1. Roland Mueser, *Long-Distance Hiking: Lessons from the Appalachian Trail* (Camden, ME: Rugged Mountain Press, 1998), 32.

2. J. J. Knapik, K. L. Reynolds, K. L. Duplantis, and B. H. Jones, "Friction Blisters: Pathophysiology, Prevention, and Treatment," *Sports Medicine* 20, no. 3 (1995): 140.

3. Karen Berger, *Advanced Backpacking* (New York: W. W. Norton & Company, 1998), 69–70.

4. The usual issues are *Backpacking* (March, the Annual Gear Guide Issue), *Outside* (May Buyer's Guide), *Runner's World* (April and September), and *Trail Runner* (spring and fall).

5. J. D. Denton, Dennis Grandy, DPM, and Tom Kennedy, "How to Find the Right Shoe for You," *Running Times* (September 1996): 16; and "How to Find a Shoe That Works," *Running Times* (March 1997): 18.

6. Tom Brunick and Bob Wischnia, "Choosing the Right Shoe" and "Know Your Foot Type," *Runner's World* (April 1997): 52.

7. Knapik, et. al., "Friction Blisters: Pathophysiology, Prevention, and Treatment": 142.

8. Twelve miles per day times 5,280 feet/mile divided by 2.5 feet/step. For each mile more than 12, add 2,100 steps. For each mile less than 12, subtract 2,100 steps.

9. Ray Jardine, *The Pacific Crest Trail Hiker's Handbook* (LaPine, OR: Adventure Lore Press, 1996), 93.

10. Daniel E. Lieberman, "Biomechanics of Foot Strikes and Applications to Running Barefoot or in Minimal Footwear," barefootrunning.fas.harvard.edu.

11. William Jungers, "Biomechanics: Barefoot Running Strikes Back," *Nature* 463, no. 7280 (January 2010): 433–34.

12. William A. Rossi, "Why Shoes Make 'Normal' Gait Impossible," Podiatry Management (March 1999): 50–61.

13. Ibid.

14. Michael Wharburton, "Barefoot Running," *Sportscience* 5, no. 3 (December 2001), sportsci.org/jour/0103/mw.htm.

15. Daniel E. Lieberman, et al., "Foot Strike Patterns and Collision Forces in Habitually Barefoot Versus Shod Runners," *Nature* 463, no. 7280 (January 2010): 531–35.

16. S. D. Perry, A. Radtke, and C. R. Goodwin, "Influence of Footwear Midsole Material Hardness on Dynamic Balance Control during Unexpected Gait Termination," *Gait and Posture* 25, no. 1 (January 2007): 94–98.

17. Dr. Jack Daniels, "How Much Does Shoe Weight Affect Performance?" *The Run S.M.A.R.T. Project* (February 6, 2012), runsmartproject.com/coaching /2012/02/06/how-much-does-shoe-weight-affect-performance.

18. W. Blattler, N. Kreis, B. Lun, J. Winiger, and F. Amsler, "Leg Symptoms of Healthy People and Their Treatment with Compression Hosiery," *Phlebology* 23, no. 5 (2008): 214–21.

19. Tim Noakes, MD, *Lore of Running* (Champaign, IL: Leisure Press, 1991), 460.

20. Rebecca Rushton, BSc (POD), *The Blister Prone Athlete's Guide to Preventing Foot Blisters* (Esperance, AU: Blister Prevention, 2015).

21. Rebecca Rushton, BSc (POD), *Blister Prevention Report: What Every Podiatrist Should Know About Blister Prevention*, (Esperance, AU: Blister Prevention, 2013).

22. Andrew Lovy, "New Blister Formula Revealed! Free!" *UltraRunning* (April 1990): 40.

23. Robert Boeder, *Beyond the Marathon: The Grand Slam of Trail Ultrarunning* (Vienna, GA: Old Mountain Press, 1996), 22.

24. Knapik, et. al., "Friction Blisters: Pathophysiology, Prevention, and Treatment": 139.

25. Colin Fletcher, *The Complete Walker III* (New York: Alfred A. Knopf, 1996), 86.

26. Richard Benyo, *The Death Valley 300: Near-Death and Resurrection on the World's Toughest Endurance Course* (Forestville, CA: Specific Publications, 1991), 142.

27. Gary Cantrell, "From the South: The Amazing Miracle of Duct Tape," *UltraRunning* (December 1988): 36–37.

28. Donald Baxter, MD; David Porter, MD, PhD; Paul Flahavan, C.Ped; and Charles May, "The Ideal Running Orthosis: A Philosophy of Design," *Biomechanics* (March 1996): 41–44.

29. T. A. Cappaert, PhD; J. A. Stone, MS; J. W. Castellani, PhD; B. A. Krause, PhD; D. Smith, ATC; and B. A. Stephens, MD, "National Athletic Trainers' Association Position Statement: Environmental Cold Injuries," *Journal of Athletic Training* 43, no. 6 (2008): 640–58.

30. Ibid.

31. Ibid.

32. Ibid.

33. Ibid.

34. Ibid.

35. M. D. Hoffman, A. Pasternak, I. R. Rogers, M. Khodaee, J. C. Hill, D. A. Townes, B. Volker Scheer, B. J. Krabak, P. Basset, and G. S. Lipman, "Medical Services at Ultra-Endurance Foot Races in Remote Environments: Medical Issues and Consensus Guidelines," *Sports Medicine* 44, no. 8 (2014): 1055–69.

36. Tim Noakes, MD, *Lore of Running*, 459.

37. Annette McGivney, "8 Survival Tips from a Grand Canyon Rescue Ranger," *Backpacker* (October 2015): 68.

38. D. Townes, MD; T. Talbot, MD; I. Wedmore, MD, and R. Billingsly, MD, "Event Medicine: Injury and Illness During an Expedition-Length Adventure Race," *Journal of Emergency Medicine* 27, no. 2 (2004): 161–65.

39. Hoffman, et al., "Medical Services at Ultra-Endurance Foot Races in Remote Environments."

40. Knapik, et. al., "Friction Blisters: Pathophysiology, Prevention, and Treatment": 136–47.

41. Id.,140.

42. Bryan Bergeron, MD, "A Guide to Blister Management," *Physician and Sportsmedicine* 23, no. 2 (February 1995): 40.

43. Id., 43.

44. William Trolan, MD, *Blister Fighter Guide* (Seattle: Outdoor Research, 1996).

45. Guy-Robert Auleley, MD, et al., "Validation of the Ottawa Ankle Rules," *Annals of Emergency Medicine* 32, no. 1 (July 1998): 14–18.

46. "The Conservative Treatment of Plantar Fasciitis: A Prospective Randomized, Multicenter Outcome Study," American Orthopaedic Foot and Ankle Society (October 1996).

47. Robert Nirschl, MD, MS, "Plantar Fasciitis—A New Perspective," *American Medical Joggers Association AMAA Quarterly* (summer 1996).

48. "Heel To Heal: New Stretch Relieves Pain from Plantar Fasciitis Source," University of Rochester Medical Center (November 13, 2006).

49. Karen Maloney Backstrom, C. Forsyth, and B. Walden, "Comparison of Two Methods of Stretching the Gastrocnemius and Their Effects on Ankle Range of Motion," University of Colorado Health Services Center (April 1994).

50. Hoffman, et al., "Medical Services at Ultra-Endurance Foot Races in Remote Environments."

51. Dean R. Focht III, MD; Carole Spicer, RN; and Mary P. Fairchok, MD, "The Efficacy of Duct Tape vs. Cryotherapy in the Treatment of Verruca Vulgaris (the Common Wart)," *Archives of Pediatric & Adolescent Medicine* 156, no. 10 (October 2002): 971–74.

Glossary

Achilles tendon—the large tendon that runs from the calf to the back of the heel

adventure racing—multisport races over difficult terrain, often done in teams over several days

arch—the curved part of the bottom of the foot

athlete's foot—a fungal infection that causes itchy, red, soggy, flaking, and cracking skin between the toes or fluid-filled bumps on the sides or sole of the foot

biomechanics—the study of the mechanics of a living body, especially of the forces exerted by muscles and gravity on the skeletal structure

blister—a fluid-filled sac between layers of skin that occurs as a result of friction

bone spur—a small, bony growth usually indicating a bone irritation

bruise—an injury in which blood vessels beneath the skin are broken and blood escapes to produce a discolored area

bunion—a bony protrusion at the base of the big toe

bunionette—a bunion on the little toe

bursitis—the formation of an inflamed, fluid-filled sac, usually where muscles or tendons glide over bone

calcaneus—the large heel bone

callus—the thickening of skin caused by recurring friction, usually on the sole of the foot, heel, or inner big toe

claw toes—toes that are contracted down at the middle joint but up at the joint at the ball of the foot

contusion—a bruising injury that does not involve a break in the skin

corn—a thickening of the skin, generally on or between the toes, usually caused by friction

dermis—the sensitive connective tissue layer of the skin located below the epidermis, containing nerve endings, sweat and sebaceous glands, and blood and lymph vessels

dislocation—a complete displacement of bone from its normal position at the joint surface

edema—the swelling of body tissues due to excessive fluid

epidermis—the outer, protective, nonvascular layer of the skin covering the dermis

eversion—movement of the foot as it rolls inward at the ankle

fibula—the outer and smaller of the two bones of the lower leg

fissure—crack in the skin, usually found on the toughened, callused skin of the heels

flat foot—a foot that has either a low arch or no arch

forefoot—the ball of the foot and the toes

friction—the force that resists one surface sliding against another

frostbite—the result of the freezing of skin tissue

Haglund's deformity—a bump in the form of an enlargement of the back of the heel bone (calcaneus) at the area of the insertion of the Achilles tendon

hallux—the great or big toe

hallux valgus—the turning in of the great toe joint that often causes bunions

hammertoes—toes that are contracted at the toe's middle joint, making the toe bend upward at its center and forcing the tip of the toe downward

heel pad—the soft tissue pad on the bottom of the heel

heel-pain syndrome—pain at the heel usually caused by overuse or repetitive stress to the foot's heel

heel spur—a small edge of bone that juts out of the calcaneus

hematoma—a swelling containing blood beneath the skin caused by an injury to a blood vessel

hot spot—a hot and reddened area of skin that has been irritated by friction

hyperhidrosis—excessive moisture

infection—condition in which a part of the body is invaded by a microorganism such as a bacteria or virus

ingrown toenail—when one or both sides of a toenail has grown into the flesh of the toe

inversion—movement of the foot as it rolls outward at the ankle

last—the form over which a shoe or boot is constructed

lateral—the outside of the foot, leg, or body

ligament—the strong, fibrous connective tissue at a joint that connects one bone to another bone

maceration—a breaking down or softening of skin tissue by extended exposure to moisture

mallet toes—toes that are contracted at the end joint only

medial—the inside of the foot, leg, or body

metatarsal—one of the five bones at the ball of the foot

metatarsalgia—pain somewhere underneath the metatarsal heads of the foot

midfoot—the mid or center part of the foot, containing the arch and five metatarsal bones

Morton's neuroma—pain on the bottom of the foot, usually under the pad of the third or fourth toe

Morton's toe—a foot type where the second toe is longer than the big toe

neuroma—the swelling of a nerve due to an inflammation of the nerve or the tissue surrounding the nerve

NSAIDs—acronym for nonsteroidal anti-inflammatory drugs; used to control pain and swelling after an injury

orthopedist—an orthopedic surgeon specializing in the treatment and surgery of bones and joint injuries, diseases, and problems

orthotic—an insert made from a mold of the bottom of the foot that is then inserted into a shoe or boot to correct a foot abnormality

pedorthist—a specialist trained to work on the fit or modification of shoes and orthotics to alleviate foot problems caused by disease, overuse, or injury

peripheral neuropathy—a painful nerve condition that can manifest itself as a burning sensation in the feet

plantar—the bottom surface of the foot

plantar fascia—the band of fibers along the arch of the foot that connects the heel to the toes

plantar fasciitis—an inflammation of the plantar fascia

plantar warts—small, hard, flesh-colored, white, or pink granulated lumps typically found on the feet and caused by a virus

podiatrist—a doctor of podiatric medicine who specializes in the treatment and surgery of the foot and ankle

pronation—the rolling of the foot toward the inside of the body when weight bearing

Raynaud's syndrome—discomfort caused by a decreased blood supply to the fingers and toes

RICE—acronym for rest, ice, compression, and elevation; describes the typical treatment of sprain and strain injuries

sesamoiditis—an inflammation of the two little bones beneath the ball of the foot and under the joint that moves the big toe

shear—a strain in the structure of a substance produced by pressure when its layers are laterally shifted in relation to each other

sole—the bottom of the foot

sprain—a joint injury in which ligament damage is sustained

sterilization—the process by which bacteria is removed

strain—muscular injury produced by overuse or abuse of a muscle

stress fracture—typically a small crack in the outer shell of the affected bone caused by sudden or repetitive stress, usually from overuse without proper conditioning

subluxation—an incomplete or partial dislocation

subungual hematoma—a hematoma under the nail plate

supination—the rolling of the foot toward the outside of the body when weight bearing

tendinitis—an inflammation of a tendon or its surrounding sheath

tendon—the elastic, tough, fibrous tissue that connects muscles to bone

toe box—the front part of a shoe or boot that covers the toes

toenail fungus—marked by nails that are thick and deformed, with a brown, white, or yellowish discoloration

transient paresthesia—a temporary nerve compression that can be caused by a gradual buildup of fluids in your feet during extended on-your-feet activity

trench foot—a serious nonfreezing cold injury that develops when the skin of the feet is exposed to a combination of moisture and cold for extended periods

turf toe—a condition of pain at the base of the big toe at the ball of the foot, usually caused from jamming the toe

ultrarunning—running distances greater than a marathon

virus—a tiny organism that causes disease

wart—a thickened, painful area of skin caused by a virus

Bibliography

Achilles Tendonitis: Prevention and Treatment. London: Peak Performance Publishing, 2002.

Copeland, Glen. *The Foot Book: Relief for Overused, Abused and Ailing Feet.* New York: John Wiley & Sons, 1992.

Davies, Clair, with Amber Davies. *The Trigger Point Therapy Workbook: Your Self-Treatment Guide for Pain Relief.* Oakland, CA: New Harbinger Publications, Inc., 2004.

Dobrowolski, Christine, DPM. *Those Aching Feet: Your Guide to Diagnosis and Treatment of Common Foot Problems,* rev. ed. San Francisco, CA: S.K.I. Publishing Co., 2005.

Ellis, Joe, DPM, with Joe Henderson. *Running Injury-Free.* Emmaus, PA: Rodale Press, 1994.

Egoscue, Pete, with Roger Gittines. *Pain Free: A Revolutionary Method for Stopping Chronic Pain.* New York: Bantam Books, 2000.

Jardine, Ray. *The Pacific Crest Trail Hiker's Handbook.* LaPine, OR: Adventure Lore Press, 1996 (out of print).

Jordan, Ryan, ed. *Lightweight Backpacking and Camping: A Field Guide to Wilderness Equipment, Technique, and Style.* Bozeman, MT: Beartooth Mountain Press, 2005.

Langer, Paul, DPM. *Great Feet for Life: Footcare and Footwear for Healthy Aging.* Minneapolis, MN: Fairview Press, 2007.

Levine, Suzanne M., MD. *My Feet Are Killing Me!* New York: McGraw-Hill Book Company, 1987 (out of print).

Maffetone, Philip, MD. *Fix Your Feet: Build the Best Foundation for Healthy, Pain-Free Knees, Hips, and Spine.* Guilford, CT: Lyons Press, 2004.

McDougall, Christopher. *Born to Run: A Hidden Tribe, Superathletes, and the Greatest Race the World Has Never Seen.* New York: Alfred A. Knopf, 2009.

McGann, Daniel M., DPM, and L. R. Robinson. *The Doctor's Sore Foot Book.* New York: William Morrow and Company, Inc., 1991 (out of print).

Noakes, Tim, MD. *Lore of Running,* 4th ed. Champaign, IL: Human Kinetics, 2003.

O'Connor, Patrick L., MD, and Thomas M. Schaller, MD. *Footworks II: The Patient's Guide to the Foot and Ankle.* Portage, MI: privately printed, 2001.

Plotkin, Stuart, DPM. *The Hiking Engine: A Hiker's Guide to the Care and Maintenance of Feet and Legs.* Birmingham, AL: Menasha Ridge Press, 2001.

Rushton, Rebecca, BSc (POD). *The Blister Prone Athlete's Guide to Preventing Foot Blisters.* Esperance, AU: Blister Prevention, 2015.

Salmans, Sandra. *Your Feet: Questions You Have . . . Answers You Need.* Allentown, PA: People's Medical Society, 1998 (out of print).

Schneider, Myles J., DPM, and Mark D. Sussman, DPM. *How to Doctor Your Feet Without a Doctor.* Washington, DC: Acropolis Books, Ltd., 1984 (out of print).

Subotnick, Steven I., DPM, MS. *The Running Foot Doctor.* San Francisco, CA: World Publications, 1977 (out of print).

———. *Sports and Exercise Injuries: Conventional, Homeopathic, and Alternative Treatments.* Berkeley, CA: North Atlantic Books, 1991.

Taliaferro Blauvelt, Carolyn, and Fred R. T. Nelson. *A Manual of Orthopaedic Terminology,* 6th ed., St. Louis, MO: Mosby, 1998.

Tremain, David M., MD, and Elias M. Awad, PhD. *The Foot and Ankle Sourcebook,* 2nd ed. Lincolnwood, IL: NTC/Contemporary Books Publishing Group, Inc., 1998.

Trolan, William, MD. *Blister Fighter Guide.* Seattle, WA: Outdoor Research, 1996 (out of print).

Weisenfeld, Murry F., MD, with Barbara Burr. *The Runner's Repair Manual.* New York: St. Martin's Press, 1980 (out of print).

Index

If you are an extreme athlete, you need this book. It's confession time: As a veteran of more than 80 marathons as well as ultramarathons up to 100 miles, and as a podiatrist for 18 years, I thought I knew it all. John's comprehensive approach of asking the so-called medical experts as well as the real experts out in the trenches for their tried-and-true advice will bring you more value for your endurance event than a podiatry degree ever will.

—**Bill Johncock, DPM fellow, American Academy of Sports Medicine Board Certified, American Board of Podiatric Surgery**

When a foot problem arises, this book's clear, concise explanations and fixes are wonderful. The book is comprehensive; every relevant topic is addressed. If you run ultras, you should have *Fixing Your Feet*.

—**Karl King, president of SUCCEED Sportsdrink, LLC, and inventor of S! Caps**

I have always had issues with blisters, particularly on long mountain runs. Since reading *Fixing Your Feet* and implementing John's techniques, I have not had any blister issues. This includes long runs in the mountains and pacing at Badwater for four years, including one double crossing and one starting at Las Vegas. For those with foot issues, this book is the solution to your foot problems.

—**Scott Morgan, ultrarunner, endurance athlete, climber, and coach for sealfit.com**

I reference *Fixing Your Feet* often when consulting with customers about their foot troubles. There simply is no replacement for the amount of relevant content introduced in *Fixing Your Feet*. The product recommendations are unbiased and based on experience with real athletes. *Fixing Your Feet* is a must-read for serious runners, hikers, and team sports athletes.

—**Jason Pawelsky, Tamarack Habilitation Technologies, ENGO Patches; goengo.com**

Through our experience as ultrarunners, we've noticed that our foot-care needs continue to change, due to different environments, changes in training and racing, and even changes in our feet. We keep coming back to *Fixing Your Feet* for the most useful and comprehensive foot advice, and we always find the answers we're looking for. This new edition keeps us up to date with the latest products and trends. We couldn't ask for anything more!

—**Gillian Robinson and Don Lundell, ultrarunners and founders of zombierunner.com**

John Vonhof literally wrote the book on foot care for ultrasports. His indispensable wisdom has made countless race finishes possible over the years, most especially at the Badwater Ultramarathon, the world's toughest foot race.

—**Chris Kostman, Chief Adventure Officer and Race Director, AdventureCORPS, Inc.**

Fixing Your Feet is the definitive guide to foot care for hikers, runners, and walkers. It has the collective wisdom of dozens of outdoor athletes who tell us what works for them. The book is well organized and full of great information. The personal anecdotes of athletes, many of whom I know either personally or by reputation, greatly enhance the readability of this reference book. The result is a smorgasbord of ideas and instructions for preventing and fixing any foot problem.

—**Flyin' Brian Robinson, first person to complete the 7,400-mile Calendar Triple Crown hikes of the Appalachian Trail, the Continental Divide Trail, and the Pacific Crest Trail in one year (2001)**

One hundred miles, 28 hours of downpours, mud, and thigh-deep rushing rivers. ZERO BLISTERS. My feet look perfect! People were crossing the finish line with their feet in tatters and crazy cases of trench foot. Everyone's been asking what my secret is, and I've been referring them to *Fixing Your Feet*!

—**Tanya Sylvan, ultrarunner and AdventureKEEN content marketing specialist**

I found *Fixing Your Feet* after a 48-hour race when my feet became so bad that I was reduced to a painful shuffle for the last 24 hours, then weeks of healing. I am now able to race 24 hours on a track without a scratch, and, as we say, "If you do not have a plan for your feet, you do not have a race plan." Thanks heaps for the help and advice you give so freely.

— **Billy Pearce, husband, father of three boys, nurse, and ultrarunner**

About the Author

John Vonhof brings a varied background and extensive experience to *Fixing Your Feet*. This sixth edition is the synthesis of 34 years of experience as a runner, hiker, and medical professional, and a never-ending quest to learn more about foot care to help athletes in extreme events.

His popular website, fixingyourfeet .com, is dedicated to providing articles, resources, links, and a blog about foot care, and it serves to inform and educate athletes about all that's new in foot care and to provide foot-care advice.

Other medical professionals recognize John's expertise too. In 2009 he was the lead author of a chapter on foot injuries in the textbook *Expedition and Wilderness Medicine* (Cambridge University Press).

Over the years John has provided volunteer medical aid at numerous sporting events around the world, patching feet, training medical staff and interested athletes, and providing advice to thousands of athletes. His expertise has taken him to Chile; Costa Rica; Brazil; British Columbia, Canada; and many states to help on medical teams. He continues to be sought out for his expertise and experience in providing answers to foot-care questions, especially for multiday events.

A runner since 1982, John discovered trail running and ultras in 1984. He has completed more than 20 ultras: 50Ks, 50-milers, 100-milers, 24-hour runs, and a 72-hour run. He ran the difficult Western States 100-mile Endurance Run three times and the Santa Rosa 24-Hour and 12-Hour Track Runs 12 times. In 1987, with fellow runner Will Uher, John fast-packed the 211-mile John Muir Trail in the Sierra Nevada in 8.5 days, carrying a 30-pound pack. He still runs and rides his road bike.

In 1992 John changed careers, becoming a paramedic, orthopedic technician, and emergency room technician. In 2013 he retired from a position as a prehospital care coordinator at an emergency medical services agency in the San Francisco Bay Area.